# SMITH'S Recognizable Patterns of Human Deformation

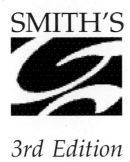

SMITH'S

*3rd Edition*

# Recognizable Patterns of Human Deformation

## John M. Graham, Jr, MD, ScD

Director, Clinical Genetics and Dysmorphology
Medical Genetics Institute
Cedars-Sinai Medical Center
Professor of Pediatrics
David Geffen School of Medicine at UCLA
Los Angeles, California

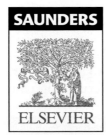

SAUNDERS

ELSEVIER

1600 John F. Kennedy Blvd, Suite 1800
Philadelphia, Pennsylvania 19103-2899

Smith's Recognizable Patterns of Human Deformation, third edition

ISBN-13: 978-0-7216-1489-2
ISBN-10: 0-7216-1489-2

**Library of Congress Cataloging-in-Publication Data**
Graham, John M.,
   Smith's recognizable patterns of human deformation. – 3rd ed. / John M. Graham, Jr.
      p. ; cm.
   Previous ed. cataloged under Smith.
   ISBN-13: 978-0-7216-1489-2
   1. Abnormalities, Human–Etiology.   2. Human mechanics.   3. Morphogenesis.   4. Birth injuries.
5. Growth disorders.   I. Smith, David W., 1926–1981. Smith's recognizable patterns of human deformation.
II. Title.   III. Title: Recognizable patterns of human deformation.
[DNLM: 1. Abnormalities. QS 675 G739s 2007]

RG627.5.S57 2007
618.92′0043–dc22                                                                                2006037457

Editor: Rebecca Schmidt Gaertner
Design Direction: Karen O'Keefe Owens

Printed in China.

Last digit is the print number: 9 8 7 6 5 4 3 2 1

To Elizabeth Spear Graham, my
wife and best friend

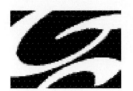# Acknowledgments

In the acknowledgment section of the first edition of this book, published in 1981, Dr. Smith wrote: "It was at an international meeting on nomenclature for birth defects, that I first heard Peter Dunn, M.D., of Bristol, England, give his impassioned plea for a clear distinction between defects due to mechanical constraint forces (deformation) as contrasted to those due to poor formation (malformation).... Since that time I have been ever more impressed by the importance, relevance, and magnitude of this deformational category of birth defects. Hence, I acknowledge Peter Dunn as the individual who set me forth on the pathway that culminated in this book."

While I was a fellow with Dr. Smith from 1978 to 1980, we investigated many of the concepts set forth in this book. This effort was greatly helped by Dr. Smith's previous fellows, to whom he dedicated the first edition of this book. Dr. Smith's dysmorphology fellows (listed in chronological order) were Drs. John Opitz, Luc Lemli, Bob Summitt, Jules LeRoy, Arlan Rosenbloom, Jaime Frias, Jon Aase, Bryan Hall, Kenneth Lyons Jones, James Hanson, Sterling Clarren, Marvin Miller, Albert Schinzel, John M. Graham, Jr., and Margot VanAllen. Drs. Judy Hall and Mike Cohen also helped to disseminate and delineate many of the concepts contained in *Recognizable Patterns of Human Deformation*. After completing the first edition of this book, Dr. Smith died on February 21, 1981. He requested that I continue his work and revise this book.

Bill Pollard prepared the vast majority of the figures for this edition of the book, and he is from the Medical Media Division of Cedars-Sinai Medical Center. Bill is a dedicated naturalist with the same love of the outdoors as Dave Smith. He scanned slides from previous illustrations, color-corrected them, constructed composites, and masterfully added color to previous line drawings. Much of the credit for the artistry of these illustrations should go to Bill Pollard.

Dr. Kathryn Donahue provided many of the anthropological observations as part of a Saul Blatman Clinical Fellowship Award. I've also appreciated the assistance of talented student volunteers Diana Oganova, Ahmed Ibrahim, and Josh Praw, medical student Tina Hong, and especially summer college student John Lee, who all helped with literature searches and retrieval of articles. I appreciate the expert review of the orthopedic sections of this book by Dr. Robert Matthew Bernstein, a skilled second-generation pediatric orthopedist at Cedars-Sinai Medical Center in Los Angeles.

I am deeply indebted to my nurse coordinator, Cathy Stoppenhagen, who organized my clinical services to patients for over 25 years, and to pediatric nurse practitioners, Dawn Earl and Jeannie Kreutzman, who provided clinical services for many of these patients and were my first nurse dysmorphology trainees. My secretary, Barbara Lawson typed and edited much of the text for this third edition. Many of the radiological images came from the International Skeletal Dysplasia Registry at Cedars-Sinai Medical Center, which is under the direction of Drs. David L. Rimoin and Ralph Lachman, who have both continued to mentor me like one of their own fellows.

Finally, I would like to express my deepest personal gratitude to my loving wife, Elizabeth, without whom none of this work would have been continued. For over three decades, she has endured the spread of research files, figures, and partially written text to virtually every flat surface in our home, and I'm sure she appreciates the return of our dining room table to its originally intended purpose. My two sons, Zachary and George, generously allowed me to use images of their own deformations as infants, emphasizing the normal nature of these findings.

The past 30 years have served to test many of the concepts advanced by Dr. Smith in the first edition of this book, and these concepts have stood the test of time. In reviewing the recent literature for this third edition, I was impressed how much data have been generated in an effort to test the concepts and theories originally advanced by Drs. David Smith and Peter Dunn.

# Preface

Ever since Peter Dunn and David Smith presented the basic concepts of deformation 30 years ago, it has become clear that unusual mechanical forces are responsible for a wide variety of structural birth defects. The impact of mechanical forces on form not only has provided an understanding of extrinsic constraint deformations but also has led to the appreciation that many of the malformation sequences can be interpreted as an initiating malformation that results in altered mechanical forces and a cascade of intrinsic deformation. Furthermore, this mechanical perspective provides a better understanding of the importance of mechanical forces in normal morphogenesis.

The major emphasis of *Smith's Recognizable Patterns of Human Deformation* is on extrinsic constraint deformations that are secondary to crowding in utero. These should, to the extent possible, be distinguished from malformations with or without secondary intrinsic deformation. Not only are there major differences in the etiology, prognosis, management, and recurrence risk for extrinsic deformations, but there are also profound differences in the prognosis that can be conveyed to the child's parents. The child with extrinsic deformation can usually be interpreted as normal, and the parents can look forward to the restoration of normal form. This attitude toward considering extrinsic deformations as a separable category of birth defects is also critical in providing better answers relative to etiology and prevention. The etiologic factors that may cause extrinsic deformation are obviously very different from those that cause malformation problems. The preventive measures for extrinsic deformations are also different and entail such considerations as external cephalic version for malpresentations and the surgical reconstruction of a malformed uterus. Furthermore, since extrinsic deformations are more common in infants of primigravida mothers and in larger fetuses, it is quite reasonable to anticipate that the incidence of extrinsic deformations might increase as a consequence of smaller families and larger babies.

The basic principles of extrinsic deformation are simple. The magnitude and direction of force have a direct impact on form. These same simple precepts are relevant to the management of deformations. With rare exceptions correction may be accomplished by the rational application of subtle forces.

Over the course of the last 25 years, since the first edition of this book, this knowledge has become an integral part of medicine because extrinsic deformations are common, and these basic concepts have become well established. The overall concepts that relate to the developmental pathology, diagnosis, and management of extrinsic deformations are simple and easily understood by primary care providers and subspecialists, as well as by parents. In recent times there has been a tendency to look for more complex answers of a biochemical, molecular, or physiologic nature and to bypass the simple mechanistic approaches. Hence this book is dedicated to bringing the mechanical aspects of morphogenesis and deformation into the mainstream of medicine, where they belong.

Very few studies of extrinsic deformation in experimental animals have been done. One reason is that few creatures other than humans tend to outgrow the uterus prior to birth and to have constraint deformations at birth. Most other animals are born at a much more mature state of development, ready to stand and run away from predators, however humans are unable to stand and run for almost a year after birth. Humans spend much of their infancy in a recumbent position, which may lead to deformation if the infant's resting position is not purposefully varied. This is one price the slowly aging, rapidly growing, large-brained human must pay for his or her present level of evolvement. One major aspect of human evolution is the prolonged period of time necessary to complete human brain development, such that the human brain continues to grow slowly over a much longer time than that necessary for other primates. It takes 6 months of postnatal growth for the human brain to reach the proportions found in a chimpanzee at birth. Thus human gestation would take an additional 7–8 months, if human neonates were to be born at the same stage of maturity as other primate infants. This continued growth of the human brain appears to leave the human cranium much more vulnerable to mechanical forces than that of other species. In order to accommodate this continued growth of the brain, the cranial sutures remain open for decades, while the plates of cranial bone continue to afford protection to the developing brain.

Congenital deformations are common, with most resolving spontaneously within the first few days of postnatal life. When such prompt resolution does not take place, further evaluation may be necessary to plan therapeutic interventions and prevent long-term negative consequences.

This book provides a rational approach for the diagnosis and management of such deformations. Information concerning unusual intrauterine positions should be transmitted to physicians caring for such newborns in the nursery. When such data are properly interpreted, it can guide further evaluation and therapy and be vastly reassuring to the parents. Prompt treatment of deformations leads to prompt resolution of such problems, while delays in treatment sometimes lead to permanent alterations and residual deformations which can have long-term implications.

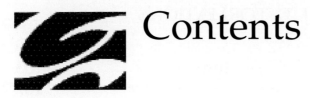# Contents

# THORACIC CAGE AND SPINAL DEFORMATIONS

# HEAD AND NECK DEFORMATIONS

# CRANIOSYNOSTOSIS

# CRANIAL BONE VARIATIONS

# ABNORMAL BIRTH PRESENTATION

## WHOLE-BODY DEFORMATION OR DISRUPTION

## MECHANICS IN MORPHOGENESIS

# SMITH'S Recognizable Patterns of Human Deformation

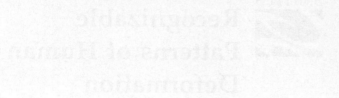

# Introduction

# 1 Clinical Approach to Deformation Problems

## MALFORMATIONS, DEFORMATIONS, DISRUPTIONS, AND DYSPLASIAS

Mechanical forces play an important role in both normal and abnormal morphogenesis. Anomalies that represent the normal response of a tissue to unusual mechanical forces are termed *deformations*, in contrast to *malformations*, which denote a primary problem in the morphogenesis of a tissue, and *disruptions*, which represent the breakdown of previously normal tissues. A fourth category of problems, termed *dysplasias*, results in abnormal structure because the tissues from which individual structures are formed are abnormal (Fig. 1-1). An isolated structural defect can arise through any of these four basic categories of morphogenesis, and clarifying the nature of the underlying defect is necessary to provide proper counseling. An isolated malformation, such as an idiopathic talipes equinovarus (rigid clubfoot), can arise as a localized error in morphogenesis with a multifactorial recurrence risk and differences in birth prevalence among various racial groups and between sexes. Prevalence ranges from a high of 6.8 per 1000 live births in Hawaiians and Maoris, to 1.2 per 1000 in Caucasians, to 0.74 per 1000 in U.S. blacks and Hispanics, to 0.39 per 1000 in Chinese populations.[1] Bilateral cases occur slightly more frequently than unilateral cases, and males are affected twice as frequently as females. Such variations in race and sex predilection occur for many different multifactorial defects, emphasizing the importance of differences in genetic background. If a clubfoot arises as part of a broader pattern of defects, it can do so through any one of these underlying categories of abnormal morphogenesis, and the recurrence risk is based on the cause of the overall pattern of abnormal morphogenesis.

A multiple *malformation syndrome* results in a primary developmental anomaly of two or more systems in which all of the structural defects are due to a single underlying etiology, which can be genetic, chromosomal, or environmental (tera-

togenic). In some cases the cause may be unknown, but as mechanisms of abnormal morphogenesis become better understood, the number of syndromes in this category has been diminishing. Multiple structural defects can also result from a *sequence* in which a single primary defect in morphogenesis produces multiple abnormalities through a cascading process of secondary and tertiary problems in morphogenesis. During the evaluation of a child with multiple anomalies, it is extremely important from the standpoint of recurrence risk counseling to distinguish a malformation syndrome from multiple defects that arose from a single localized error in morphogenesis, such as spina bifida malformation sequence (when a failure in neural tube closure results in secondary clubfeet and bladder/bowel problems). Examples of different types of structural defects are discussed in the next paragraph.

In Fig. 1-1, *A*, an infant with camptomelic syndrome has a cleft palate, hypospadias, abnormal skeletal development, and talipes equinovarus due to a mutation in *SOX9*, which resulted in a malformation syndrome. In Fig. 1-1, *B*, an infant was born at 36 weeks after amniotic membranes ruptured prematurely at 26 weeks, resulting in oligohydramnios deformation sequence. This may have occurred spontaneously, or it could have been caused by an underlying genetic connective tissue disorder such as Ehlers-Danlos syndrome, which predisposes the fetus toward early amnion rupture, ligamentous laxity, and hernias. The fetus in Fig. 1-1, *C* has been affected by the disruption of previous normal structures due to early amnion rupture during the first trimester, resulting in strands of amnion damaging facial structures. The infant in Fig. 1-1, *D* has an autosomal recessive skeletal dysplasia (diastrophic dysplasia) that resulted in cleft palate, malformed pinna with calcification of ear cartilage, hitchhiker thumbs, synphalangism, and talipes equinovarus with progressive

3

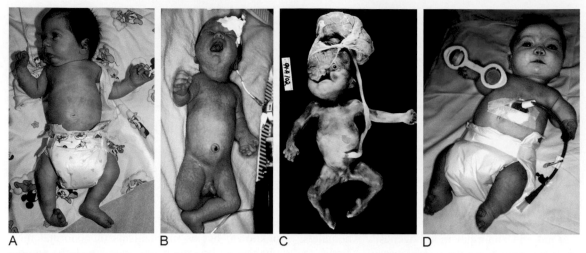

FIGURE 1-1. The four major types of problems in morphogenesis: malformation, deformation, disruption, and dysplasia. **A,** An infant with camptomelic dysplasia syndrome, which results in a multiple malformation syndrome due to a mutation in *SOX9*. **B,** An infant with oligohydramnios deformation sequence due to premature rupture of membranes from 17 weeks of gestation until birth at 36 weeks; the infant was delivered from a persistent transverse lie. **C,** A fetus with early amnion rupture sequence with attachment of the placenta to the head and resultant disruption of craniofacial structures with distal limb contractures. **D,** An infant with diastrophic dysplasia due to inherited autosomal recessive mutations in a sulfate transporter protein.

scoliosis, which is particularly refractory to treatment. This condition results from a mutant sulfate transporter protein gene, which is inherited from each parent, with no signs evident in the carrier parents. In order to offer appropriate genetic counseling, it is important to distinguish such underlying malformation syndromes, skeletal dysplasias, and genetic connective tissue disorders from isolated defects that resulted solely from fetal disruption or late gestational constraint. Syndromes and dysplasias often have a genetic basis.

Deformations often involve either the craniofacial region or the limbs, and they are usually attributed to intrauterine molding and termed *positional defects*. The mechanical pressure causing the molding can either be intrinsic (e.g., neuromuscular imbalance) or extrinsic (e.g., fetal crowding). When a prolonged decrease in fetal movement occurs due to either type of problem, joints may develop contractures because joints require movement in order to form in a normal way. Thus, there are predominantly two types of deformational problems: those in which the causative forces are due to an intrinsic problem within the developing fetus (such as a neuromuscular insufficiency or a central nervous system developmental defect) and those in which the deformation was produced by mechanical forces that were extrinsic to an otherwise normal fetus.

The two predominant types of deformation are depicted in Fig. 1-2, and the distinctions between

these two types are based on historical and physical findings. In Fig. 1-3, the overall pattern of intrinsic deformation due to neuromuscular insufficiency is quite similar for both congenital myotonic dystrophy (Fig. 1-3, *A*), an autosomal dominant disorder with a 50% recurrence risk, and Pena-Shokeir syndrome (Fig. 1-3, *B*), an autosomal recessive disorder with a 25% recurrence risk. Myotonic dystrophy results from amplification of a trinucleotide repeat in the 3 untranslated region of a protein kinase gene on chromosome 19. Normally, there are 5 to 30 repeat copies of this repeat. When there are 50 to 80 repeats, the result is mild disease; when there are more than 2000 repeats, infants are severely affected with congenital myotonic dystrophy, as depicted in Fig. 1-3, *A*. This severe pattern is seen in the offspring of affected women only and becomes more likely as the mutant allele is transmitted through successive generations, a phenomenon termed *anticipation*.

The pattern of intrinsic neuromuscular deformation is recognizably different from the pattern seen with extrinsic deformation due to oligohydramnios deformation sequence, as demonstrated in Fig. 1-1, *B*. In Fig. 1-3, *C*, the facial effects of intrinsic deformation due to Möbius sequence (deficient cranial nerve VI and VII function) also differ from the extrinsic facial deformations seen in Fig. 1-3, *D*, in which prolonged oligohydramnios and a persistent transverse lie resulted

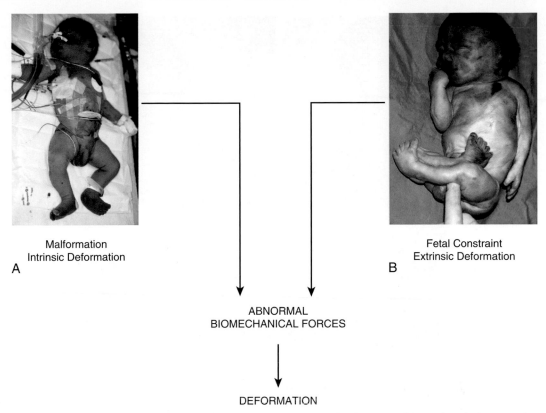

Malformation
Intrinsic Deformation
A

Fetal Constraint
Extrinsic Deformation
B

ABNORMAL
BIOMECHANICAL FORCES

DEFORMATION

FIGURE 1-2. Unusual mechanical forces resulting in deformation may be the consequence of extrinsic constraint of a normal fetus, or they may be the result of an intrinsic malformation of the fetus. **A,** An infant with oligohydramnios deformation sequence due to bilateral renal agenesis. **B,** An infant with oligohydramnios deformation sequence due to prolonged leakage of amniotic fluid. Both infants died shortly after birth from associated pulmonary hypoplasia.

in marked facial compression. Disruptive defects occur when a previously normally formed structure is partly or completely destroyed. This can result from either amniotic bands (see Fig. 1-1, C) or an interruption of blood supply (Fig. 1-4, A); in some cases of early amnion rupture, both mechanisms may occur (see Fig. 1-4, C). When one monozygotic, monochorionic twin dies in utero, interruption of blood supply to fetal structures can lead to infarction, necrosis, hypoplasia, and/or resorption of tissues distal to where thromboembolic debris lodges in the circulation of the surviving twin (see Fig. 1-4, A).

Extrinsic forces may result in a single localized deformation, such as a positional foot deformation, or they may cause a deformation sequence. A *deformation sequence* refers to the manifold molding effects of a given deforming situation. A good example of one such deformation sequence is the oligohydramnios sequence, in which oligohydramnios is responsible for a number of associated deformations (see Figs. 1-1, B, 1-2, B, and 1-3, D).

The major cause of such deformations is uterine constraint of the rapidly growing, malleable fetus in late gestation. Most of these molded deformations have an excellent prognosis once the fetus is released from the constraining environment. However, they usually merit prompt treatment at the appropriate time in order to achieve the best result (usually the earlier, the better). Such treatment often involves the use of gentle mechanical forces to attempt to reshape the deformed structure into a more normal form.

A clear distinction between deformation and malformation is critical to providing parents with a clear understanding of their infant's problem and its prognosis, management, and recurrence risk. Such a clear distinction may not always be possible, and the study of structural defects in twins demonstrates the complexity of making such distinctions. Twin studies represent a unique approach to understanding both genetic and environmental etiologic contributions to the development of congenital anomalies.[2,3] Twins

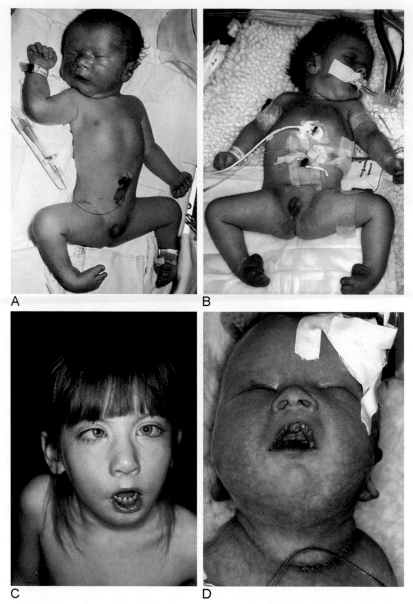

FIGURE 1-3. The overall pattern of intrinsic deformation due to neuromuscular insufficiency is quite similar for both congenital myotonic dystrophy (**A**), an autosomal dominant disorder with a 50% recurrence risk, and Pena-Shokeir syndrome (**B**), an autosomal recessive disorder with a 25% recurrence risk. In **C**, note the facial effects of intrinsic deformation due to Möbius sequence (deficient cranial nerve VI and VII function), which differ from the extrinsic facial deformations seen in **D**, in which prolonged oligohydramnios and a persistent transverse lie resulted in marked facial compression.

share identical intrauterine environments, but their genetic constitutions are either homogeneous, as in monozygotic twins, or heterogeneous, as in dizygotic twins. Monozygotic twins often share the same placenta and placental vasculature, which makes them more vulnerable to vascular disruption. Late fetal crowding makes deformations much more common in twins, and deformations are equally likely in both types of twinning. Because the fetal head accounts for much of the volume in late gestation, it is particularly susceptible to extrinsic, constraint-related deformations.

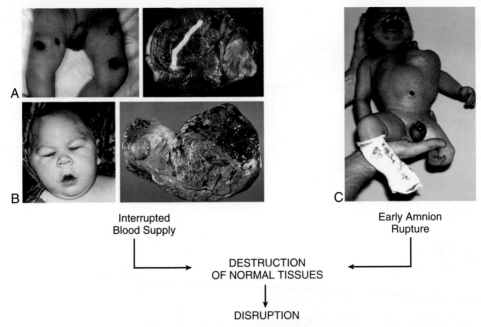

Interrupted
Blood Supply

Early Amnion
Rupture

DESTRUCTION
OF NORMAL TISSUES

DISRUPTION

FIGURE 1-4. The two predominant types of fetal disruption are demonstrated. Disruptive defects occur when there is destruction of a previously normally formed part. This can result from interruption of blood supply (**A** and **B**) or from amniotic bands. In some cases of early amnion rupture, both mechanisms may occur (**C**). When one monozygotic, monochorionic twin dies in utero, interruption of blood supply to fetal structures can lead to infarction, necrosis, hypoplasia, and/or resorption of tissues distal to where thromboembolic debris lodges in the circulation of the surviving co-twin (**A** and **B**). A deceased co-twin is evident on examination of the placentas for an infant born with cutis aplasia over the knees (**A**) and for an infant with hydranencephaly (**B**).

Among 801 infants with deformational plagiocephaly who were treated with an external orthotic device, 69 (8.6%) were of multiple-birth origin.[4] Because there is less space within the lower portion of the uterus, the bottom twin in vertex presentation is most likely to develop torticollis-plagiocephaly deformation sequence (Fig. 1-5).

Monozygotic twinning results when a fertilized zygote splits into two embryos during the first 14 days after fertilization; this splitting process is associated with an increased likelihood of early malformations, many of which lead to the three-fold higher mortality rate in monozygotic twins compared with dizygotic twins or singletons.[2] Among craniofacial anomalies, structural defects of the malformative or disruptive type occur more frequently in monozygotic twins compared with dizygotic twins. Malformations are often concordant, whereas disruptions and deformations are not. Among 35 twin pairs in which one or both twins exhibited craniofacial anomalies, 21 pairs were monozygotic and 14 pairs were dizygotic.[3] Malformations were more common among monozygotic twins as compared with dizygotic twins, and concordance occurred predominantly in the

monozygotic group, with 7 of 8 pairs being concordant. Among 20 twin pairs with discordant anomalies for whom there was information regarding fetal position, the affected infant was usually vertex and inferior in the pelvis, and deformational craniofacial anomalies were often associated with early fetal head descent during the third trimester.[3]

Monozygotic twins with placental vascular interconnections may be predisposed toward vasculodisruptive defects in the surviving twin when one twin dies in utero (termed *twin disruption sequence*). Among monochorionic twin pregnancies with one dead twin (see Fig. 1-4, *A* and *B*), only 57% of the co-twin survivors were unaffected, with 19% of the co-twins dying in utero or during the neonatal period and 24% surviving with serious sequelae (e.g., cerebellar infarcts, porencephaly, hydranencephaly, microcephaly, spinal cord infarcts, hemifacial microsomia, gastroschisis, limb reduction defects, renal cortical necrosis, atresia of small bowel, and cutis aplasia).[5] Among 18 twins with twin disruption sequence, most deaths occurred in the second or third trimesters, and intrauterine death in the first

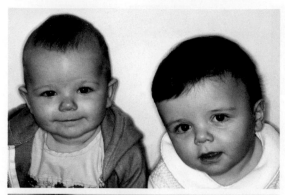

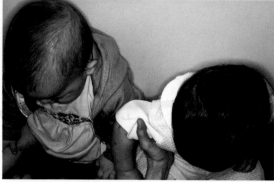

FIGURE 1-5. Torticollis-plagiocephaly deformation sequence is more frequent in twins, and it is usually the bottommost twin who is most likely to develop torticollis and secondary craniofacial deformation. The twin on the right was on the bottom and has residual plagiocephaly at age 10 months due to untreated torticollis and an asymmetric postnatal resting position.

trimester rarely caused damage to the surviving co-twin. Survivors had a poor prognosis due to microcephaly, spastic tetraplegia, severe mental retardation, and therapy-resistant epilepsy.[6]

In general, deformations have a much more favorable prognosis than malformations. The collective frequency of all types of extrinsic deformations of late fetal origin is about 2% of live births.[7-9] This frequency is based on the work of neonatologist Peter Dunn, who correlated clinical records of 4754 infants born in the Birmingham Maternity Hospital (United Kingdom) with maternal medical history and infant follow-up. This population study documented a 3.6% incidence of malformation, with or without deformation, and among the malformed infants in Dunn's sample, 7.6% were also deformed.[7-9] The deformation rate was 26.7% for infants with urinary tract malformations and 100% for those with bilateral renal agenesis. Of 11 infants born to mothers with premature rupture of membranes, none were malformed, but 10 were deformed. Among the group

of infants with postural deformations, Dunn noted that 33% had two or more deformations and that there were significant associations between facial deformity, plagiocephaly, mandibular asymmetry, muscular torticollis, scoliosis, developmental dysplasia of the hip, and talipes equinovarus.[9] About one third (32%) of the deformed infants had been in breech presentation. First-born infants were significantly more likely to be deformed than subsequently born infants (54% versus 35%). Thus, it is particularly important to look for deformations in the infants of primigravida mothers and in infants with malpresentation.

In a study of 1,455,405 Spanish infants born alive between 1976 and 1997, 26,290 (1.8%) had major or minor anomalies detected at birth; of this group, 3.67% also had deformations. Deformations were found four times more frequently (14.62%) among stillborn infants with anomalies.[10] The authors of this study distinguished three distinct patterns of deformation. One pattern featured polyhydramnios, thin skin without dermal ridges, and multiple deformations resulting from fetal akinesia-hypokinesia sequence due to various intrinsic neuromuscular defects. A second pattern resulted in oligohydramnios with redundant thick skin and multiple deformations due to intrinsic renal or urinary tract defects or to extrinsic loss of amniotic fluid. A third pattern of deformation was associated with normal amounts of amniotic fluid and was caused by various types of extrinsic fetal compression.[10] Differences between the 0.07% frequency of extrinsic deformations in this latter study and the 2% frequency noted by Dunn reflect major differences in the classification of minor postural deformations. In Dunn's earlier studies, 90% of the postural deformations he observed resolved spontaneously, and such transient defects were probably not counted in the Spanish study. Alternatively, with more accurate gestational dating and size determination, the incidence of large-for-gestational-age and postmature infants has been decreasing, thereby lowering the risk for late-gestational constraint.

This text is primarily concerned with extrinsic deformations produced by unusual or excessive constraint of an otherwise normal fetus. Individual deformations in this book are presented in an atlas format along with deformation sequences. Because it may sometimes be difficult to exclude an underlying connective tissue dysplasia, examples of such problems are also discussed as part of the differential diagnosis. Because the major emphasis of this text is extrinsic deformations due to uterine constraint, this category will be considered first. Next, consideration will be given to the interaction between extrinsic and intrinsic factors in the genesis of some deformations. Finally, intrinsic deformations due to a fetal neuromuscular insufficiency are discussed.

## EXTRINSIC DEFORMATIONS DUE TO UTERINE CONSTRAINT

The presumption in this category is that there is no primary problem within the fetus and that the deformations are secondary to extrinsic forces that have deformed an otherwise normal fetus. The most common cause of extrinsic deformation is uterine constraint. About 2% of babies are born with an extrinsic deformation, 90% of which resolve spontaneously; hence, these are relatively common problems.[7-9] Usually, the amount of amniotic fluid is adequate to cushion the fetus, allowing for normal growth and mobility prior to 36 to 37 weeks of gestation. Thus, one of the major functions of the amniotic fluid is to distend the uterus and enable the fetus to move freely and to grow with equal pressure in all regions with no excessive or localized constraint.[11] As the fetus becomes more crowded within the uterus during late gestation, it will usually settle into a position in which the largest moving fetal parts, the relatively bulky legs, have more room in the upper portion of the uterus. Thus, the fetus tends to assume a vertex presentation. The implication that most extrinsic deformations are produced during late fetal life is supported by the observations of Nishimura, who found that both hip dislocation and clubfoot are rare findings in aborted fetuses prior to 20 weeks of gestation.[12]

After about 35 to 38 weeks of gestation, the human fetus tends to grow out of proportion to the size of the uterine cavity (Fig. 1-6). During this period of rapid late fetal growth, the relative proportion of amniotic fluid decreases, causing the fetus to become increasingly constrained. Uterine constraint of rapidly growing, malleable fetal structures may result in mechanically induced deformations. Because the cause of one deformation may often have led to other constraint-related problems in the pliable fetus, there may be a non-random occurrence of more than one deformation in the same child. Dunn[8] found that 33% of newborn infants with one deformation problem had additional deformations (Fig. 1-7). In this text, the combination of multiple deformations resulting from the same extrinsic cause is termed a *deformation sequence.*

Uterine constraint tends also to reduce the rate of late fetal growth and is one cause of prenatal

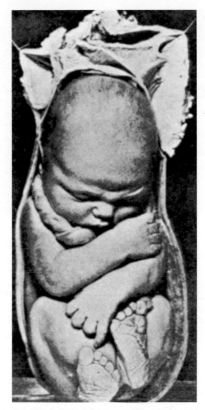

FIGURE 1-6. A primigravida's term fetus in breech position illustrates the uterine constraint that is a feature of late fetal life and this mode of presentation. The mother was killed in a motor vehicle accident, and the fetus was dead on arrival at the hospital.

(Courtesy of Peter Dunn, Southmead Hospital, Bristol, United Kingdom.)

growth deficiency.[13] Such newborn babies frequently show deformational evidence of uterine constraint other than growth deficiency alone. Any situation that tends to overdistend the uterus may be associated with early onset of labor and premature birth. This is a major concern for multiple-gestation infants, who simply distend the uterus prematurely, and also for the woman with uterine structural malformations or extensive uterine myomas. When fetal growth has been constrained during late gestation, catch-up growth is usually initiated promptly after delivery so that most term fetuses reach their genetically determined growth percentiles by age 6 to 8 months.[14]

If the basic type of deformation is not clearly determined at the time of birth, then the early postnatal course usually provides valuable clues as to whether the deformations noted at birth are extrinsic or intrinsic in causation. The otherwise normal infant who has been constrained in late

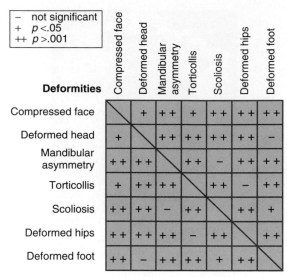

| Deformities | Compressed face | Deformed head | Mandibular asymmetry | Torticollis | Scoliosis | Deformed hips | Deformed foot |
|---|---|---|---|---|---|---|---|
| Compressed face | | + | + + | + | + + | + + | + + |
| Deformed head | + | | + + | + + | + + | + + | – |
| Mandibular asymmetry | + + | + + | | + + | – | + + | + + |
| Torticollis | + | + + | + + | | + + | – | + + |
| Scoliosis | + + | + + | – | + + | | + + | + |
| Deformed hips | + + | + + | + + | – | + + | | + + |
| Deformed foot | + + | – | + + | + + | + | + + | |

Legend:
– not significant
+ p<.05
++ p>.001

FIGURE 1-7. The non-random clinical association among deformations.

(Adapted from Dunn PM: Congenital postural deformities: further perinatal associations, *Proc R Soc Med* 65:735, 1972.)

fetal life tends to show progressive improvement in growth and form after being released from the deforming situation upon delivery. If growth has been slowed by constraint in late fetal life, the infant tends to show catch-up growth toward his or her genetic potential in early infancy, beginning within the first 2 months. If the growth of particular structures has been restrained, they tend to show catch-up growth toward normal form, such as with the nasal and mandibular growth restriction seen following prolonged face presentation. Joints that have been externally constrained prenatally tend to show progressive increases in their range of motion after birth, often showing more dramatic resolution with neonatal physical therapy. This is clearly evident with positional torticollis or positional foot deformations but not with structural neck malformations (e.g., Klippel-Feil malformation) or rigid clubfoot. If there is a lack of catch-up growth and/or little or no return toward normal form after birth, then further evaluation is indicated to search for a more intrinsic problem that might be responsible for the deformation(s).

## Historical Perspective

As long ago as Hippocrates, it was known that uterine constraint could cause fetal deformation. Aristotle carried out experiments demonstrating that crowding of development caused limb deformations in chicks; however, little was written about constraint deformations until the Renaissance era. In 1573 Ambroise Paré[15] of France wrote "Narrowness of the uterus produces monsters by the same manner that the Dame of Paris carried the little dog in a small basket to the end that it didn't grow." In 1921 von Reuss's text *Diseases of the Newborn* contained an entire chapter on postural deformations,[16] but modern texts about the newborn have more limited coverage of this subject. Full understanding of the mechanisms and types of fetal deformation is vitally important for clinicians who deal with problems of aberrant morphogenesis. A number of investigators made major contributions to the knowledge and understanding of extrinsic deformations during the past century. A few brief summations and quotations from representative investigators will serve to emphasize some of their important observations and interpretations.

Thompson[17]: This Scottish naturalist and mathematician held the Chair of Natural History in St. Andrews for 64 years. He wrote: "We are ruled by gravity.... There is freedom of movement in the plane perpendicular to gravitational force.... Gravity affects stature and leads to sagging of tissues and drooping of the mouth."

von Reuss[16]: This early Viennese neonatologist made the following statement about contractural deformities: "... the deformities occur probably most frequently from pressure on the part of the uterine wall; sometimes marks of pressure may be observed on the skin."

Chapple and Davidson[18]: These pediatricians noted that the "position of comfort" of the deformed infant soon after birth tends to be that which had existed in utero, and repositioning the baby into the "position of comfort" might allow the clinician to more readily deduce the causative compressive factors that resulted in the deformation.

Browne[19,20]: Denis Browne, an orthopedist at Great Ormond Street Children's Hospital in London, recognized that deformed infants were often the product of an "uncomfortable" pregnancy, implying uterine constraint. He emphasized the need for controlled forces, using functional growth, in the correction of such deformations.

Dunn[7-9]: This English neonatologist was responsible for resurrecting and extending knowledge regarding the importance of extrinsic deformation. He stated that "intrauterine forces capable of moulding the fetus increase throughout pregnancy as the infant grows, the mother's uterus and abdominal wall are stretched, and the volume of amniotic fluid diminishes. At the same time the ability of the infant to resist deformation increases as the rate of fetal growth slows, the skeleton ossifies, and leg movements become more powerful. All these factors are, of course, themselves directly or indirectly under the influence of heredity and are involved in a dynamic interplay throughout fetal life. Nature plays her hand to the limit. The price paid for a larger and more mature infant at birth, better able to withstand the stresses of extra uterine life, is a 2% incidence of deformities."

## Factors That Enhance Fetal Constraint in Utero

Box 1-1 summarizes some of the factors that increase the likelihood of fetal constraint in utero; these factors are presented in more detail in this section.

### Primigravida

The first fetus usually experiences more constraint than later offspring because it is the first to distend the mother's muscular uterus and abdominal wall. As a consequence, constraint-related deformations are more common in infants born to primigravidas than to multigravidas. Fig. 1-8 shows the form of the uterus in a primigravida compared with a multigravida, emphasizing the difference in shape and size of the structures surrounding the fetus. The greater magnitude of late fetal constraint in the primigravida is considered to be one major reason why the first-born infant is normally smaller at

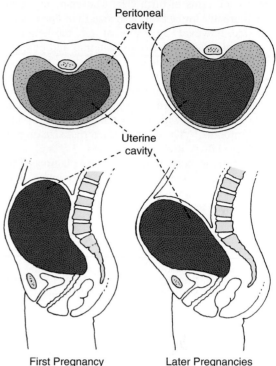

Primigravida Versus Multigravida

First Pregnancy          Later Pregnancies

FIGURE 1-8. Transverse and sagittal section diagrams of the abdomens of primigravida and multigravida women illustrate the impact of the unstretched abdominal muscles on the shape of the uterine cavity during the later weeks of pregnancy.
(Adapted from Dunn PM: Perinatal observations on the etiology of congenital dislocation of the hip, *Clin Orthop* 119:11, 1976.)

birth than later-born offspring. Even though the first-born infant tends to be 200 to 300 g smaller than later offspring at birth, they are of comparable size by 1 year of age. Thus, the mild late fetal growth deficiency in the offspring of a primigravida is transient, and such infants tend to catch up to their genetically determined rate of growth within the first few months after birth.[13,14] The first-born infant is also more likely to become constrained in an unusual position, such as a breech presentation, and to have consequent deformations relating to malpresentation.

### Small Maternal Size

The smaller the mother in relation to fetal size, the greater the likelihood of deforming uterine constraint in late fetal life. Deformations are more

---

**BOX 1-1.   Risk Factors for Fetal Constraint**

**Maternal Risk Factors**
 Primigravida
 Small maternal size
 Small uterus
 Uterine malformation
 Uterine fibromata
 Small maternal pelvis

**Fetal Risk Factors**
 Oligohydramnios
 Large fetus
 Multiple fetuses

common in offspring born to small women than in those born to larger women. This impact is readily evident in terms of birth size. Maternal size has a much greater impact on birth size than does paternal size; however, by 1 year of age, the length of the infant relates equally to maternal and paternal stature. Much of this maternal impact on birth size appears to relate to the transient effect of small maternal size in restraining late fetal growth. After birth, the infant moves into his or her own genetic pace of growth, which is usually evident by age 6 to 8 months.[14] The effect of maternal size on prenatal growth is illustrated in Figs. 1-9 and 1-10. Many infants born with torticollis-plagiocephaly deformation sequence are born to parents with obvious size discrepancies (i.e., small mothers and large fathers).

## Uterine Malformation

Limitation in the capacity of the uterus to accommodate a term-size fetus may result in early miscarriage, stillbirth, prematurity, and/or offspring who survive to be born with sufficient constraint to give rise to deformation(s). Such reproductive problems are particularly likely to occur with uterine malformations such as a bicornuate or

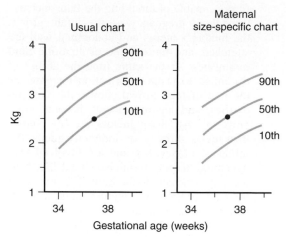

FIGURE 1-10. The weight of a 2.3-kg newborn baby born to a small mother with a weight of 40 kg and height of 150 cm, plotted on the usual growth chart *(left)* and on one that is specific for maternal size *(right)*.

(Adapted from Winick M: Biologic correlations, *Am J Dis Child* 120:416, 1970. Standards for the chart on the right are from Thomson AM, Billewicz WZ, Hytten FE, et al: The assessment of fetal growth, *J Obstet Gynecol Br Comm* 75:903, 1968.)

unicornuate uterus. About 1% to 2% of women have a uterine malformation, and the likelihood of a deformation problem in a fetus reared in a bicornuate uterus has been crudely estimated to be about 30%.[21] Many of the genetic factors that result in a bicornuate uterus also affect renal morphogenesis, which leads to renal dysplasia and resultant oligohydramnios, further increasing the likelihood of fetal deformation. The recognition that a malformation of the mother's uterus has caused a fetal problem may lead to corrective surgery on that uterus, thus providing a better opportunity for the next fetus to grow without as much constraint.

## Uterine Fibromata

A large fibroid of the uterus may limit intrauterine space and therefore have a gestational impact similar to that of a bicornuate uterus. Surgical removal of the fibroid may allow for better fetal space, and this merits consideration if it will not weaken the structure of the uterus. Fortunately, most uterine fibromata develop relatively late in reproductive life and are an infrequent cause of fetal deformation; however, a small fibroma may grow rapidly during gestation under the influence of increased levels of maternal estrogen.

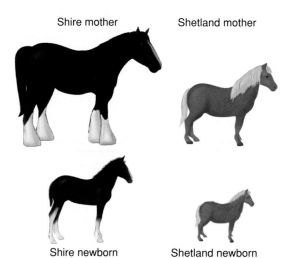

FIGURE 1-9. The cross between a shire horse and a Shetland pony dramatically illustrates influence of maternal size on the size of the offspring at birth. Although the genetic situation is the same, the foal of the small mother is much smaller at birth than that of the large mother, presumably because of the smaller space within which to rear this fetus.

(Adapted from Hammond J: Growth in size and body proportions in farm animals. In Zarrow MX, ed: *Growth in living systems*, New York, 1961, Basic Books, p 321.)

## Small Maternal Pelvis

Vaginal delivery through a pelvic outlet that is small in relationship to the size of the fetus may result in appreciable molding of the craniofacies. This molding is usually transient; however, if there has been prolonged engagement of the fetal head, the degree of molding can be severe, and there may be a slower resolution toward normal form after birth. Early treatment via appropriate positioning can facilitate a more complete return to normal form.

## Early Pelvic Engagement of the Fetal Head

During labor, the fetal head usually engages in an occiput transverse (OT) position as the head enters and passes through the pelvic inlet. In the typical female pelvis (gynecoid), this results more commonly in a left-oriented occiput position than in a right-oriented position (58.5% versus 40.5%).[22-24] Progressive descent of the fetal head occurs as it traverses the pelvic inlet with the sagittal suture in the transverse diameter of the pelvic inlet and the biparietal diameter (BPD) parallel to the anteroposterior diameter of the pelvic inlet. With progressing decent of the fetal head, internal rotation occurs and the fetal head usually passes the ischial spines in an occiput anterior or posterior position. As the head descends, it encounters resistance from the cervix, the walls of the pelvis, and/or the pelvic floor, resulting in further flexion of the fetal head. Engagement of the fetal head is considered to have occurred when the BPD, the largest transverse diameter of the fetal head, has traversed the pelvic inlet. In nulliparous patients, engagement may occur by 36 weeks, but most nulliparous women present in labor without the fetal head engaged; in multiparous patients, engagement occurs significantly later and often only intrapartum.[25]

Early descent of the fetal head into the maternal pelvis is an unusual event and often accompanied by maternal symptoms of marked pelvic pressure and pubic discomfort that sometimes include pains radiating down the back of the legs. It is very unusual for the fetal head to descend more than 6 weeks before term, and it rarely does so more than 1 month before delivery. Early fetal head descent is more common in the primigravida. When the symptoms are severe, pain may make it difficult for the mother to walk during late gestation. Fetal head descent usually takes place shortly before birth, and the head in vertex presentation rotates into the left occiput transverse position in 58.5% of cases in order to pass through the mother's pelvis (Fig. 1-11). Consequences of early fetal head descent can include congenital muscular torticollis, craniotabes, craniosynostosis, and persistent vertex molding.[26] The fetal head is particularly susceptible to deforming forces because it is a relatively large and rapidly growing structure. One manifestation is vertex craniotabes secondary to prolonged compression of the top of the calvarium, resulting in poorly mineralized, malleable bone in the region of compression.[27] Another potential consequence is lateral constraint of the fetal head, resulting in a lack of growth stretch across the sagittal suture. If there is a lack of growth stretch across a given suture, then that suture can become ossified, resulting in craniosynostosis.[26,28] The most common problem after early fetal head descent is congenital muscular torticollis, which can lead to deformational plagiocephaly without appropriate therapy. Some degree of transient vertex head molding always occurs in most infants in cephalic presentation, but this usually resolves within a few days. It is rare, even with prolonged engagement of the fetal head, for such molding to persist, and corrective postnatal positioning can facilitate a return to normal head shape.

## Fetal Position

Prior to 36 to 37 weeks, when the fetus usually has adequate room for movement in its aquatic environment, it is not unusual for the fetus to be in varying positions, most commonly breech presentation. As the fetus becomes more crowded, he or she tends to shift into the vertex presentation position, there being more room in the fundal portion of the uterus for the bulkier legs. Unusual late fetal position in utero may result from all the factors that increase the risk for fetal constraint (see Fig. 11-1), as well as from a primary fetal neuromuscular problem or malformation, which limits the ability of the fetus to move (Fig. 1-12). The most common reason for an aberrant position is fetal constraint that has limited the capacity of the fetus to move into a vertex presentation. Abnormal fetal position during late fetal life may result in unusual constraint forces and significantly affect craniofacial structures. Examples include breech presentation, face presentation, brow presentation, and transverse lie. Breech presentation, although occurring in only 4% of pregnancies, was associated with 32% of all extrinsic deformations in Dunn's early studies.[7-9]

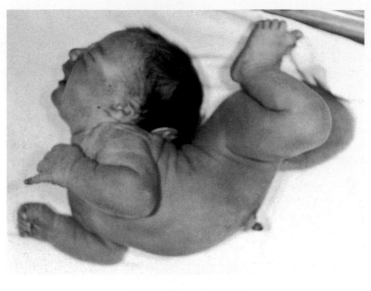

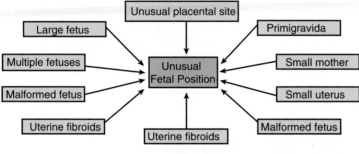

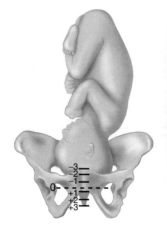

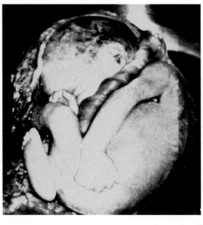

FIGURE 1-11. This drawing shows the left occiput transverse position, which occurs most commonly in vertex presentations. The top figure and the bottom right figure show aberrant fetal positions, which can result from any of the factors shown in this diagram.

(Courtesy of Jan Norbisrath, Medical Illustrator, Dept. of Obstetrics and Gynecology, University of Washington School of Medicine, Seattle.)

## Large Fetus with Rapid Growth

The fetus normally manifests a rapid rate of growth. For example, it normally doubles in weight between 28 to 34 weeks of gestation. The faster the growth rate, the larger the fetus becomes, and the greater the likelihood of all types of external constraint-related deformations. In a prospective study of 801 pregnancies that resulted in the birth of an infant weighing 4100 g or more, shoulder dystocia and perinatal lacerations were related to increasing birth weight. Difficult deliveries leading to clavicular fractures, brachial plexus injuries, or facial trauma resulted in an 11.4% perinatal morbidity rate. Asphyxia was observed in 7.7% and hypoglycemia in 5.2%, suggesting a need for close surveillance of infants of obese or diabetic mothers.[29] The male is normally larger

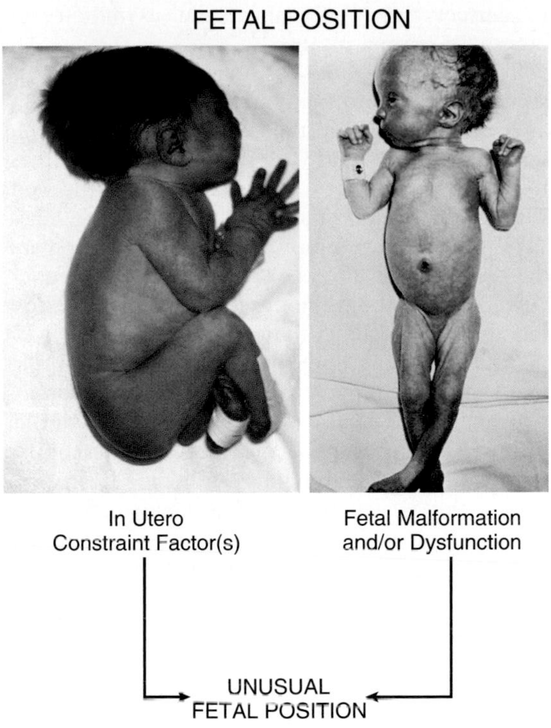

## FETAL POSITION

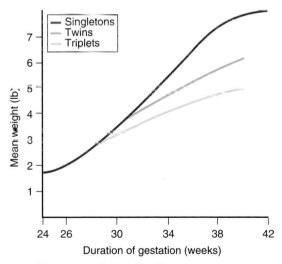

In Utero
Constraint Factor(s)

Fetal Malformation
and/or Dysfunction

UNUSUAL
FETAL POSITION

FIGURE 1-12. Unusual fetal position in utero may be the result of constraint factors to a normal fetus, or it may be the consequence of a primary fetal malformation and/or neuromuscular dysfunction.

and grows more rapidly in late fetal life than does the female.[14] Many extrinsic deformations are more common in the male than in the female, with the exceptions of developmental dysplasia of the hip and other similar joint-dislocation deformations that appear to be related to greater connective tissue laxity in females. Although torticollis-plagiocephaly deformation sequence is more common in males, this does not appear to be due to size differences at birth.[30] The effects of relaxing hormones and hormone receptors in the female fetus may affect their connective tissues so as to allow for cervical dilatation, increase their susceptibility to congenital hip dislocation, and protect them from torticollis. Testosterone may also accentuate muscular development in males, increasing susceptibility to torticollis and protecting them from hip dislocation.

### Multiple Fetuses

Multiple fetuses fill out the uterine cavity more quickly than does a singleton fetus, and the average uterus is capable of handling a maximum of 4 kg of fetal mass. For twins, this combined size is usually achieved by approximately 34 weeks of gestation, after which there tends to be a slowing in growth as the uterine cavity becomes filled,[31] as shown in Fig. 1-13. Postural deformations and transient growth deficiency are more common in twins, especially malpositioning of the feet and molding of the cranium.[4,20,30,31] Torticollis-plagiocephaly deformation sequence occurs particularly frequently in multiple births, and usually the bottom-most twin is more likely to develop torticollis and secondary craniofacial deformation (see Fig. 1-5). Because of these factors, monozygotic twins may not appear to be identical at the time of birth. One twin may have been constrained in a different manner and to a different degree than the other twin. Some differences may also relate to aberrant fetal positioning in one of the twins.

### Oligohydramnios

A deficit of amniotic fluid in late fetal life may be due to a variety of causes such as early rupture of the amnion with chronic leakage of amniotic fluid, lack of urine flow into the amniotic space, or maternal hypertension. Regardless of the cause, a lack of amniotic fluid tends to give rise to an unusual degree of uterine constraint, which adversely affects fetal growth and pulmonary maturation

FIGURE 1-13. The mean fetal weights of singletons as compared with twins and triplets. Although the initial growth rate is the same, the combined size of twins or triplets leads to earlier uterine constraint and late fetal slowing of growth.

(Adapted from Bulmer MG: *The biology of twinning in man*, Oxford, 1970, Clarendon Press.)

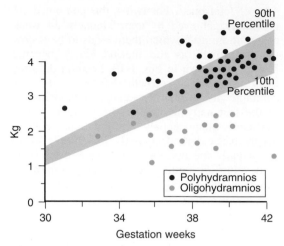

FIGURE 1-14. Impact on birth weight in kilograms of oligo-hydramnios due to renal insufficiency *(green dots)* versus polyhydramnios *(blue dots).*

(Adapted from Dunn PM: Growth retardation of infants with congenital postural deformities, *Acta Med Auxol* 7:63, 1975.)

and results in craniofacial and limb deformations.[32] The consequences of a prolonged deficit of amniotic fluid are referred to as the *oligohydramnios deformation sequence.* The impact of oligohydramnios versus polyhydramnios on birth size is shown in Fig. 1-14.

## Management, Prognosis, and Counsel

When a deformation is due to external constraint in late fetal life in an otherwise normal infant, the prognosis for a return to normal form is usually excellent, but this does not imply that the clinician caring for such infants should do nothing. The management of extrinsic deformations varies with the cause and type of deformation, and early treatment is the key to a successful outcome. Sometimes it is worthwhile to observe the neonate for spontaneous changes for several days after birth before making a decision as to whether any further therapy is indicated. Treatment often uses corrective mechanical forces similar to those that gave rise to the deformation, in an effort to reshape the deformed structures into a more normal form. When possible, this mechanical therapy should take advantage of the normal rapid rate of postnatal growth. This is particularly true for torticollis-plagiocephaly deformation sequence. When deformational plagiocephaly cannot be corrected with repositioning, use of orthotic management while the head is still growing rapidly has repeatedly been documented

to correct deformational cranial asymmetry in otherwise normal infants.[30,32,33-35]

The precise modes of management for constraint-related deformations may vary appreciably and yet accomplish the same purpose. Simple manual manipulation with molding and stretching toward a normal form may be all that is needed. This is a common practice in India, where "massage women" are employed to mold and shape the neonate's head and extremities. These women come to the infant's home daily for the first few months or as long as indicated. By massage with oil and stretching, they form the baby into a normal shape and remove any extrinsic deformations that may have been present at birth. In a similar fashion, parents can be instructed to accomplish such molding or stretching at home. Reshaping forces can be applied to foot deformations by frequent adhesive taping, resulting in gradual improvement in form. When such benign measures do not adequately correct the deformation, more rigorous means of molding and stretching, such as casting of the limbs or orthotic molding of the head, may be used. The current epidemic of torticollis-plagiocephaly deformation sequence is due to underrecognition of signs of positional torticollis at birth and failure to institute corrective measures of physical therapy of the neck and repositioning of the infant's head in a timely manner.[30] When a joint is seriously dislocated or malpositioned and conservative measures have not been successful in correcting the joint into normal alignment, surgical intervention may be indicated. Ideally, this should be done as soon as it is established that conservative measures are not working. The tendency toward earlier surgery for such defects is especially important for developmental dysplasia of the hip and for severe equinovarus deformity in which the calcaneus and talus are, at least, partially dislocated. Proper bony alignment is necessary to foster normal subsequent joint development.

The counseling given to parents of a baby with an extrinsic deformation problem can usually be quite optimistic. With rare exceptions, the parents may be counseled in the following manner: "I believe your baby is normally formed. He (she) became crowded in the uterus before birth, and this resulted in some unusual features at birth. Having been released from this constraint, the baby's features should return toward normal with proper neonatal management. It is for this reason that I say your baby is normal but requires some consistent management." Any treatment that is merited should be explained to the parents, and appropriate demonstrations of how to manage the infant should be provided. This is particularly important when it comes to infant sleeping positions and the early, frequent establishment of "tummy time" while the infant is awake and under observation. The switch from prone to supine infant sleep position has decreased the frequencies of sudden infant death syndrome (SIDS), tibial torsion, and intoeing while increasing the frequency of deformational plagiocephaly, which is usually preventable.[30] The recurrence risk depends on the cause of the extrinsic deformation. For most deformations, the recurrence risk is low. However, it may be quite high if the cause is a persisting one, such as a uterine malformation. Obviously, it is important to distinguish extrinsic deformation from intrinsic deformation, which may be secondary to a genetic neuromuscular problem, because this distinction has a major impact on the prognosis and management of the child and on the recurrence risk for the parents.

### Prevention

The prevention of extrinsic deformation seems an unlikely possibility due to the immaturity, pliability, and size of the human fetus. However, several examples of preventive measures already exist, and more may be developed in the future. Surgical repair of a malformed uterus that has previously resulted in serious deformation problems and decreased fetal survival may result in a greatly improved prognosis for a normal offspring. The prevention of pulmonary hypoplasia by instilling replacement fluid for leaking amniotic fluid or by fetal surgery for diaphragmatic hernia or urethral obstruction malformation sequence may lead to improved fetal viability.

External version of a fetus in an abnormal presentation is now an accepted mode of therapy in maternal-fetal medicine. This is usually accomplished between 35 and 37 weeks from conception. After 37 weeks, it is more difficult to accomplish external version of the fetus into the vertex presentation, and before 35 weeks, the fetus may revert to a breech presentation. The most common indication for external version is breech presentation, and routine use of external version for fetal malpresentation reduced the usual 3.5% incidence of breech presentation at term to 0.54%.[36] Since breech presentation was responsible for almost one third of the extrinsic deformations and one half of the cases of dislocation of the hip in Dunn's series, any reduction in the frequency of breech presentation at term would have a significant impact on the frequency of deformations. Contraindications to external version include multiple pregnancy, placenta previa, malformation of the uterus, and gross obesity. Version is accomplished by gently manipulating the fetus through the abdominal wall and uterus while monitoring the fetal heart.

Prevention of more serious problems secondary to constraint deformation merits additional commentary. One example is the dolichocephalic head with prominent occiput that may develop following prolonged breech presentation in late fetal life.[37] Breech head deformation sequence is itself usually a benign deformation that tends to resolve after birth. However, the contour of this head can pose serious problems during vaginal delivery because it tends to become arrested during the second stage of labor. This complication increases the likelihood of damage to the brachial plexus and cervical spinal cord during vaginal delivery. Detection of the breech head by ultrasonography is now an indication for cesarean section delivery of a fetus in breech presentation. Thus, prenatal detection of such a deformation may influence management toward the prevention of serious birth trauma.

## INTERACTIONS BETWEEN EXTRINSIC AND INTRINSIC FACTORS

A given deformation might relate to both extrinsic and intrinsic factors, representing an interaction between the two categories. One example is congenital hip dislocation (Fig. 1-15). Most instances

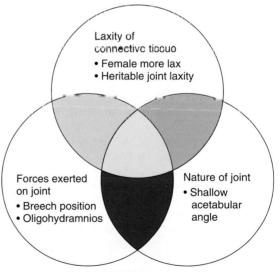

FIGURE 1-15. Interacting factors may relate to the likelihood of developing a deformation such as developmental dysplasia of the hip.

of developmental dysplasia of the hip (DDH) are secondary to external constraint, which forces the head of the femur out of its socket and stretches the joint capsule and ligamentum teres. DDH is more common in the female because of increased connective tissue laxity in the female due to the impact of relaxing hormones and the relative deficiency of testosterone during the perinatal period.[38] DDH may also result from an intrinsic abnormality in the fetus with unusually lax connective tissues due to a genetic connective tissue dysplasia, such as Ehlers-Danlos syndrome or a malformation syndrome like Larsen syndrome. Ehlers-Danlos syndrome can be suspected clinically by noting laxity in multiple joints and/or detecting joint laxity in a parent.

Another example of the interaction between intrinsic and extrinsic factors in creating a deformation is the fetus who has an intrinsic neuromuscular abnormality that limits the ability of the fetus to turn into the vertex position before birth. Such a fetus is more likely to be caught in the breech position and to be born with such problems as breech head, DDH, and other deformations that occur more frequently in the fetus presenting in breech position.

## INTRINSIC CAUSATION OF DEFORMATION

Intramembranous bones are usually flat, and they primarily comprise the bones in the cranial vault and facial region. They arise directly from mesenchyme and differ from endochondral bones, which are formed initially from cartilage models.[39] The axial and appendicular skeletal bones form primarily through endochondral ossification and are of mesodermal origin, whereas some membranous bones originate from neural crest and others originate from mesoderm.[39] The clavicle is formed through a combination of both endochondral and intramembranous ossification. Type I and type XI collagens are involved in bone formation, and types II, IX, X, and XI collagen are involved in cartilage formation.[40] In addition to these structural proteins, other genes play critical roles in osteogenesis, such as transcription factors and various growth factors and their receptors. Mutations in these genes account for a wide variety of genetic connective tissue disorders, many of which are associated with an increased risk of deformation.[40]

The cause of a given deformation may be due to altered mechanical forces that are the consequence of a more primary problem within the fetus, such as

a malformation. Although these intrinsic deformations are not the main subject of this text, it is important to consider them in the differential diagnosis of extrinsic deformations. Some deformations may be caused by either extrinsic or intrinsic factors. For example, the same type of malposition of the foot may result from external constraint, a neurologic deficit, or a muscle disorder. The judgment of the clinician is required to determine the primary causation of such deformations. The overall diagnosis, prognosis, and recurrence risk for a child with a malpositioned foot may differ widely if the deformation is secondary to uterine constraint rather than the result of a primary neuromuscular problem. Several types of intrinsic fetal problems

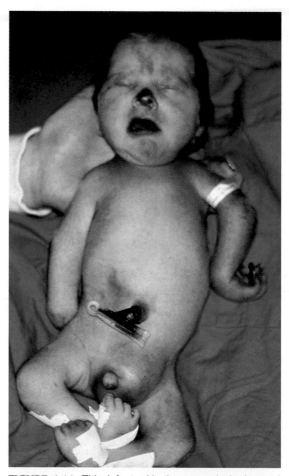

FIGURE 1-16. This infant with the amyoplasia form of arthrogryposis experienced early loss of motor nerve function to limbs (possibly due to disruption of blood supply to the spinal cord), resulting in replacement of muscle with fibrous tissue and fat and causing joints to become fixed in an early fetal position.

may result in altered mechanics and thereby give rise to deformation of otherwise normal tissues. Examples include neuromuscular disorders, aberrant growth of a tissue, and obstruction of a hollow organ. Examples of each are described in this section.

## Neuromuscular Problems

Any deficit of neuromuscular function may result in multiple deformations. When the primary problem is neural, a secondary loss of muscle mass may occur (Fig. 1-16). As a consequence of

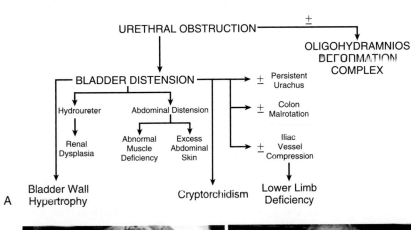

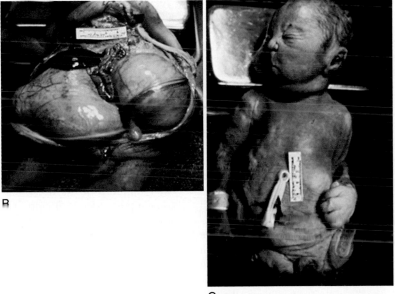

FIGURE 1-17. **A,** Urethral obstruction malformation sequence stems from the initiating malformation of urethral obstruction, which usually occurs at the level of the prostatic urethra (hence, it is nine times more frequent in males than females). Most of the other features are deformations due to the backpressure in the urinary system. Sometimes the distended bladder **(B)** disrupts iliac vessel blood flow to the legs. In order to survive to a term birth, the distended bladder must decompress, thus yielding the "prune belly" abdomen **(C)**.

(**A,** From Pagon RA, Smith DW, Shepard TH: Urethral obstruction malformation complex: a cause of abdominal muscle deficiency and the "prune belly," *J Pediatr* 96:900–906, 1979.)

diminished movement, there may be joint fixations, and with a lack of stress, the bone grows more slowly in breadth, tending to become more slender and fragile. This phenotype has been termed *fetal akinesia deformation sequence*.[41,42] Sites of muscle attachment to bone, which are normally prominent, may be less prominent or even lacking as a result of such neuromuscular deficiency. Excessive neuromuscular function, such as is seen with spasticity, may give rise to an unusual magnitude and direction of muscle forces with consequent mechanical effects on the spine, hips, and feet. These unusual neuromuscular forces may require repeated injections of neuromuscular toxins such as botulinum toxin or orthopedic surgical management to reduce the magnitude of the excessive neuromuscular forces.

## Localized Growth Deficiency

Localized growth deficiency within one tissue may give rise to subsequent deformational problems in adjacent tissues, as can be seen with localized growth deficiency of the mandible. If this occurs during early morphogenesis, it tends to place the tongue in a posterior location in the oropharynx (termed *glossoptosis*). If this happens prior to 9 to 10 weeks of gestation, before closure of the posterior palate, the tongue may obstruct posterior palatal closure, yielding a U-shaped palatal defect. Once the baby is born, there may be upper airway obstruction secondary to the retroplaced tongue. These combined findings are referred to as the *Pierre Robin malformation sequence*.[43] Deficient mandibular growth may result from any of the types of abnormal morphogenesis described in Fig. 1-1. Beyond the initiating malformation of a small mandible, the remaining features are the consequences of altered biomechanics engendered by the small mandible. When the mandibular growth deficiency occurs as part of a malformation syndrome or connective tissue dysplasia, it carries a much worse prognosis than does the isolated Robin sequence. Isolated Robin sequence is associated with twinning in 9% of cases and is usually discordant.[44]

## Localized Overgrowth

A localized overgrowth may cause mechanical problems in the adjacent region. This is apparent with many tumors. One example is a cervical teratoma, which can obstruct palatal closure and partially occlude the upper airway, yielding deformational features similar to those noted for the Robin sequence.[45]

## Obstruction of a Hollow Viscus

Obstruction of a hollow organ will result in altered mechanic forces with increased pressures causing deformations or disruptions of the expanded tissue, as well as distortion of tissues that surround the enlarging hollow structure. Examples include obstructive hydrocephalus, intestinal obstruction, and obstruction in the urogenital system. One dramatic illustration is the urethral obstruction sequence shown in Fig. 1-17, which has been more commonly termed *prune belly syndrome*.[46,47] Usually, the primary malformation is an obstruction in the development of the penile urethra. This results in massive enlargement of the bladder and the ureters, and the back-pressure adversely affects renal morphogenesis. The enlarging bladder distends the abdomen, causing diminished abdominal musculature. It also prevents full rotation of the gut, resulting in malrotation; obstructs the descent of the testes; and may compress vessels to the legs, resulting in hypoplastic legs.[47] The horrendous compressive effects of the distended bladder are usually lethal in early fetal life unless the bladder is decompressed, either by rupturing an obstructing urethral valve or by draining through a patent urachus (which tends to remain patent as a consequence of the pressure). Once the bladder is decompressed, the fetus is left with a lax abdomen and redundant folds of excess skin, the so-called prune belly. Thus, all of these deformations are secondary to one primary intrinsic malformation, early urethral obstruction. Similar distension and muscular thinning of the abdomen can be seen with congenital ascites, which may result from a variety of causes.

## References

1. Moorthi RN, Hashmi SS, Langois P, et al: Idiopathic talipes equinovarus (ITEV) (clubfeet) in Texas, *Am J Med Genet* 132A:376–380, 2005.
2. Schinzel AA, Smith DW, Miller JR: Monozygotic twinning and structural defects, *J Pediatr* 95:921–930, 1979.
3. Keusch CF, Mulliken JB, Kaplan LC: Craniofacial anomalies in twins, *Plast Reconstr Surg* 87:16–23, 1991.
4. Littlefield TR, Kelly KM, Pomatto JK, et al: Multiple-birth infants at higher risk for development of deformational plagiocephaly, *Pediatrics* 103:565–569, 1999.
5. Nicolini U, Poblete A: Single intrauterine death in monochorionic twin pregnancies, *Ultrasound Obstet Gynecol* 14:297–301, 1999.

6. Zankl A, Brooks D, Boltshauser E, et al: Natural history of twin disruption sequence, *Amer J Med Genet* 127A: 133–138, 2004.

7. Dunn P: Congenital postural deformities: perinatal associations, *Proc R Soc Med* 67:1174–1178, 1974.

8. Dunn P: Congenital postural deformities: further perinatal associations, *Proc R Soc Med* 65:735–738, 1972.

9. Dunn PM: Congenital postural deformities, *Br Med Bull* 32:71–76, 1976.

10. Martinez-Frias ML, Bermejo E, Frias JL: Analysis of deformations in 26,810 consecutive infants with congenital defects, *Am J Med Genet* 84:365–368, 1999.

11. Harrison RG, Malpas P: The volume of human amniotic fluid, *J Obstet Gynaec Br Emp* 60:632–639, 1953.

12. Nishimura H: Etiological mechanism of congenital abnormalities. In Fraser FC, McKusick VA, eds: *Congenital malformations* (International Congress Series, no. 204), Amsterdam, 1970, Excerpta Medica, p 275.

13. Alkalay AL, Graham JM Jr, Pomerance JJ: Evaluation of neonates born with intrauterine growth retardation: review and practice guidelines, *J Perinatol* 18:142–151, 1998.

14. Harvey MA, Smith DW, Skinner AL: Infant growth standards in relation to parental stature, *Clin Pediatr* 18:602–603, 611–613, 1979.

15. Tarruffi C: *Storia della teratologia [History of teratology]*, Bologna, 1881, Regia Tipografia.

16. von Reuss AR: *The disease of the new born*, 1921, William Wood.

17. Thompson DW: *On growth and form. A new edition*, Cambridge, 1942, Cambridge University Press.

18. Chapple CC, Davidson DT: A study of the relationship between fetal position and certain congenital deformities, *J Pediatr* 18:483–493, 1941.

19. Browne D: Talipes equinovarus, *Lancet* 224:969–974, 1934.

20. Browne D: Congenital deformities of mechanical origin, *Arch Dis Child* 30:37–41, 1955.

21. Miller ME, Dunn PM, Smith DW: Uterine malformation and fetal deformation, *J Pediatr* 94:387–390, 1979.

22. Caldwell WE, Moloy HC, D'Esopo DA: A roentgenologic study of the mechanism of engagement of the fetal head, *Am J Obstet Gynecol* 28:824–841, 1934.

23. Sherer DM, Miodovnik M, Bradley KS, et al: Intrapartum fetal head position I: comparison between transvaginal digital examination and transabdominal ultrasound assessment during the active stage of labor, *Ultrasound Obstet Gynecol* 19:258–263, 2002.

24. Sherer DM, Miodovnik M, Bradley KS, et al: Intrapartum fetal head position II: comparison between transvaginal digital examination and transabdominal ultrasound assessment during second stage of labor, *Ultrasound Obstet Gynecol* 19:264–268, 2002.

25. Sherer DM, Abulafia O: Intrapartum assessment of fetal head engagement: comparison between transvaginal digital and transabdominal ultrasound determinations, *Ultrasound Obstet Gynecol* 21:430–436, 2003.

26. Graham JM Jr: Craniofacial deformation, *Balliere's Clinical Paediatrics* 6:293–315, 1998.

27. Graham JM, Smith DW: Parietal craniotabes in the neonate: its origin and relevance, *J Pediatr* 95:114–116, 1979.

28. Graham JM, deSaxe M, Smith DW: Sagittal craniostenosis: fetal head constraint as one possible cause, *J Pediatr* 95:747–750, 1979.

29. Golditch IM, Kirkman K: The large fetus: management and outcome, *Obstet Gynecol* 52:26–30, 1978.

30. Graham JM Jr, Gomez M, Halberg A, et al: Management of deformational plagiocephaly: repositioning versus orthotic therapy, *J Pediatr* 146:258–262, 2005.

31. Graham JM Jr, Kneutzman J, Earl D, et al: Deformational brachycephaly in supine-sleeping infants, *J Pediatr* 146:258–262, 2005.

32. Thomas IT, Smith DW: Oligohydramnios, cause of the nonrenal features of Potter's syndrome, including pulmonary hypoplasia, *J Pediatr* 84:811–814, 1974.

33. Littlefield TR, Beals SP, Manwarring KH, et al: Treatment of craniofacial asymmetry with dynamic orthotic cranioplasty, *J Craniofacial Surg* 9:11–17, 1998.

34. Kelly KM, Littlefield TR, Pomatto JK, et al: Importance of early recognition and treatment of deformational plagiocephaly with orthotic cranioplasty, *Cleft Palate Craniofac J* 36:127–130, 1999.

35. Mulliken JB, Vander Woude DL, Hansen M, et al: Analysis of posterior plagiocephaly: deformational versus synostotic, *Plast Reconstr Surg* 103:371–380, 1999.

36. Ranney B: The gentle art of external cephalic version, *Am J Obstet Gynecol* 116:239–248, 248–251 [comments], 1973.

37. Haberkern CM, Smith DW, Jones KL: The "breech head" and its relevance, *Am J Dis Child* 133:154–156, 1979.

38. Fernando J, Arena P, Smith DW: Sex liability to single structural defects, *Am J Dis Child* 132:970–972, 1978.

39. Cohen MM: Merging the old skeletal biology with the new. I. Intramembranous ossification, endochondral ossification, ectopic bone, secondary cartilage, and pathologic considerations, *J Craniofac Genet Dev Biol* 20:84–93, 2000.

40. Cohen MM: Merging the old skeletal biology with the new. II. Molecular aspects of bone formation and bone growth, *J Craniofac Genet Dev Biol* 20:94–106, 2000.

41. Moessinger AC: Fetal akinesia deformation sequence: an animal model, *Pediatrics* 72:857–863, 1983.

42. Hall JG: Analysis of the Pena-Shokeir phenotype, *Am J Med Genet* 25:99–117, 1986.

43. Hanson JW, Smith DW: U-shaped palatal defect in the Robin anomalad: developmental and clinical relevance, *J Pediatr* 87:30–33, 1975.

44. Holder-Espinasse M, Abadie V, Cormier-Daire V, et al: Pierre Robin sequence: analysis of 117 consecutive cases, *J Pediatr* 139:588–590, 2001.

45. Kerner B, Flaum E, Mathews H, et al: Cervical teratoma: prenatal diagnosis and long-term follow-up, *Prenatal Diagnosis* 10:51–59, 1998.

46. Pagon RA, Smith DW, Shepard TH: Urethral obstruction malformation complex: a cause of abdominal muscle deficiency and the "prune belly," *J Pediatr* 94:900–906, 1979.

47. Perez-Aytes A, Graham JM Jr, Hersh JH, et al: The urethral obstruction sequence and lower limb deficiency: evidence for the vascular disruption hypothesis, *J Pediatr* 123:398–405, 1993.

# Patterns of Deformation

# 2 Foot Deformations

## FOOT CONTRACTURES, POSITIONAL FOOT ABNORMALITIES

Any cause of prolonged immobilization of a joint tends to give rise to joint fixation with contracture. This can result from immobilization due to external constraint, intrinsic neuromuscular problems, defects in the formation of the joint, or joints formed from abnormal connective tissue (Figs. 2-1 and 2-2). When the problem is the result of external constraint, the position of a given joint reflects the nature of the forces that resulted in the deformation. The most common region affected is the foot, although fixations of other joints may also occur. The differential diagnosis of foot anomalies includes the following: metatarsus adductus (deformation or malformation), talipes equinovarus (deformation or malformation), talipes calcaneovalgus (deformation), pes planus (often connective tissue dysplasia), and vertical talus (malformation).[1-3]

Foot deformation usually originates during fetal life, but in China, the practice of foot binding in young girls became widespread during the 12th century (Fig. 2-3). This practice was initiated around age 3 years, when all toes but the first toes were broken and bound with tight cloth over the next 2 years so as to keep the feet less than 10 cm in length with a marked concavity of the sole.[4]

Through contact with Western culture, this practice ceased at the beginning of the 20th century, but even in the contemporary Chinese population, 38% of women older than 80 years and 18% of women between ages 70 and 79 years had their feet bound. An additional 17% of women older than 70 years had their feet bound, but the binding was released early. Women with deformed feet due to such foot binding are more prone to falling, are less able to rise from a chair, are unable to squat, and suffer severe, lifelong disability.[4]

When fixations of multiple joints are present at birth, the term *arthrogryposis* is used (Fig. 2-4). This term designates a descriptive category and should not be considered a diagnosis. Arthrogryposis is a sign that can be associated with many specific conditions or syndromes.[5] Decreased fetal movement results in arthrogryposis, although the cause of such *fetal akinesia* may not always be known with certainty. Multiple congenital contractures (arthrogryposis) occurs in 1 in 3000 live births, and in 1 in 200 newborns there is some form of joint contracture, with clubfeet (1:500) and dislocated or subluxing hips (1:200 to 1:500) being most frequent.[6] The decreased fetal movements that result in arthrogryposis can be caused

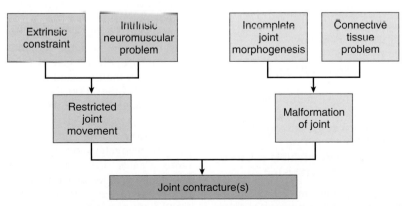

FIGURE 2-1. Joint contracture at birth may be the consequence of a number of modes of developmental pathology, of which in utero constraint is the most common.

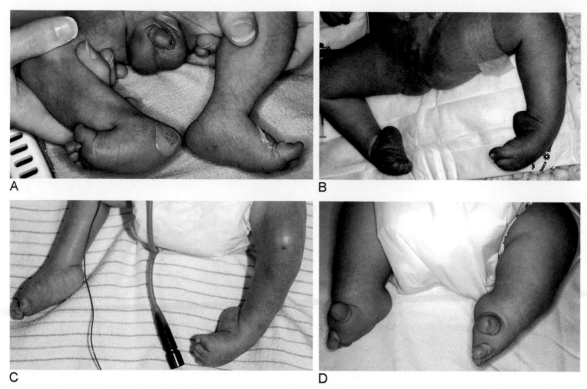

FIGURE 2-2. **A,** This infant has bilateral equinovarus foot deformations due to prolonged oligohydramnios resulting from leaking amniotic fluid from 17 weeks of gestation until birth. This is an example of extrinsic deformation. **B,** This infant with type I Pena-Shokeir syndrome demonstrates bilateral equinovarus foot deformities due to fetal akinesia deformation sequence (intrinsic deformation). **C,** Neurogenic clubfeet due to an unknown neuromuscular disorder. **D,** These equinovarus feet resulted from a connective tissue abnormality in an infant with diastrophic dysplasia. This is an example of a connective tissue dysplasia that has given rise to malformation of a joint.

by either fetal abnormalities or maternal abnormalities, and the earlier the onset of decreased fetal movement, the more severe the resultant contractures. Hall has delineated six major causes of decreased fetal movements[5]:

1. Neuropathic abnormalities (e.g., spina bifida or Marden-Walker syndrome [Fig. 2-5])
2. Muscle abnormalities (e.g., congenital myopathies)
3. Abnormalities of connective tissue (e.g., diastrophic dysplasia [see Fig. 1-1, *A*] and some forms of distal arthrogryposis [see Fig. 3-6])
4. Space limitations (e.g., multiple gestation, uterine structural abnormalities)
5. Vascular disruption (e.g., amyoplasia [see Figs. 1-16 or 2-4])
6. Maternal diseases (e.g., multiple sclerosis, diabetes, or myasthenia gravis)

The sorting of presentations into three major categories can be helpful in identifying underlying conditions or syndromes: (1) disorders with mainly limb involvement (e.g., amyoplasia or distal arthrogryposis); (2) limbs plus other body areas (e.g., multiple pterygium syndrome or diastrophic dysplasia); and (3) limbs plus central nervous system dysfunction (e.g., trisomy 18 [see Fig. 1-12], Pena-Shokeir syndrome [see Fig. 1-2, *B*], or Marden-Walker syndrome [see Fig. 2-5]).[5]

According to Ruth Wynne-Davies, congenital malposition of the foot occurs with a frequency of about 4.0 to 5.6 per 1000 live births.[6,7] The most serious subtype is talipes equinovarus (clubfoot), which is difficult to treat, manifests a tendency to recur within families, and occurs with a frequency of 1.2 to 1.3 per 1000 live births (males, 1.6 per 1000; females, 0.8 per 1000).[6,7] Postural talipes equinovarus occurs in 0.5 per 1000 live births (males, 1.6 per 1000; females, 0.8 per 1000), talipes calcaneovalgus occurs in 1.1 per 1000 live births (males, 0.1 per 1000; females, 0.3 per 1000), and metatarsus varus occurs in 1.2 per 1000 live births (males, 1.0 per 1000; females 0.2 per 1000).[4] Many congenital malpositions of the foot represent deformations due to external constraint

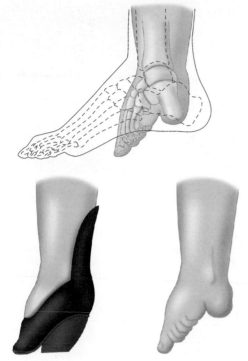

FIGURE 2-3. For almost 1500 years, certain young Chinese girls were subjected to the harrowing experience of foot binding for several years in order to produce the desired small feet, which were considered physically attractive. The form into which the deformed feet were molded is shown above, along with the special shoes and resultant foot position.

(From Levy HS: *Chinese footbinding*, New York, 1966, Walton Rawls.)

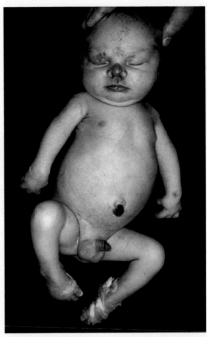

FIGURE 2-4. This infant has the amyoplasia form of arthrogryposis, a sporadic condition attributed to spinal cord damage (possibly with a vascular basis) in early gestation. Fetal movement is limited, with joint ankylosis and absent flexion creases. The posture of this condition is quite characteristic, with the hands fixed in external rotation and extension of the elbows (the "policeman's tip" position). This is an example of intrinsic deformation due to vascular disruption.

in utero, and the treatment prognosis is much better for postural deformations than for other types of congenital joint contractures.

Evaluation of the foot includes determination of the full range of its mobility, inspection of its usual position or posture with notation of unusual skin creases, and palpation of the dorsalis pedis pulse because the anterior tibial vascular tree is often poorly developed in children with neuromuscular clubfoot.[8] Radiographs are of little value in early infancy because feet are best evaluated radiographically when bearing weight and the bones are not sufficiently ossified to allow for the relevant assessment; however, magnetic resonance imaging has been used for research purposes in congenital talipes equinovarus.[9,10] In a prospective study of 2401 newborns, 4% were found to have foot contractures, of which three fourths were various forms of adductus anomalies. These children were followed through age 16 years, when they were examined by dynamic foot pressure and gait analysis. Only those children with clubfeet showed persistent abnormalities. By age 6 years, 87% of adductus anomalies had resolved, and by age 16 years, 95% had resolved.[11] Congenital clubfoot and congenital vertical talus tend to persist and cause disability unless treated aggressively; thus, early referral and treatment is extremely important. Such joint contractures are usually released operatively in the first year of life.

Among the associated anomalies that tend to occur with postural equinovarus or calcaneovalgus types of foot deformities are joint laxity (10%) and inguinal hernia (7%). These findings suggest that minor connective tissue problems may enhance the tendency toward positional deformation of the foot. Postural deformations that began in utero may be perpetuated by prone sleeping postures in early infancy. Consequently, the incidence of these postural deformations has decreased in cultures using supine sleeping positions. Hence, consideration of sleeping posture and whether it is augmenting or ameliorating the deformation may be an important part of the

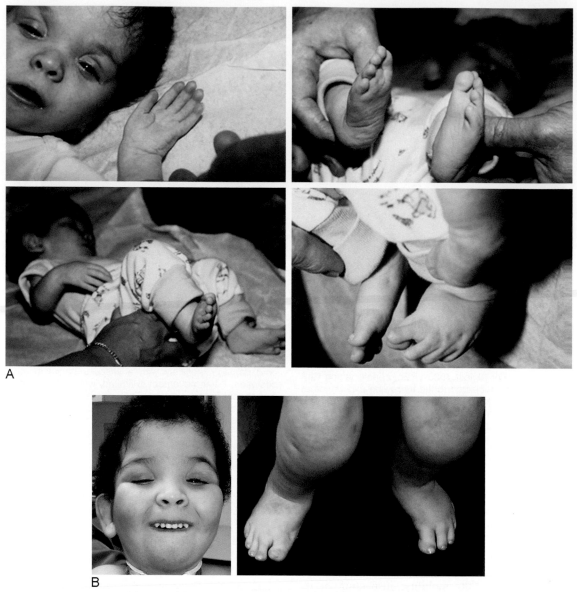

FIGURE 2-5. Marden-Walker syndrome is an autosomal recessive malformation syndrome. **A,** This infant was born with severe congenital contractures, Dandy-Walker malformation, cleft palate, blepharophimosis, tethered spinal cord, and severe growth and developmental delay. Note diminished finger creases from lack of movement in utero. **B,** By age 6 years, the child's contractures had responded well to early intermittent splinting to reduce contractures and physical therapy, followed by surgical correction.

infant's initial evaluation. Postural foot deformations are common and are often considered physiologic variations in foot shape; these include metatarsus adductus, calcaneovalgus, and flexible flatfeet. Similar physiologic variations affecting the shape of the legs include genu varum, genu valgum, femoral anteversion, and tibial torsion. On the other hand, cavus feet are usually a manifestation of muscle imbalance from an underlying neuromuscular disorder, which might be static

(cerebral palsy), recurrent after initial stabilization (spina bifida), or progressive (Charcot-Marie-Tooth disease).

Several modes of management have been used in the attempt to restore the foot to its usual position. These are summarized in Table 2-1. In infants who are born prematurely, contractures can be splinted using silicone rubber dental-impression material, which is held in place with Velcro strips (Fig. 2-6).[12] Such splints can easily

## TABLE 2-1.   MANAGEMENT STRATEGIES FOR FOOT CONTRACTURES

| METHOD | COMMENT |
| --- | --- |
| Manual stretching | Performed at each feeding and diaper change |
| Adhesive taping | Sometimes alternated with physical therapy to increase joint range of motion |
| Splinting | Devices such as the Denis-Browne splint and reversed-last shoes may be used, particularly at night, to maintain desired position. Newer, lightweight fiberglass splints may be used with physical therapy |
| Plaster cast | Used initially with stretching and taping to correct position and facilitate surgery. Also used after surgery to maintain position |
| Surgery | Merits consideration if more conservative measures have not resulted in improvement of foot position during early infancy |

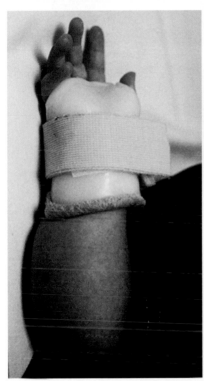
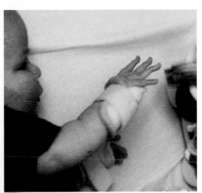
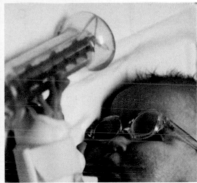

FIGURE 2-6. Use of custom hand splints held in place with Velcro fasteners in a child with congenital contractural arachnodactyly due to Beals syndrome. Fingers are left free to encourage their use in grasping and reaching, and the splints can be removed for physical therapy.

be removed for passive stretching exercises or intravenous access and then replaced just as easily. Each type of foot contracture should be considered individually with regard to both prognosis and management. For example, the prognosis for calcaneovalgus with manipulative stretching alone is usually excellent, whereas at least half the cases of equinovarus contracture resist correction by conservative measures. In general, initial corrective surgery is accomplished through soft tissue releases to align the joints and osteotomies to correct residual deformities, with arthrodesis reserved for the older child or adult with established degenerative arthrosis of a joint or with severe problems that

cannot be corrected with releases and osteotomies. For the child with arthrogryposis, additional management strategies are overviewed and comprehensively illustrated in a patient-oriented text by Staheli et al.[13]

### References

1. Furdon SA, Donlon CR: Examination of the newborn foot: positional and structural abnormalities, *Adv Neonatal Care* 2:248–258, 2002.
2. Gore AI, Spencer JP: The newborn foot, *Am Fam Physician* 69:865–872, 2004.
3. Sass P, Hassan G: Lower extremity abnormalities in children, *Am Fam Physician* 68:461–468, 2003.

4. Cummings SR, Ling X, Stone K: Consequences of foot binding among older women in Beijing, China, *Am J Pub Health* 87:1677–1679, 1997.
5. Hall JG: Arthrogryposis multiplex congenita: etiology, genetics, classification, diagnostic approach, and general aspects. Part B, *J Pediatr Orthop* 6:159–166, 1997.
6. Wynne-Davies R: Family studies and aetiology of clubfoot, *J Med Genet* 2:227–232, 1965.
7. Boo NY, Ong LC: Congenital talipes in Malaysian neonates: incidence, pattern and associated factors, *Sing Med J* 31:539–542, 1990.
8. Muir L, Laliotis N, Kutty S, et al: Absence of the dorsalis pedis pulse in the parents of children with clubfoot, *J Bone Joint Surg Br* 77:114–116, 1995.
9. Downey DJ, Drennan JC, Garcia JF: Magnetic resonance image findings in congenital talipes equinovarus, *J Pediatr Orthop* 12:224–228, 1992.
10. Grayhack JJ, Zawin JK, Shore RM, et al: Assessment of calcaneocuboid joint deformity by magnetic resonance imaging in talipes equinovarus. Part B, *J Pediatr Orthop* 4:36–38, 1995.
11. Widhe T: Foot deformities at birth: a longitudinal prospective study over a 16-year period, *J Pediatr Orthop* 17:20–24, 1997.
12. Bell E, Graham EK: A new material for splinting neonatal limb deformities, *J Pediatr Orthop* 15:613–616, 1995.
13. Staheli LT, Hall JG, Jaffe KM, et al: *Arthrogryposis: a text atlas*, 1998, Cambridge, Cambridge University Press.

# 3 Calcaneovalgus (Pes Planus)

## GENESIS

Sometimes called "flexible flatfoot," calcaneovalgus has a reported frequency of 1.1 per 1000 live births,[1] although some authors indicate that more than 30% of newborns have calcaneovalgus deformity of both feet.[2] It is usually the result of uterine constraint having forced the foot into a dorsiflexed position against the lower leg and is especially common after prolonged breech position with extended legs. Associated congenital hip dislocation occurs in 5% of patients with calcaneovalgus[1,3] and should be searched for in any newborn with this foot deformity. Congenital hip dislocation is more frequent among infants in breech presentation (0.9%), and minor anomalies comprising the breech head deformation complex are also much more frequent with breech presentation, regardless of the mode of delivery.[4,5]

Among infants with frank breech presentation, the extended leg is particularly susceptible to calcaneovalgus foot deformation and genu recurvatum of the knee. Calcaneovalgus is more common in first-born infants, with 75% of affected infants being primiparous,[6] and it is much more common in females than in males (4:1).[1,3] A greater degree of joint laxity occurs in females, which may explain this finding. There is also a 2.6% frequency of this deformity in parents and siblings by history.[1]

## FEATURES

Calcaneovalgus is usually the result of extrinsic deformation. The foot is dorsiflexed toward the fibular side of the lower leg (Figs. 3-1 and 3-2). This often results in posterior displacement of

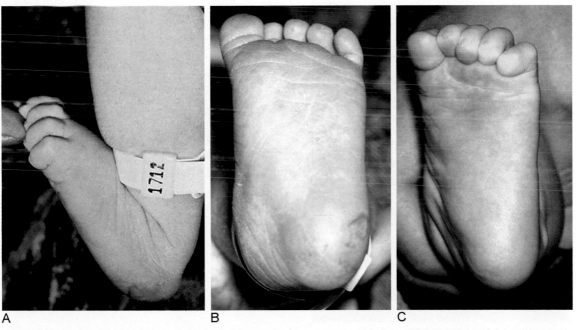

A     B     C

FIGURE 3-1. **A,** Gentle pressure recreates the presumed in-utero position of this foot, which engendered the calcaneovalgus positioning. The foot dorsiflexes quite easily at birth because of a stretched elongated heel cord. **B,** The valgus deviation of the heel is evident in this view, and the heel deviates laterally. **C,** The same foot, treated with simple manipulation at age 12 weeks.

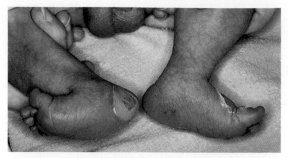

FIGURE 3-2. Bilateral calcaneovalgus feet (more significant in right foot than left foot) after prolonged oligohydramnios due to prolonged leakage of amniotic fluid.

the lateral malleolus in association with pressure-induced deficiency of subcutaneous adipose tissue at the presumed site of folding compression. In unusual cases, the heel may be in valgus position relative to the ankle, but the bones of the foot itself are usually in normal alignment. Posteromedial bowing of the tibia is sometimes associated with

calcaneovalgus foot deformity (Fig. 3-3). It is important to rule out congenital vertical talus (Fig. 3-4), which is a malformation resulting in a rigid congenital flat foot.

## MANAGEMENT, PROGNOSIS, AND COUNSEL

The foot is usually flexible, and, with no therapy or with passive stretching toward a normal position, there should be a rapid return toward normal form. If the improvement is not rapid, then taping may be used. If the situation has not resolved within the first few postnatal months, then the use of splinting, night braces, and/or casting merits consideration. Therefore, serial examinations are useful to confirm the progress of resolution. When casted, the foot is positioned in an equinovarus position with a mold placed under the arch to relax the plantar ligaments and posterior tibialis muscle, which repositions the foot in normal alignment

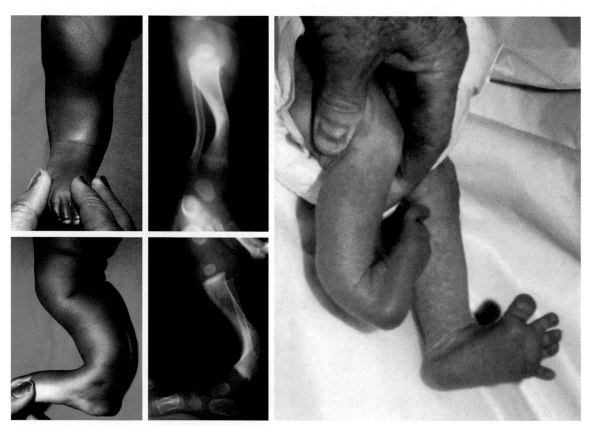

FIGURE 3-3. Posteromedial bowing of the tibia can be associated with calcaneovalgus foot deformation and usually corrects spontaneously, although it may lead to a clinically significant leg length discrepancy requiring epiphysiodesis of the opposite proximal tibia prior to maturation.

(Courtesy of Saul Bernstein and Robert M. Bernstein, Cedar Sinai Medical Center, Los Angeles, Calif.)

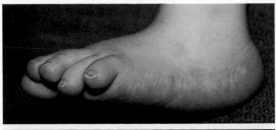

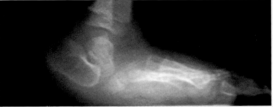

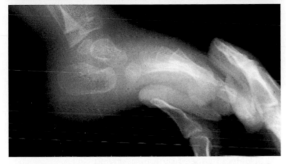

FIGURE 3-4. Congenital vertical talus results in a rigid flat foot with a rocker-bottom appearance, and the head of the talus is palpable medially in the foot. In the calcaneovalgus foot, plantar flexion reduces the navicular on the talus, but in these radiographs of congenital vertical talus, the relationship of the dorsally displaced talus is not changed, and the navicular remains in its dislocated position on the dorsum of the talus.

(Courtesy of Robert M. Bernstein, Cedar Sinai Medical Center, Los Angeles, Calif.)

and allows the stretched ligaments to tighten.[7] Calcaneovalgus was diagnosed in 13 (0.5%) of 2401 examined newborns, and all 13 had normal feet at age 16 years. Dynamic foot pressure showed no tendency to planus or increased outward rotation of the feet.[8] When associated posterior medial bowing occurs, it usually resolves during postnatal life, suggesting intrauterine fracture or fetal deformation as the cause; thus, corrective osteotomy should be delayed to allow for spontaneous correction. Although the posteromedial bowing usually corrects, there may be a 2- to 5-cm leg length discrepancy at maturation (with the degree of shortening proportional to the initial deformity). Hence, this deformity usually requires epiphysiodesis of the opposite proximal tibia prior to full growth attainment in order to result in equalization of leg length by adulthood.

## DIFFERENTIAL DIAGNOSIS

Congenital vertical talus is a rare malformation that may yield a foot in similar position to calcaneovalgus at birth, but this defect is associated with muscle atrophy, and the foot is stiff with a concave outer border as compared with the flexible flatfeet of calcaneovalgus foot deformity (see Fig. 3-4). With congenital vertical talus, the calcaneus is in equinus and the forefoot is in dorsiflexion, resulting in a midfoot break. The definitive abnormality is fixed dorsal dislocation of the navicular on the neck of the talus. The term *vertical talus* refers to the classic radiographic appearance of the affected foot in lateral view, which results in a rocker-bottom foot when viewed from the side. Congenital vertical talus can be inherited as a variable autosomal dominant trait with no evidence of associated malformations or neuromuscular disease. One family spanning four generations included 11 individuals with isolated congenital vertical talus evident at infancy; during their teenage years, a few of these individuals developed cavo-varus foot deformities that resembled Charcot-Marie-Tooth disease.[9] This family was found to have a HOXD10 mutation segregating with this foot malformation.[10] Other associated congenital anomalies often occur, such as arthrogryposis, myelodysplasia, or sacral agenesis (Fig. 3-5). Congenital vertical talus is particularly common in patients with distal arthrogryposis (Fig. 3-6). Different types of distal arthrogryposis (nonprogressive congenital contractures of two or more body areas) are caused by mutations in different genes that encode proteins of the contractile machinery of fast-twitch myofibers. These neuromuscular problems are

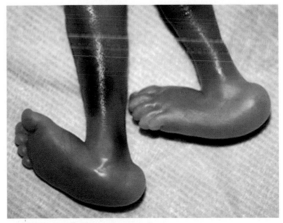

FIGURE 3-5. Bilateral congenital vertical talus in a fetus with trisomy 18.

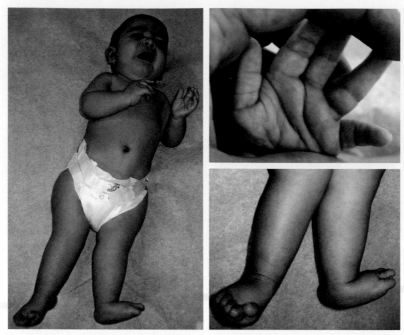

FIGURE 3-6. This child has congenital vertical talus rather than talipes equinovarus, and she demonstrates classic features of distal arthrogryposis. In this case, there was involvement of both hands and feet with no facial involvement, suggesting distal arthrogryposis type 1. Note the rocker-bottom feet with hand contractures and absent distal finger flexion creases; these features underline the fact that congenital vertical talus can be part of a broader pattern of defects caused by an underlying neuromuscular disorder. Distal arthrogryposis type 1 can result from autosomal dominant mutations in the tropomyosin gene (TPM2).

extremely difficult to treat and benefit little from casting; early surgery with extensive soft tissue release is required to achieve a functional foot.

## References

1. Wynne-Davies R: Family studies and aetiology of clubfoot, *J Med Genet* 2:227–232, 1965.
2. Sullivan JA: Pediatric flatfoot: evaluation and management, *J Am Acad Orthop Surg* 7:44–53, 1999.
3. Nunes D, Dutra MG: Epidemiological study of congenital talipes calcaneovalgus, *Braz J Med Biol Res* 19:59–62, 1986.
4. Gunther A, Smith SJ, Maynard PV, et al: A case-control study of congenital hip dislocation, *Public Health* 107:9–18, 1993.
5. Hsieh Y-Y, Tsai F-J, Lin C-C, et al: Breech deformation complex in neonates, *J Reprod Med* 45:933–935, 2000.
6. Aberman E: The causes of congenital clubfoot, *Arch Dis Child* 40:548–554, 1965.
7. Furdon SA, Donlon CR: Examination of the newborn foot: positional and structural abnormalities, *Adv Neonatal Care* 2:248–258, 2002.
8. Widhe T: Foot deformities at birth: a longitudinal prospective study over a 16-year period, *J Pediatr Orthop* 17:20–24, 1997.
9. Levinsohn EM, Shrimpton AE, Cady RB, et al: Congenital vertical talus and its familial occurrence: an analysis of 36 patients, *Skeletal Radiol* 33:649–654, 2004.
10. Shrimpton AE, Levinsohn EM, Yozawitz JM, et al: A HOX gene mutation in a family with isolated congenital vertical talus and Charcot-Marie-Tooth disease, *Am J Hum Genet* 75:92–96, 2004.

# 4 Metatarsus Adductus (Metatarsus Varus)

## GENESIS

Compression of the forefoot with the legs flexed across the lower body in late gestation is a frequent cause of metatarsus adductus (also known as *metatarsus varus*), which has a frequency of about 1.2 per 1000 live births and an 80% predilection for males.[1] Metatarsus adductus is associated with congenital hip dislocation in 5% to 10% of infants, further implicating fetal constraint as an important etiologic factor.[2] Such constraint takes place late in gestation, and metatarsus adductus is rarely found in premature infants delivered prior to 30 weeks of gestation.[3]

## FEATURES

Metatarsus adductus may be due to either deformation or malformation. The predominant feature is adduction of the forefoot, often with some supination and inability to abduct the forefoot past neutral. The feet turn inward, but the ankle and heel are generally in normal position with a flexible heel cord (Fig. 4-1). Metatarsus adductus with significant hindfoot valgus is termed *skew foot* or *serpentine foot*; however, this is a fairly rare condition. Normally, the lateral border of the foot is straight, but in metatarsus adductus, the lateral border of the foot is convex, with a concave inner border (i.e., kidney bean shaped) when viewed from the sole with the infant lying prone with the knees flexed. The adduction occurs at the tarsal-metatarsal joint, leaving a wider space between the first and second toes and often resulting in a deep crease on the medial midfoot (see Fig. 4-1). The shape and direction of the sole of the foot can be detected by projecting a line along the longitudinal axis of the foot. Normally, a line bisecting the heel should traverse the space between the first and second toes. In patients with metatarsus adductus, this line is directed toward the lateral toes. The line passes through the third toe with mild deformity and between the fourth and fifth toes with severe deformity. This deformity may be aggravated by the infant sleeping on his or her abdomen

with the knees tucked up and the lower legs and feet rolled inward (Fig. 4-2); hence, its frequency is reduced in supine sleeping infants. To discriminate between positional metatarsus adductus and structural metatarsus adductus, try to abduct the forefoot past midline without using excessive pressure or causing pain. Structural metatarsus adductus is fixed and does not abduct beyond neutral, making it difficult to distinguish from talipes equinovarus.[4]

## MANAGEMENT, PROGNOSIS, AND COUNSEL

Approximately 85% to 90% of cases resolve without treatment, and treatment is based on the severity of the condition (Fig. 4-3).[4,5] In mild and flexible cases, manipulative stretching of the tight medial soft tissues and avoidance of sleeping postures that tend to augment the deformity may be all that are required. If the sleeping posture is perpetuating the deformity, then attempts to change this posture may be of value. Several practical suggestions may be useful. One is putting the child in a heavy sleeper garment, which keeps the child warm and causes him or her to sprawl rather than tuck in the legs. The leggings of the sleeper may be pinned or sewn together at the knees, making it difficult to achieve the deforming posture. If this garment is not helpful, a pair of open-toed, straight-last shoes with the heels tied together may be placed on the child. If simpler measures fail, then reversed-last, open-toed shoes tied at the heels may be tried for nighttime wear, or the shoes may be connected by a short Denis-Browne or Fillauer splint to provide mild outward rotation (see Fig. 4-2). It may be necessary to augment this by early reversed-last shoes in order to maintain the corrected form.

If the foot cannot be passively placed in the neutral position, it is generally wiser to achieve initial correction by very careful casting. If there is associated internal tibial torsion, as frequently happens, a long leg cast may be used; however, if there is no internal tibial torsion, a short leg cast is usually adequate. The hindfoot and midfoot

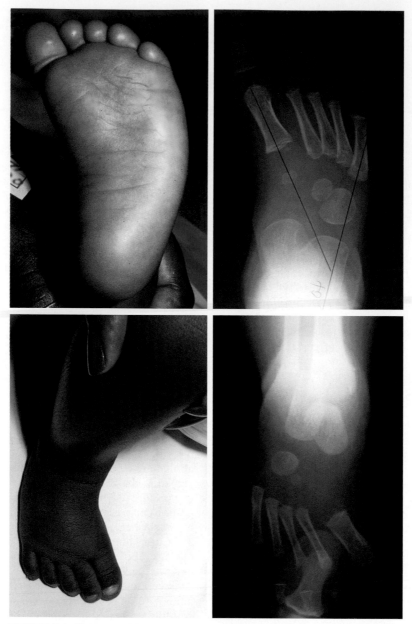

FIGURE 4-1. The normal lateral border of the foot is straight, but in metatarsus adductus, the lateral border of the foot is convex, with a concave inner border, when viewed from the sole with the infant lying prone with the knees flexed. This results in a kidney bean–shaped sole. Forefoot adduction occurs at the tarsal-metatarsal joint, leaving a wider space between the first and second toes and often resulting in a deep crease on the medial midfoot. When a line is projected along the longitudinal axis of the foot from the heel, it should traverse the space between the first and second toes, but in metatarsus adductus, this line is directed toward the lateral toes.

(Courtesy of Saul Bernstein and Robert M. Bernstein, Cedar Sinai Medical Center, Los Angeles, Calif.)

should be carefully maintained in their neutral positions during the casting. Early management may be critical because the metatarsus adductus tends to become less flexible with time, and excessive compensation at the level of the medio-tarsal joint can lead to the development of bunions, hammer toes, and other conditions.[5] In some instances, surgical treatment such as antero-medial soft tissue release may be needed, but this remains controversial.[6-11]

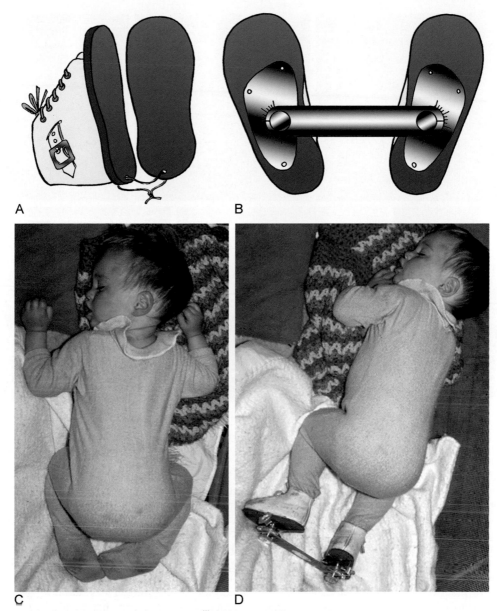

A

B

C

D

FIGURE 4-2. Simple methods for controlling sleeping posture by using open toed, straight-last shoes and tying the heels together with a shoelace through holes punched in the heels (**A**) and Denis-Browne splint (**B**) placed on sleeping shoes to prevent the deforming sleeping posture. **C,** This infant characteristically slept on his stomach with his knees flexed and his toes turned inward, accentuating metatarsus adductus. **D,** Management was directed toward trying to correct sleeping posture by turning the feet out with a Fillauer bar.

One study evaluated treatment of metatarsus adductovarus with a hinged, adjustable shoe orthotic during infancy and reported that 96% of the 120 cases resolved with use of the orthotic alone, 3% required additional casting, and 1% required both a bar and shoes for complete correction.[8] Another study of 795 patients used a straight metal bar and attached reverse-last shoe protocol and

reported that 99% achieved full correction, with surgery necessary in less than 1% of cases.[9] A long-term study of patients who received either no treatment or serial manipulation and application of plaster holding casts during infancy showed uniformly good results in adulthood, with no need for surgery.[10] In another long-term study of 2401 infants, 3.1% were found to have adductus

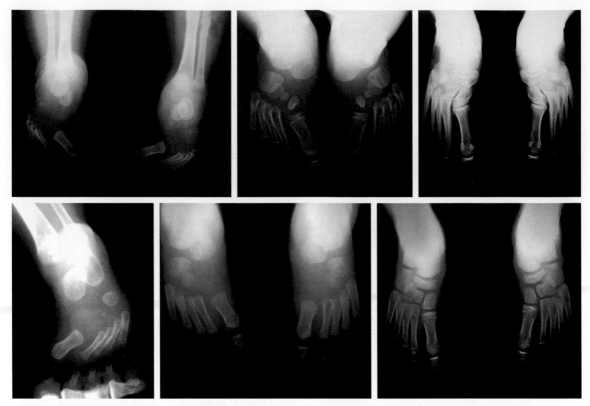

FIGURE 4-3. Serial radiographs from two individuals with spontaneous correction of metatarsus adductus without casting or bracing.
  (Courtesy of Saul Bernstein and Robert M. Bernstein, Cedar Sinai Medical Center, Los Angeles, Calif.)

deformities. By age 6 years, 87% of adductus anomalies had resolved, and by age 16 years, 95% had resolved.[11] Dynamic foot pressure and gait analyses at age 16 years showed no differences between the group with adductus deformities and the group with normal feet at birth. These studies also showed that in the vast majority of cases, there were no differences between treatment with orthotics or braces and no treatment at all. Metatarsus adductus is considered to be a multifactorial defect, and the recurrence risk in first-degree relatives is 1.8%.[1]

## DIFFERENTIAL DIAGNOSIS

When metatarsus adductus is accompanied by heel cord rigidity and varus positioning of the heel, the most likely diagnosis is talipes equinovarus (clubfoot), which requires prompt referral to a pediatric orthopedist if early treatment is to be maximally effective before soft tissue contractures become fixed and more resistant to treatment. Another common cause of intoeing is internal tibial torsion, which occurs when the tibia is medially rotated on its long axis at birth; however, this may not be noticed until the child begins to walk. This condition tends to spontaneously resolve by age 2 to 3 years unless accentuated by sleeping in the prone, intoed position, or sitting in the "reverse tailor" position. Neither special shoes nor shoe modifications alter the course of internal tibial torsion resolution. Another common cause of intoeing is femoral anteversion, which results from medial rotation of the femur at birth. This condition is at its peak in children ages 1 to 3 years, and it resolves spontaneously by late adolescence. Use of special shoes or bracing does not hasten this process, but continuation of adverse sleeping or sitting positions will slow or prevent resolution. Surgery is usually only contemplated in skeletally mature individuals with insufficient spontaneous correction.

### References

1. Wynne-Davies R: Family studies and aetiology of clubfoot, *J Med Genet* 2:221–232, 1965.
2. Kumar SJ, MacEwen GD: The incidence of hip dysplasia with metatarsus adductus, *Clin Orthop* 164:234–235, 1982.

3. Katz K, Naor N, Merlob P, et al: Rotational deformities of the tibia and foot in preterm infants, *J Pediatr Orthop* 10:483–485, 1990.
4. Furdon SA, Donlon CR: Examination of the newborn foot: positional and structural abnormalities, *Adv Neonatal Care* 2:248–258, 2002.
5. Gore AI, Spencer JP: The newborn foot, *Am Family Physician* 69:865–872, 2004.
6. Ghali NN, Abberton MJ, Silk FF: The management of metatarsus adductus and supinatus, *J Bone Joint Surg Br* 66:376–380, 1984.
7. Bohne W: Metatarsus adductus, *Bull N Y Acad Med* 63:834–838, 1987.
8. Allen WD, Weiner DS, Riley PM: The treatment of rigid metatarsus adductovarus with the use of a new hinged adjustable shoe orthosis, *Foot Ankle* 14:450–454, 1993.
9. Pentz AS, Weiner DS: Management of metatarsus adductovarus, *Foot Ankle* 14:241–246, 1993.
10. Farsetti P, Weinstein SL, Ponseti IV: The long-term functional and radiographic outcomes of untreated and non-operatively treated metatarsus adductus, *J Bone Joint Surg Am* 76:257–265, 1994.
11. Widhe T: Foot deformities at birth: a longitudinal prospective study over a 16-year period, *J Pediatr Orthop* 17:20–24, 1997.

# 5 Talipes Equinovarus (Clubfoot)

## GENESIS

Talipes equinovarus (clubfoot) is often a serious foot defect, with more than 50% of cases requiring surgical intervention, but predicting severity and response to treatment in the newborn has been notoriously difficult. The stiffer the foot, the less likely it will be corrected by manipulation, but early treatment with gentle foot manipulation and serial casting is extremely important. The term *idiopathic talipes equinovarus* is used to describe the most common type of isolated clubfoot that is not part of a syndrome. The birth prevalence varies among racial groups, with 1.12 per 1000 live births among Caucasians; it is lowest among Chinese (0.39 per 1000) and highest among Hawaiians and Maoris (6.8 per 1000).[1-4] Males are affected twice as often as females among all ethnic groups, and bilateral involvement occurs slightly more often than unilateral involvement, with the right side more frequently involved than the left side.[2-4] Postural equinovarus occurs in 0.5 per 1000 live births and is two to three times more common among females than males.[1-4] Talipes equinovarus (TEV) can be either a positional deformation or a structural malformation resulting from a wide variety of causes (intrauterine compression, abnormal myogenesis, neurologic abnormalities, vascular insufficiency, and/or genetic factors).[2]

Structural TEV can be either isolated or syndromic, and such syndromes can result from genetic, chromosomal, or teratogenic causes. Whenever TEV occurs as part of a broader pattern of altered morphogenesis, strong consideration should be given to various genetic connective tissue disorders and skeletal dysplasias that affect the tissues forming the foot (e.g., Larsen syndrome, diastrophic dysplasia, or camptomelic dysplasia), neuromuscular disorders that result in diminished foot movement, and various types of vascular disruption as possible causes. Isolated TEV is seen more frequently in large-for-gestational age (LGA) infants, as is congenital hip subluxation.[5] TEV also occurs 3.1 times more frequently in infants born to obese diabetic women than in those born to non-obese, non-diabetic women.[6] Part of this increased risk may be due to macrosomia associated with poor glucose homeostasis in late gestation, causing positional TEV, but poor diabetic control in early gestation is associated with an increased risk for skeletal defects, central nervous system defects, and caudal axis defects, all of which can lead to structural TEV.

It is not always possible to determine whether idiopathic TEV is due to constraint-related foot deformations, and a multifactorial cause encompassing both environmental and genetic factors seems most likely. Positional TEV can result from uterine constraint due to factors such as oligohydramnios, multiple gestation, or breech presentation (Figs. 5-1 and 5-2). Recent studies support

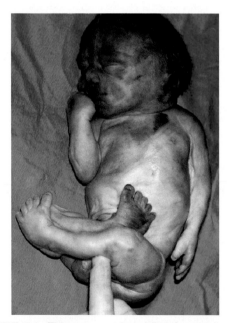

FIGURE 5-1. This term newborn died from pulmonary hypoplasia following 6 weeks of oligohydramnios due to premature rupture of membranes. He was in complete breech presentation with breech head deformation sequence and oligohydramnios deformation sequence. When folded into his in-utero position of comfort, his feet demonstrate bilateral positional equinovarus foot deformations.

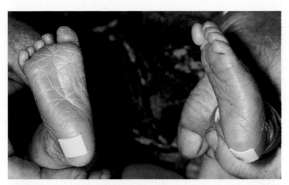

FIGURE 5-2. This flexible equinovarus left foot was associated with a maternal bicornuate uterus.

the importance of a major dominant gene in the causation of idiopathic TEV among the Polynesian population, which comprises the largest group of patients with nonsyndromic congenital clubfoot.[4,7-11] One study noted a positive family history for idiopathic TEV in 24.4% of all patients studied, and in 20.8% pedigrees studied, parent-to-child transmission occurred.[11] There is also evidence that the anterior tibial vascular tree is poorly developed in children with clubfoot, with a significantly greater prevalence of absence of the dorsalis pedis pulse in the parents of such children.[12] Other studies in patients with idiopathic TEV demonstrate abnormal muscle fiber grouping within a smaller calf, suggesting either a neurogenic etiology or localized scar-contracture formation.[13,14] Parental smoking is a risk factor for this multifactorial defect,[15,16] and a family history of a first-degree relative with TEV, combined with maternal smoking, increases the risk for isolated

TEV, thereby suggesting a gene/environment interaction.[17]

Oligohydramnios and early amnion rupture are associated with TEV, and there is a higher incidence of TEV with early amniocentesis at 11 to 12 weeks of gestation (1.3%) compared with second trimester amniocentesis at 15 to 17 weeks (0.1%).[18,19] This may relate to the relatively larger proportion of total amniotic fluid volume withdrawn for early amniocentesis (15.7% versus 7.3% at mid-trimester) at a time when the fetal foot is assuming its normal position from a previous physiologic equinus position. This period may be unusually sensitive to constraint and/or vascular disruption.[19] Amniotic fluid leakage before 22 weeks was the only significant factor associated with clubfoot, there being a 15% risk with leakage but only a 1.1% risk without leakage (Fig. 5-3). No case of clubfoot had persistent leakage at 18 to 20 weeks. Such a transient fluid leak suggests that a disruptive process might have resulted in a developmental arrest of the foot as it moved from the normal equinus position at 9 weeks to the neutral position at 12 weeks. Vascular disruption may be a final common pathway for environmentally induced TEV, which has also been caused by maternal hyperthermia.[20] The use of misoprostol, as well as other unsuccessful early pregnancy termination attempts that result in vascular disruption and hypoxic-ischemic insults to the spinal cord and brainstem, can result in structural TEV, arthrogryposis, Möbius sequence, and cranial nerve damage.[21] Neuromuscular toxins administered during gestation or neuromuscular defects such as arthrogryposis, spinal muscular atrophy, meningomyelocele, and sacral dysgenesis are all associated with structural TEV.

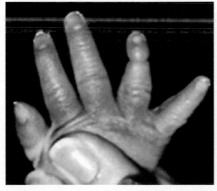
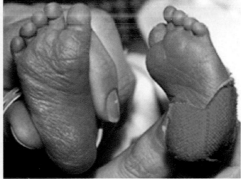

FIGURE 5-3. This rigid equinovarus left foot deformity was associated with an amniotic band around the fourth finger and a history of amniotic fluid leakage at 11 to 12 weeks.

## FEATURES

Idiopathic TEV, or true clubfoot, is an isolated congenital deformity of the foot and lower leg resulting in fixation of the foot into four positional components: cavus and adduction of the forefoot, along with varus and equinus positioning of the hindfoot, which are associated with concomitant soft tissue abnormalities. The forefoot is inverted, as are the heel and the whole foot, which is in plantar flexion, with a characteristic single posterior skin crease and a medial midfoot crease (Figs. 5-4 to 5-8). Clubfoot is characterized by the inability to dorsiflex, medial deviation of the heel, and a sole that is kidney shaped when viewed from the bottom. There is often a varus deformation of the neck of the talus and a medial shift of the navicular on the head of the talus. The calf muscles may be deficient with shortening and tapering. The fibrous capsule of the joint may be thickened on the lateral aspect of the foot. If there has been a long-term compression over the lateral margin of the foot, that site may have thin skin

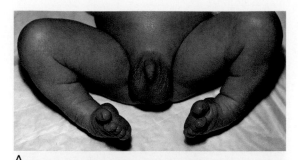

A

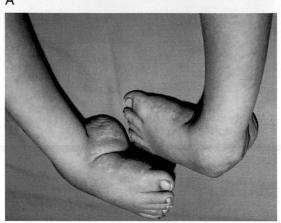

B

FIGURE 5-5. Bilateral talipes equinovarus feet at birth **(A)** and later in childhood (without treatment) **(B)**. Note the heel varus (medial deviation) and rigid foot posture with inability to dorsiflex.
(Courtesy of Robert M. Bernstein, Cedar Sinai Medical Center, Los Angeles, Calif.)

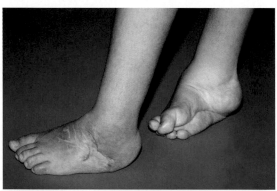

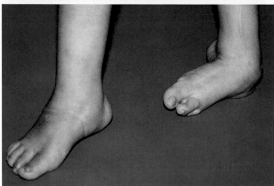

FIGURE 5-4. This rigid left equinovarus foot in an 18-year-old was untreated, resulting in the individual walking on the outside edge of this foot.
(Courtesy of Robert M. Bernstein, Cedar Sinai Medical Center, Los Angeles, Calif.)

with deficient subcutaneous tissue. The depth of skin creases on the medial side of the foot is indicative of the severity of the deformity, and the more rigid the foot, the poorer the prognosis. TEV is unilateral in 45% of cases and more commonly affects the right foot (1.2:1.0).[17]

## MANAGEMENT, PROGNOSIS, AND COUNSEL

Neonates with TEV should be referred immediately to an experienced pediatric orthopedist for corrective serial casting during the first week so as to take advantage of residual neonatal ligamentous laxity. If there is flexibility to the foot, initial manipulation and stretch taping toward dorsiflexion of the foot with eversion of the heel should be attempted (Fig. 5-9). Maintenance of the corrected position may sometimes need to be fostered by casting and/or Denis-Browne splints in order to prevent a lapse toward the deformed position. If

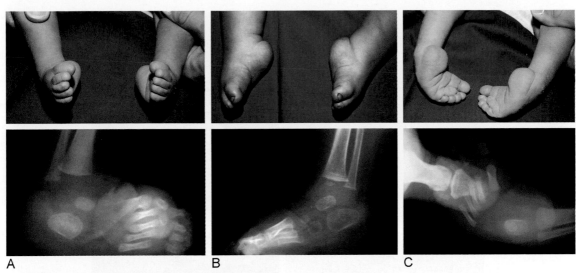

FIGURE 5-6. These neurogenic equinovarus feet resulted from a lumbosacral meningomyelocele. Note varus deformation **(A)**, equinus position **(B)**, and adductus deformation **(C)**.
   (Courtesy of Robert M. Bernstein, Cedar Sinai Medical Center, Los Angeles, Calif.)

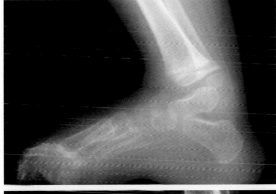

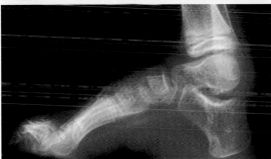

FIGURE 5-7. Cavus foot deformity can result from muscular imbalance due to deficient gastrocnemius function in spina bifida.
   (Courtesy of Saul Bernstein and Robert M. Bernstein, Cedar Sinai Medical Center, Los Angeles, Calif.)

continued improvement does not occur after 3 months of conservative management or if there is little or no flexibility in the foot (especially in the ability to bring the hindfoot equinus into a normal position), then early surgical intervention

may be merited. Long-term results of manipulation and serial casting using the Ponseti method suggest that when properly performed, surgical release is indicated in less than 1% of cases, primarily those with a short, rigid forefoot or with severe deformity that does not respond to proper manipulation.[22]

Prognostic classification in older studies was usually based on the reducibility of the equinovarus deformity by manipulation. Mild TEV that can be manipulated to or beyond neutral had an 89% success rate with serial casting as compared with 46% for moderate deformity that could only be manipulated to within 20 degrees of neutral and 10% for more severe deformity.[23] The initial treatment is usually nonsurgical regardless of severity, with serial casting favored in North America and vigorous physical therapy with splinting favored in Europe. This latter approach reported good results in as many as 77% of cases.[24] Early correction usually begins distally and is accomplished in the following order: adduction, varus, and then equinus. With moderately severe cases, some type of soft tissue release surgery may be required in more than half of such cases, usually between ages 6 and 12 months.[13] In the past, limited posterior release procedures were performed, followed by more extensive releases, and currently more limited releases are favored.[13] Good results were reported in most cases in a prospective study of congenital equinovarus foot among 20,000 neonates.[25] If full correction is not obtained by 1 year of age, it is unlikely to be achieved, and surgical correction is more difficult

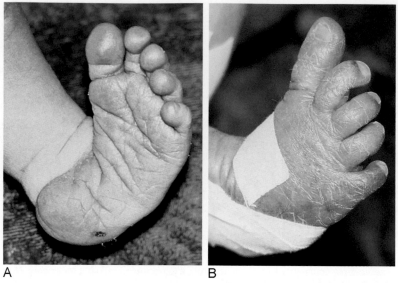

A                                B

FIGURE 5-8. **A,** Plantar view of an equinovarus foot. Note the inward rotation of the heel and forefoot with the whole foot deviated inward at the ankle. **B,** At the site of in-utero compression over the left lateral ankle, the skin was very thin, erythematous, and stretched as a result of prolonged pressure. Outward pressure on the heel and forefoot via taping resulted in a partial correction toward a neutral foot position. Taping and manipulation alone corrected this foot.

when there is an associated neurologic syndrome or underlying genetic connective tissue disorder.

Because vertical transmission has been seen in 20.8% of idiopathic TEV, prenatal diagnosis with ultrasonography may provide useful information when a parent is affected. Among 103 patients with clubfoot diagnosed at birth, 26 had positive prenatal scans, and the diagnosis was made as early as 15 weeks.[26] In one 1999 series of prenatally diagnosed clubfoot, it was diagnosed in 0.43% of prenatal ultrasound exams, with one third of cases being isolated and two thirds associated with other anomalies, further complicating prenatal counseling.[27] A 1998 study of 68 fetuses with apparently isolated clubfoot detected on prenatal ultrasonography noted that 5.9% of these fetuses had abnormal karyotypes, suggesting that chromosome analysis was indicated whenever an isolated clubfoot was detected prenatally.[28] In a 1999 study of 13 fetuses with clubfoot born to 12 Israeli couples, there were 9 bilateral and 4 unilateral cases of clubfoot, and the ultrasound diagnosis was made at the average menstrual age of 21.6 weeks from conception (range, 15–34 weeks).[29] Of these 13 fetuses, 23% had other associated anomalies, causing parents to terminate the pregnancies in 2 cases, while a third fetus died 2 weeks after birth from cardiac complications.

One other fetus was found to have normal feet at birth. Of these 22 cases of clubfoot diagnosed prenatally, 14 did not respond to serial casting and required surgical correction.[29]

As prenatal ultrasonography has improved, it has become more reliable in distinguishing isolated TEV from clubfoot that occurs as part of a broader pattern and from rocker-bottom feet. Chitty and Pajkrt[30] searched a computerized database of the Fetal Medicine Unit at University College London Hospitals and ascertained 364 cases of fetal joint contractures seen between January 1999 and February 2004. Outcomes were available for 299 cases (82%), and all 87 cases of isolated TEV (29%) had a good outcome and a normal karyotype. Rocker-bottom feet were never isolated and always carried a poor prognosis. The same was true for clenched hands and flexed wrists, and complex joint deformities were always manifestations of a broad spectrum of conditions that included aneuploidies, myopathies, neuropathies, and genetic syndromes. A careful search for associated anomalies demonstrated that associated anomalies (e.g., spina bifida, multiple anomalies, arthrogryposis, radial club hand, clenched hand, or generalized joint deformities) were present and the risk of adverse fetal outcome and chromosome abnormalities (20%) was significantly

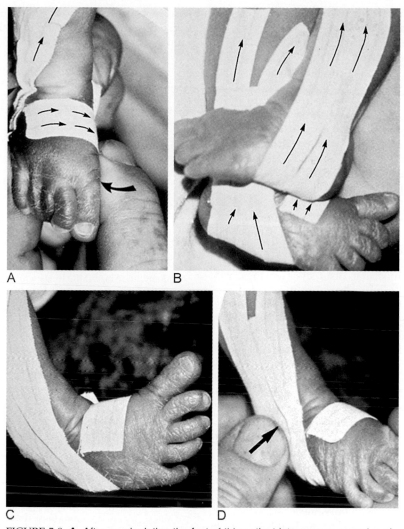

FIGURE 5-9. **A,** After manipulating the foot of this patient into a more normal position, several layers of adhesive tape are applied (tincture of benzoin on skin), starting over the dorsum of the foot and bringing the tape medially under the sole and up the lateral aspect of the leg. **B,** After taping, the feet tend to return partially to their pretaped position. When the foot is taped and partially corrected, it is possible for the parents to repeatedly manipulate the foot toward the ideal position (**C** and **D**) a mode of management that is not possible when the foot is in a cast.

increased. Postmortem examinations and genetic consultations helped further define the diagnosis and subsequent genetic counseling.[30]

Although there has not been a clear separation of postural TEV from other types of TEV, the prognosis for restoration toward normal form is much better when the cause is uterine constraint in an otherwise normal child. The general recurrence risk for an equinovarus defect is 2%, and when only postural equinovarus cases are considered, the recurrence risk is 3%.[1] If the propositus is a male, the recurrence risk for siblings is 6.3%; if the propositi is female, the recurrence risk for siblings is 1.9%, with 4.2% of patients having an affected first-degree relative.[2]

## DIFFERENTIAL DIAGNOSIS

Congenital vertical talus, or rocker-bottom foot, is a severe malformation that results in a rigid foot with a convex plantar surface rather than a cavus arch and with a deep crease on the lateral dorsal side of the foot (see Fig. 5-4). The forefoot is abducted (turned outward) and dorsiflexed, while the heel is also turned outward with the toes pointing down, resulting in the "rocker-bottom foot" configuration.[31,32] With congenital vertical talus, the talus is rigidly fixed in a vertical position in plantar flexion, and the forefoot cannot be plantar flexed. There is dorsal dislocation of the navicular on the talus, and the calcaneocuboid joint is irreducible. The Achilles tendons are contracted, and hypoplasia of the talar head can be palpated on the medial sole. Early casting to stretch soft tissues and tendons starts at birth and continues until surgical reconstruction, but the foot usually remains abnormal. Congenital vertical talus can be isolated or part of a broader pattern of malformation due to chromosomal or neuromuscular disorders (see Figs. 3-5 and 3-6).[31,32]

Pronounced tightness of the Achilles tendon, with very little dorsiflexion, differentiates TEV from metatarsus adductus. The etiology for idiopathic TEV, which has a predilection for males and varies in racial incidence, is unknown, but it tends to be more rigid than constraint-induced deformation, with more associated atrophy of calf muscles. The talus tends to be hypoplastic and altered in form, and there is some question as to whether the primary defect is in talonavicular development, possibly on a vascular basis.[7-12] When TEV is a feature of intrinsic deformation, the prognosis for achieving a normal foot form is usually poor. TEV may accompany certain neurologic deficiencies, especially those affecting the spinal cord, such as occurs so frequently with meningomyelocele. An infant with TEV should be checked for spinal defects and the lower spine should be closely inspected for hemangiomata, hairy nevus, or other subtle clues that might suggest occult spinal dysraphism. A neurologic evaluation is also indicated because partial degrees of equinovarus position occur in a number of neuromuscular and cerebral palsy disorders.

Deficiency of the tibia (tibial hemimelia) often results in an equinovarus foot defect, and amniotic bands around the leg, proximal to the foot, may also result in TEV. This defect may also be part of an arthrogrypotic disorder such as amyoplasia, in which the inward rotation of the hands and shoulders may allow an overall diagnosis (see Fig. 2-4) or Marden-Walker syndrome (see Fig. 2-5). Finally, TEV may be one feature of a skeletal dysplasia, such as diastrophic dysplasia, an autosomal recessive genetic connective tissue dysplasia (see Figs. 1-1, *D* and 2-2, *D*). This

represents an example of an underlying connective tissue dysplasia leading to malformation of a joint.

## References

1. Wynn-Davies R: Family studies and aetiology of clubfoot, *J Med Genet* 2:227–232, 1965.
2. Moorthi RN, Hashmi SS, Langois P, et al: Idiopathic talipes equinovarus (ITEV) (clubfeet) in Texas, *Amer J Med Genet* 132A:376–380, 2005.
3. Chung CS, Nemechek RW, Larson IJ, et al: Genetic and epidemiological studies of clubfoot in Hawaii, *Hum Hered* 19:321–342, 1969.
4. Lochmiller CL, Johnston D, Scott A, et al: Genetic epidemiology study of idiopathic talipes equinovarus, *Amer J Med Genet* 79:90–96, 1998.
5. Lapunzina P, Camelo JS, Rittler M, et al: Risks of congenital anomalies in large for gestational age infants, *J Pediatr* 140:200–204, 2002.
6. Moore LL, Singer MR, Bradlee ML, et al: A prospective study of risk of congenital defects associated with maternal obesity and diabetes mellitus, *Epidemiology* 11:689–694, 2000.
7. Andrade M, Barnholtz JS, Amos CI, et al: Segregation analysis of idiopathic talipes equinovarus in a Texan population, *Amer J Med Genet* 79:97–102, 1998.
8. Rebbeck TR, Dietz FR, Murray JC, et al: A single-gene explanation for the probability of having idiopathic talipes equinovarus, *Amer J Hum Genet* 53:1051–1063, 1993.
9. Wang JH, Palmer RH, Chung CS: The role of major gene in clubfoot, *Amer J Hum Genet* 42:772–776, 1988.
10. Yang HY, Chung CS, Nemechek RW: A genetic analysis of clubfoot in Hawaii, *Genet Epidem* 4:299–306, 1987.
11. Chapman C, Stott NS, Port RV, et al: Genetics of club foot in Maori and Pacific people, *J Med Genet* 37:680–683, 2000.
12. Muir L, Laliotis N, Kutty S, et al: Absence of the dorsalis pedis pulse in the parents of children with clubfoot, *J Bone Joint Surg* B77:114–116, 1995.
13. Roye DP, Roye BD: Idiopathic congenital talipes equinovarus, *J Am Acad Orthop Surg* 10:239–248, 2002.
14. Alderman BW, Takahashi ER, LeMier MK: Risk indicators for talipes equinovarus in Washington State, 1987–1989, *Epidemiology* 2:289–292, 1991.
15. Skelly AC, Holt VL, Mosca VS, et al: Talipes equinovarus and maternal smoking: a population-based case-control study in Washington State, *Teratology* 66:91–100, 2002.
16. Honein MA, Paulozzi LJ, Moore CA: Family history, maternal smoking, and clubfoot: an indication of a gene-environment interaction, *Am J Epidemiol* 152:658–665, 2000.
17. Anonymous: Randomized trial to assess safety and fetal outcome of early and midtrimester amniocentesis. The Canadian Early and Mid-trimester Amniocentesis Trial (CEMAT) Group, *Lancet* 351:242–247, 1998.
18. Farrell SA, Summers AM, Dallaire L, et al: Clubfoot, an adverse outcome of early amniocentesis: disruption or amniocentesis? *J Med Genet* 36:843–846, 1999.
19. Tredwell SJ, Wilson D, Wilmink MA: Review of the effect of early amniocentesis on foot deformity in the neonate, *J Pediatr Orthop* 21:636–641, 2001.
20. Graham JM Jr, Edwards MJ, Edwards MJ: Teratogen update: gestational effects of maternal hyperthermia due to febrile illnesses and resultant patterns of defects in humans, *Teratology* 58:209–221, 1998.
21. Gonzales CH, Marques-Dias MJ, Kim CA, et al: Congenital abnormalities in Brazilian children associated with miso-

prostol misuse in first trimester of pregnancy, *Lancet* 351:1624–1627, 1998.

22. Morcuende JA: Congenital idiopathic clubfoot: prevention of late deformity and disability by conservative treatment with the Ponseti technique, *Pediatr Ann* 35:128–136, 2006.

23. Harold AJ, Walker CJ: Treatment and prognosis in congenital club foot, *J Bone Joint Surg Br* 65:8–11, 1983.

24. Souchet P, Bensahel H, Themar-Noel C, et al: Functional treatment of clubfoot: a new series of 350 idiopathic clubfeet with long-term follow-up, *J Pediatr Orthop B* 13:189–196, 2004.

25. Vadivieso-Garcia JL, Escassi-Gil A, Zapatero-Martinez M, et al: Prospective study of equinovarus foot in 20,000 live newborn infants, *An Esp Pediatr* 28:325–326, 1988.

26. Burgan HE, Furness ME, Foster BK: Prenatal ultrasound diagnosis of clubfoot, *J Pediatr Orthop* 19:11–13, 1999.

27. Treadwell MC, Stanitski CL, King M: Prenatal sonographic diagnosis of clubfoot: implications for patient counseling, *J Pediatr Orthop* 19:8–10, 1999.

28. Shipp TD, Benacerraf BR: The significance of prenatally identified isolated clubfoot: is amniocentesis indicated? *Am J Obstet Gynecol* 178:600–602, 1998.

29. Katz K, Meizner I, Mashiach R, et al: The contribution of prenatal sonographic diagnosis of clubfoot to preventive medicine, *J Pediatr Orthop* 19:5–7, 1999.

30. Chitty LS, Pajkrt E: Fetal joint contractures: sonographic diagnosis, management and prognosis, Presented at the 11th Manchester Birth Defects Conference, Manchester, United Kingdom, November 9–12, 2004.

31. Furdon SA, Donlon CR: Examination of the newborn foot: positional and structural abnormalities, *Adv Neonatal Care* 2:248–258, 2002.

32. Gore AI, Spencer JP: The newborn foot, *Am Family Physician* 69:865–872, 2004.

# 6 Deformed Toes

## GENESIS

Constraint of the feet while the legs are in a flexed and folded position can result in medial overlapping of the toes, especially the fifth, fourth, and third toes.

## FEATURES

The fifth, fourth, and third toes tend to overlap medially with mild to moderate incurvature (Fig. 6-1). There may be accentuated longitudinal creasing in the sole of the foot, where the sole has been "folded" by external compression.

## MANAGEMENT AND PROGNOSIS

If the toes do not readily tend to realign after birth, then manipulative lateral stretching and/or taping is merited. Rarely is surgery necessary.

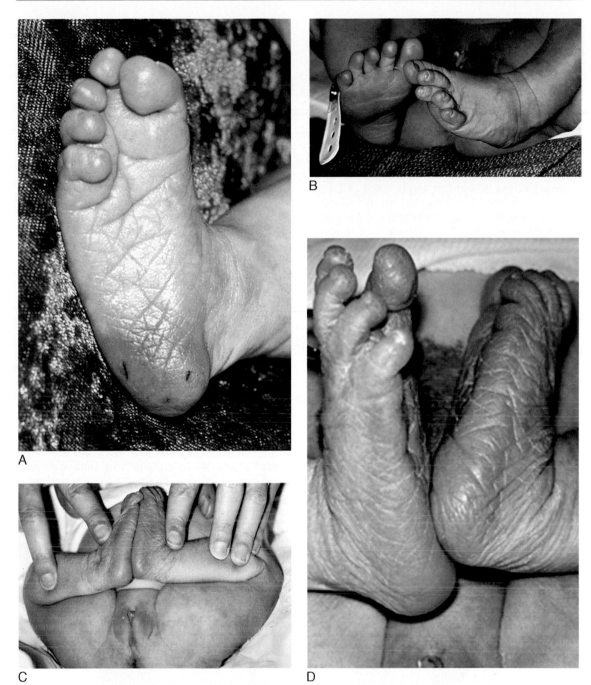

FIGURE 6-1. **A,** Deformed toes. **B,** Presumed position in utero, in which uterine constraint from oligohydramnios compressed the forefoot, resulting in overlapping of the toes. **C,** Presumed positioning in utero, in which uterine constraint compressed the feet, yielding unilateral, partially folded forefoot and deformation of toes. **D,** Note the thin, wrinkled skin over the lateral malleolus *(left)*, which is a strong clue that constraint induction of the deformation occurred.

# 7 Flexible Flatfoot

## GENESIS

Flexible flatfoot is common and is noted in 7% to 22% of children.[1,2] This deformity usually becomes evident with weight bearing and is often caused by ligamentous laxity, hence it is strongly associated with genetic connective tissue disorders such as Marfan syndrome and Ehlers-Danlos syndrome. When flexible flatfeet are part of such a broader pattern of connective tissue dysplasia, there is usually hyperextension of fingers, elbows, and knees with a positive family history because such disorders are often genetic. Children with flexible flatfeet are generally asymptomatic as adults, and the development of the arch occurs with growth and is not related to the use of external supports or shoes.[3] The prevalence of flatfeet decreases with increasing age. There is a higher prevalence of flatfeet in children who wear shoes versus those who wear no shoes at all, and closed-toe shoes inhibit development of the arch more than do slippers and sandals.[4] The support of the longitudinal arch is primarily ligamentous, with muscle supporting and stabilizing the arch during heavy loading.[3]

## FEATURES

All children have a minimal arch filled with fatty tissue at birth, but more than 30% of neonates have a calcaneovalgus deformity of both feet that is not painful and usually resolves without treatment.[3] The arch develops slowly by about age 4 to 5 years, and most children presenting to an orthopedist for evaluation of flatfeet have flexible flatfeet that only become apparent after the child begins to walk.[3,4] Ligamentous laxity allows the foot to collapse medially with weight bearing, and the heel rolls into a medially deviated valgus position. The ankle and foot are sufficiently strong, and the child with flexible flatfeet can form a good arch when asked to stand on tiptoe and when the heel goes into mild varus (Fig. 7-1). The ability to stand on the heel implies that the heel cord is not excessively tight. The ability to stand first on the outer border of the foot and then on the inner border of the foot implies normal function of the posterior tibialis, anterior tibialis, and peroneal musculature, with normal subtalar function. Foot muscle strength and passive range of motion of the ankle and subtalar joint are examined in the seated position.[3] Examination of shoe wear can yield important clues. Normally, there is heel wear on the lateral aspect, with no heel wear implying tight heel cords. Wear on the medial portion of the heel may be associated with a pronated flexible flatfoot. An abnormal gait may suggest a skeletal dysplasia or neuromuscular disorder. Radiographs are indicated when the flatfoot is symptomatic and painful, particularly if a skeletal dysplasia is suspected.

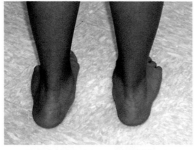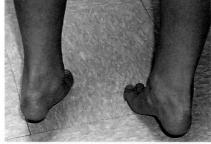

FIGURE 7-1. Ligamentous laxity allows the foot to collapse medially with weight bearing; the heel rolls into a medially deviated valgus position, and the arch disappears. The ankle and foot are sufficiently strong, and the child with flexible flatfeet can form a good arch when asked to stand on tiptoe, when the heel goes into mild varus.
(Courtesy of Robert M. Bernstein, Cedar Sinai Medical Center, Los Angeles, Calif.)

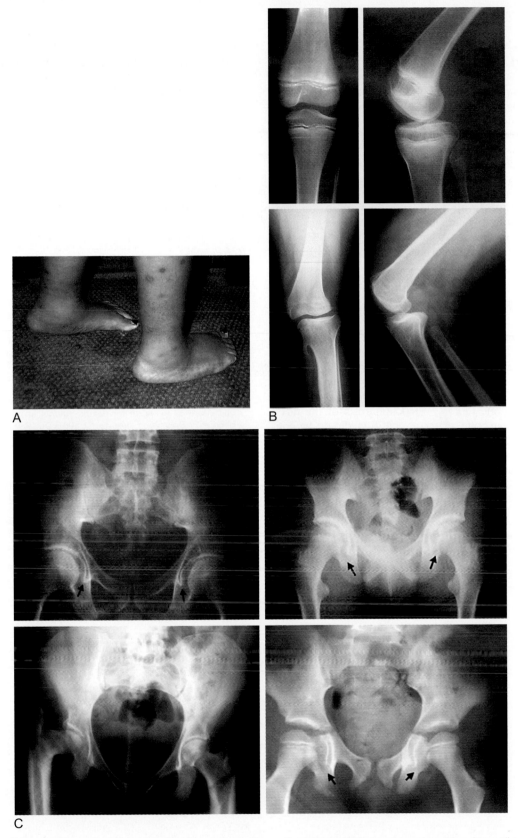

FIGURE 7-2. **A,** Typical rigid, painful flatfeet in a patient with small patella syndrome and tarsal coalition. In small patella syndrome, there is absence or hypoplasia of the patella **(B)**, with diagnostic pelvic features consisting of hypoplasia of the descending pubic rami and of the ischiopubic synchondrosis, congenital coxa vara, and so-called ax-cut notching *(arrows)* **(C)**.

# MANAGEMENT, PROGNOSIS, AND COUNSEL

Treatment of flexible flatfeet is controversial as to whether corrective shoes or custom orthotics provide demonstrable benefit. In 1979 most pediatricians and orthopedists did not prescribe orthotic inserts or corrective shoes.[5] A prospective study of 129 children with flexible flatfoot revealed no benefit from such treatment, and many physicians now recommend use of running or basketball shoes with good arch support and a shoe design that is straight with adequate room for the toes; special shoes are used only for cases with severe deformity or persistent pain.[4,6,7] Surgery is rarely indicated.[3]

# DIFFERENTIAL DIAGNOSIS

Flexible flatfoot can also occur with tight heel cords in various neurologic disorders, such as muscular dystrophy or mild cerebral palsy. It is unusual for a flatfoot to be stiff and painful, and in such cases, trauma, occult infection, a foreign body, bone tumors, osteochondrosis of the tarsal navicular bone, or tarsal coalition should be considered.[1,2,6] In these circumstances, radiographic studies using standard and oblique views of the foot and ankle with orthopedic evaluation is merited. Tarsal coalition can be part of a broader pattern of skeletal dysplasia, such as small patella syndrome (Fig. 7-2), an autosomal dominant condition caused by mutations in TBX4.[8,9] This condition combines absence or hypoplasia of the patella with diagnostic pelvic features (hypoplasia of the descending pubic rami and hypoplasia of the ischiopubic synchondrosis, with congenital coxa vara). Patients with tarsal coalition manifest a familial tendency and may not present until they approach skeletal maturity, when they experience pain in the midtarsal region with activity. Talocalcaneal coalitions are rarely diagnosed on plain radiographs but are easily demonstrated using computed tomography. As opposed to flexible flatfeet, treatment usually requires surgical resection of a middle-facet coalition.[3]

## References

1. Barry RJ, Scranton PE Jr: Flat feet in children, *Clin Orthop Rel Res* 181:68–75, 1983.
2. Churgay CA: Diagnosis and treatment of pediatric foot deformities, *Am Fam Physician* 47:863–889, 1993.
3. Sullivan JA: Pediatric flatfoot: evaluation and management, *J Am Acad Orthop Surg* 7:44–53, 1999.
4. Rao UB, Joseph B: The influence of footwear on the prevalence of flat foot: a survey of 2300 children, *J Bone Joint Surg Br* 74:525–527, 1992.
5. Staheli LT, Giffin L: Corrective shoes for children: a survey of current practice, *Pediatrics* 65:13–17, 1980.
6. Wenger DR, Maudlin D, Speck G, et al: Corrective shoes and inserts as treatment for flexible flatfoot in infants and children, *J Bone Joint Surg Am* 71:800–810, 1989.
7. Wenger DR, Leach J: Foot deformities in infants and children, *Pediatr Clin North Am* 33:1411–1427, 1986.
8. Bongers EM, van Bokhoven H, van Thienen M-N, et al: The small patella syndrome: description of five cases from three families and examination of possible allelism with familial patella aplasia-hypoplasia and nail-patella syndrome, *J Med Genet* 38:209–213, 2001.
9. Bongers EM, Duijf PH, van Beersum SE, et al: Mutations in the human TBX4 gene cause small patella syndrome, *Am J Hum Genet* 74:1239–1248, 2004.

# Other Lower Extremity Deformations

# 8 Tibial Torsion

## GENESIS

*Rotation* refers to the twist of the tibia along its long axis. Normal rotation in direction and magnitude is termed *version*, and normal values are determined according to age. Abnormal rotation is termed *torsion*, and the degree of rotation is determined by the angle between the transmalleolar axis at the ankle and the bicondylar axis of the proximal tibia at the knee. Rotational abnormalities of the lower extremities (intoeing and outtoeing) are common in young children. These abnormalities vary by site with advancing age and usually respond to conservative treatment. Intoeing is caused by one of three types of deformity: metatarsus adductus (during the first year), internal tibial torsion (in toddlers), and increased femoral anteversion (in early childhood). Internal tibial torsion may occur in combination with metatarsus adductus, and it can be accentuated by postures such as prone sleeping with the toes turned in (see Fig. 4-2) or sitting in a W position.

Torsion of the tibia is sufficiently common in the normal newborn to be considered a normal variant; however, more severe variations are seen in about 3% of infants. Tibial torsion is especially likely with fetal constraint of the legs in a folded and flexed position, and it is frequently associated with positional equinovarus deformity and metatarsus adductus, each of which derive from similar types of mechanical constraint.[1-4] During the seventh week of gestation, the lower limb buds rotate internally, bringing the great toe to the midline from its initial lateral position.[5] During fetal life, the legs are molded so that the femurs rotate externally and the tibiae rotate internally. Internal tibial torsion averaging 4 degrees is normal at birth, after which the tibiae rotate externally to an average of 23 degrees in adulthood (as measured by the transmalleolar axis). In support of the concept that tibial torsion occurs late in gestation due to fetal constraint, this deformation is not encountered in premature infants born before 30 weeks of gestation.[6]

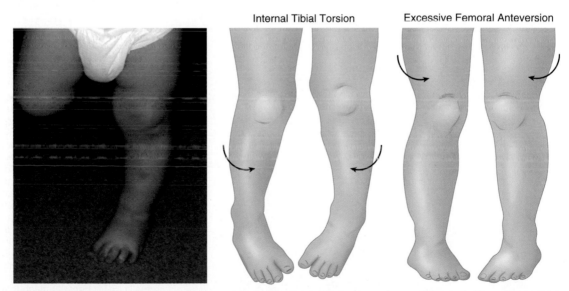

Internal Tibial Torsion      Excessive Femoral Anteversion

FIGURE 8-1. Internal tibial torsion usually presents as intoeing during the second year of life, and with persistent tibial torsion, the patellae point forward with walking or standing while the feet point inward. The diagrams compare the patellae and feet in tibial torsion and femoral anteversion. With excessive femoral anteversion, both the patellae and the feet point inward with walking.

(Courtesy of Robert M. Bernstein, Cedar Sinai Medical Center, Los Angeles, Calif.)

## FEATURES

In fetal life the hips are positioned in flexion and lateral rotation while the feet are in medial rotation, resulting in lateral hip rotation that is greater than medial hip rotation and causing internal tibial torsion, most of which corrects by the second year of life.[1-9] The tibia is medially rotated on its long axis at birth, with the most acute incurving occurring distally (Fig. 8-1). Internal tibial torsion usually presents as intoeing during the second year of life, and thus it may not be noticed until the child begins to walk. Tibial torsion tends to resolve spontaneously unless accentuated by sleeping in a prone, intoed position, hence this deformation and metatarsus adductus have decreased in frequency with the adoption of a supine sleeping position. Intoeing in an infant is usually due to metatarsus adductus, and after age 3 years, intoeing is usually due to excessive femoral anteversion, but a combination of causes is often present. With persistent tibial torsion, the patellae point forward with walking or standing while the feet point inward (see Fig. 8-1). With excessive femoral anteversion, both the patellae and the feet point inward with walking. Tibial torsion tends to angle the plantar surfaces of the feet toward each other, hence there may also be mild to moderate metatarsus adductus in association with tibial torsion.[1-3] Tibial torsion is usually bilateral, but when it is unilateral, the left side is more often involved.[7]

Rotational problems should be evaluated by determining the rotational profile.[5] Intoeing is quantified by estimating and following the foot-progression angle, which is the angular difference between the long axis of the foot and the line of

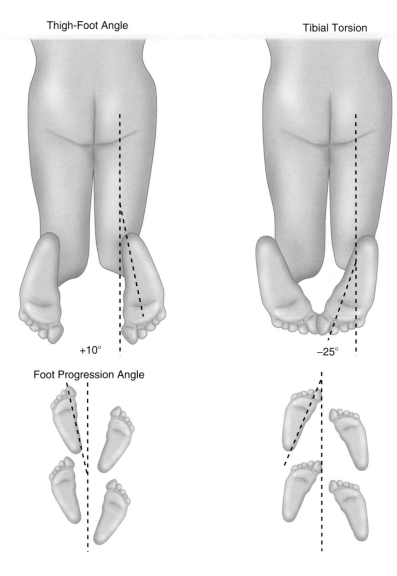

Thigh-Foot Angle

Tibial Torsion

+10°

−25°

Foot Progression Angle

FIGURE 8-2. Diagrams demonstrating normal and abnormal thigh-foot angles and foot-progression angles. The normal foot-progression angle is +10 degrees, with a range from −3 to +20 degrees. Tibial rotation is determined by measuring the thigh-foot angle, which is the angular difference between the axis of the foot and the axis of the thigh when the patient is in prone position with the knees flexed 90 degrees and the foot in neutral position. A negative (−) value means the tibia is rotated internally (internal tibial torsion), and a positive (+) value means the tibia is rotated externally (external tibial torsion). An infant normally has a negative thigh-foot angle that becomes progressively positive with age, resulting in a mean thigh-foot angle during childhood of +10 to +15 degrees (normal range, −5 to +30 degrees).

progression with ambulation (Fig. 8-2). Intoeing is denoted by a minus (−) sign and out-toeing by a plus (+) sign. The normal foot-progression angle is +10 degrees, with a range of −3 to +20 degrees. Hip rotation in femoral anteversion is measured by having the child lie prone on the examination table with the knees flexed 90 degrees and allowing the legs to fall inward and outward by gravity alone. The amount of internal and external rotation of the hip should be similar, inscribing a total arc of about 90 degrees; medial rotation in excess of 70 degrees suggests excessive femoral anteversion. Tibial rotation is determined by measuring the thigh-foot angle, which is the angular difference between the axis of the foot and the axis of the thigh when the patient is in prone position with the knees flexed 90 degrees and the foot in neutral position (see Fig. 8-2). A negative value means the tibia is rotated internally (internal tibial torsion), and a positive value means the tibia is rotated externally (external tibial torsion). An infant normally has a negative thigh-foot angle that becomes progressively positive with age, resulting in a mean thigh-foot angle during childhood of +10 to +15 degrees (normal range, −5 to +30 degrees). Quantification of rotational abnormalities is usually done by physical examination, and imaging is used only when a significant rotational abnormality does not resolve with time. Pelvic radiographs may be taken to rule out hip dysplasia as a cause of femoral anteversion, but tibial radiographs are not helpful in assessing tibial torsion.

## MANAGEMENT, PROGNOSIS, AND COUNSEL

Because spontaneous resolution occurs in 95% of cases by 7 to 8 years of age, management is seldom required. The use of shoe modifications or night splints is not indicated, and parents should be informed that after release from the constraining intrauterine position, progressive straightening of the legs tends to occur.[1-9] However, certain sleeping postures may tend to foster persistence of the tibial torsion, and the same preventive measures for adverse sleeping postures as mentioned for metatarsus adductus may be used. Following the torsional profile over time, with regular examinations and measurements to confirm improvement, can be extremely reassuring to parents.[2,7-9] Tibial torsion persisting after age 8 years, especially with a family history of rotational anomalies that persist into adulthood, is less likely to resolve spontaneously. The only effective treatment for residual internal tibial torsion is tibial osteotomy, which is usually not performed until after 8 to 10 years of age. Surgery is usually only contemplated in skeletally mature individuals with insufficient spontaneous correction. In such cases, an underlying disorder such as cerebral palsy,

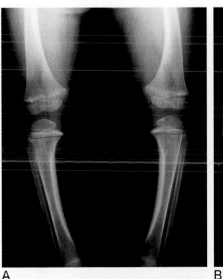
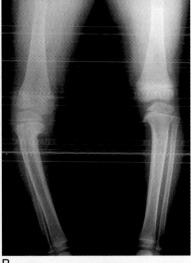

A                                    B

FIGURE 8-3. **A,** Physiological bowing in an otherwise normal child. **B,** Tibia vara (Blount disease) results from disordered growth of the proximal medial metaphyses, and a medial metaphyseal lesion is evident on these radiographs in the proximal tibias. Blount disease may be associated with obesity, and it must be distinguished from physiologic bowing **(A).**

(Courtesy of Saul Bernstein, Cedar Sinai Medical Center, Los Angeles, Calif.)

hip dysplasia, or skeletal dysplasia should be evaluated.

## DIFFERENTIAL DIAGNOSIS

Three causes of intoeing affect otherwise normal children: metatarsus adductus, internal tibial torsion, and excessive femoral anteversion resulting from medial rotation of the femur. Internal tibial torsion is at its peak in children ages 1 to 3 years and resolves spontaneously by late adolescence. Rotational anomalies, even if severe, are not painful; therefore, any history of pain should prompt a search for another cause. Sometimes a rotational problem is a manifestation of an

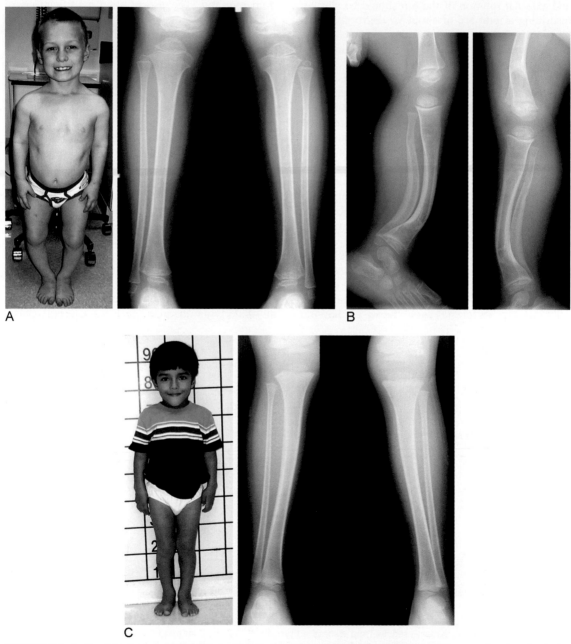

FIGURE 8-4. **A,** Persistent genu varum (bowlegs) can result from skeletal dysplasias, such as pseudoachondroplasia, presumably as a result of excessive ligamentous laxity. Pseudoachondroplasia can be caused by mutations in cartilage oligomeric matrix protein (COMP). **B,** Persistent genu varum can also result from hypophosphatemic rickets. **C,** Pseudoachondroplasia can also result in genu valgum (knock-knees) due to ligamentous laxity.

underlying disorder such as cerebral palsy, hip dysplasia, or a skeletal dysplasia. Any clinical findings such as abnormal muscle tone, gait abnormality, limited hip abduction, leg length discrepancy, or disproportionate short stature should prompt a more intensive evaluation. A child with mild cerebral palsy may walk with mild equinus and intoeing, whereas hip dysplasia is suggested by a leg length discrepancy and a Trendelenburg gait (i.e., the pelvis tilts toward the normal hip when the affected side bears weight due to weak hip abductors).

Out-toeing is much less common than intoeing. Femoral retroversion can be caused by external rotation contracture of the hip. It is common in early infancy and becomes apparent prior to walking when the infant stands with feet turned out nearly 90 degrees in a "Charlie Chaplin" stance. It occurs more commonly in obese children, and when unilateral, it is more commonly right-sided.[8] Another cause of out-toeing in the obese child is a slipped capital femoral epiphysis, which requires hip radiographs if suspected. If femoral retroversion persists beyond age 2 to 3 years, referral to an orthopedist is indicated. External tibial torsion is seen between 4 and 7 years of age. External tibial torsion may be unilateral (more commonly right-sided), causing patellofemoral instability and pain. Tibial torsion may require surgical osteotomy if it persists beyond age 10 years.[8] Flexible flatfeet may also result in out-toeing.[8,9]

The lower legs may be more bowed than usual because of a variety of generalized neuromuscular or skeletal disorders, many which require surgical management. Physiologic bowing confined to the tibia occurs during the first year and usually resolves (Fig 8-3, A). When it occurs during the second year and involves both the tibia and the distal femur, it is often associated with medial tibial torsion. Physiologic bowing usually resolves spontaneously, and bracing does not affect the natural history.

Tibial vara, or Blount disease, results from abnormal proximal tibial metaphyseal growth, often in association with medial tibial torsion (Fig. 8-3, B). It is often associated with obesity and is caused by osteochondrosis due to mechanical stress, with a medial metaphyseal lesion evident on radiographs in the proximal tibia. In its early stages, this disorder is treated with corrective osteotomy.

Angular deformities, such as genu varum (bowlegs) and genu valgum (knock-knees) need to be distinguished from rotational abnormalities (Fig. 8-4).[8] Genu varum is seen from birth to age 2 years, whereas genu valgum peaks between ages 2 and 4 years. Measurements of the intercondylar and intermalleolar distance taken over time have confirmed gradual spontaneous resolution in some cases.[8] Failure to resolve, particularly when there is associated short stature, may suggest the presence of a skeletal dysplasia or metabolic bone disease such as metaphyseal chondrodysplasia, hypophosphatemic rickets, multiple epiphyseal dysplasia, or pseudoachondroplasia.[8]

Limited hip abduction or leg length discrepancy should prompt a search for developmental dyspla-

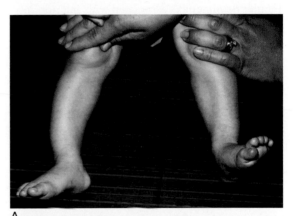

A

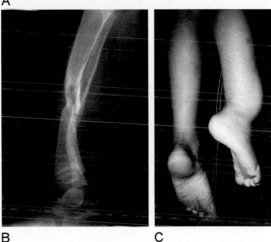

B                                    C

FIGURE 8-5. Anterolateral bowing is a dangerous form of bowing that is usually associated with pseudarthrosis of the tibia. **A,** Pseudarthrosis is often associated with type 1 neurofibromatosis. Radiographs may show a radiolucent lesion at the apex of the bow, but usually only narrowing and sclerosis are seen. Fracture can lead to pseudarthrosis, resulting in nonunion of the fracture and requiring eventual amputation, thus bracing is often attempted to prevent such a fracture. When fracture occurs (**B** and **C**), the ends of the bone are tapered and sclerotic, with the presence of disorganized bone impairing bone strength.

(Courtesy of Saul Bernstein, MD, Cedar Sinai Medical Center, Los Angeles, Calif.)

sia of the hip. An abnormal neurologic exam should prompt consideration of mild cerebral palsy, spinal dysraphism, hydrocephalus, or hereditary motor-sensory neuropathies. Anterior bowing with a cystic, narrowed, or sclerotic medullary canal may progress to pseudarthrosis in neurofibromatosis or fibrous dysplasia; therefore, it is very important to search for café-au-lait spots that might suggest the presence of such an underlying generalized disorder (Fig. 8-5). Various problems in bone formation may also result in malleable or fragile bones, such as occur with hypophosphatasia or osteogenesis imperfecta; these bones can lead to bowing. Fibular hemimelia is associated with anterior bowing, dimpling of the skin at the apex of the curve, ipsilateral shortening of the long bones (especially the fibula), and an equinovalgus foot position. The tibial cortex is thickened on the concave side of the deformity, and the medullary canal may be partly obliterated. In certain skeletal dysplasias, there is characteristic bowing of the long bones (e.g., camptomelic dysplasia, achondroplasia, or thanatophoric dysplasia), and a complete skeletal survey can help distinguish between these skeletal dysplasias. Osteotomies to correct bowing in skeletal dysplasias (e.g., achondroplasia) are usually not done until ages 8 to 10 years.

## References

1. Staheli LT, Corbett M, Wyss C, et al: Lower extremity rotational problems in children, *J Bone Joint Surg Am* 67:39–47, 1985.
2. Staheli LT: Rotational problems in children, *J Bone Joint Surg Am* 75:939–949, 1993.
3. Heirich SD, Sharps CH: Lower extremity torsional deformities in children: a prospective comparison of two treatment modalities, *Orthopedics* 14:655–659, 1991.
4. Bruce RW Jr: Torsional and angular deformities, *Pediatr Clin North Am* 43:867–881, 1996.
5. Guidera KJ, Ganey TM, Keneally CR, et al: The embryology of lower-extremity torsion, *Clin Orthoped Relat Res* 302:17–21, 1994.
6. Li YH, Leong JCY: Intoeing gait in children, *Hong Kong Med J* 5:360–366, 1999.
7. Sass P, Hassan G: Lower extremity abnormalities in children, *Am Fam Physician* 68:461–468, 2003.
8. Lincoln TL, Suen PW: Common rotational variations in children, *J Am Acad Orthop Surg* 11:312–320, 2003.
9. Greene WB: Genu varum and genu valgum in children: differential diagnosis and guidelines for evaluation, *Compr Ther* 22:22–29, 1996.

# 9 Femoral Anteversion

## GENESIS

*Femoral rotation* describes the normal twist present in the femur, and excessive femoral anteversion results from medial rotation of the femur after birth. Normal rotation in direction and magnitude is termed *version*, with normal values determined according to age.[1-8] Abnormal rotation is termed *torsion*, and the rotation of a given bone is determined by the angle between the axis of the head and neck of the femur and the axis of the distal condyles at the most posterior points. If the angle between the proximal and distal axes is positive (+), the femur is considered "anteverted," and if it is negative (−), the femur is "retroverted." Excessive femoral anteversion is the most common cause of intoeing that develops after age 3 years, and it usually resolves spontaneously by late adolescence.[1-8] Femoral anteversion can be familial, is more common in females, and is usually symmetric. Excessive intoeing during the second year is usually caused by tibial torsion, and severe intoeing may be due to a combination of causes.[6] Use of special shoes or bracing does not hasten resolution, but continuation of adverse sleeping or sitting positions may slow or prevent progress. Surgery is usually only contemplated in skeletally mature individuals with insufficient spontaneous correction.[1-9] Out-toeing is much less common than intoeing. Femoral retroversion can be caused by external rotation contracture of the hip. It becomes apparent prior to walking when the infant stands with feet turned out nearly 90 degrees in a "Charlie Chaplin" stance. It occurs more commonly in obese children, and when unilateral, it is more commonly right-sided.[7] Another cause of out-toeing in the obese child is a slipped capital femoral epiphysis, which requires hip radiographs if suspected. If femoral retroversion persists beyond ages 2 to 3 years, referral to an orthopedist is indicated.

## FEATURES

Normal femoral anteversion decreases from about 30 to 40 degrees at birth to 10 to 15 degrees by early adolescence, with most of this improvement occurring before age 8 years.[1,9] Internal tibial torsion is normal at birth, after which the tibiae rotate externally to about 15 degrees in adolescence. Excessive femoral anteversion usually presents as a cause of intoeing at ages 3 to 4 years, increases in magnitude through ages 5 to 6 years, and then gradually decreases thereafter.[7] With excessive femoral anteversion, both the patellae and the feet point inward with walking, whereas with persistent tibial torsion, the patella points forward with walking or standing, while the foot points inward. The child may trip and fall easily because of crossing over of the feet, and the child prefers to sit in the W or reversed tailor position (Fig. 9-1).

Rotational problems should be evaluated by determining the rotational profile.[5] Intoeing is quantified by estimating and following the foot-progression angle, which is the angular difference between the long axis of the foot and the line of progression with ambulation. Intoeing is denoted by a minus (−) sign and out-toeing by a plus (+) sign. The normal angle is +10 degrees, with a range of −3 to +20 degrees. Hip rotation is measured by having the child lie prone on the examination table with knees flexed 90 degrees and allowing the legs to fall inward and outward by gravity alone (see Fig. 9-1). The amount of internal and external rotation of the hip should be similar, inscribing a total arc of about 90 degrees. Internal rotation in excess of 70 degrees suggests excessive femoral anteversion. With mildly excessive femoral anteversion, there are 70 to 80 degrees of internal rotation and 10 to 20 degrees of external rotation. With severe problems, there is no external rotation and internal rotation is greater than

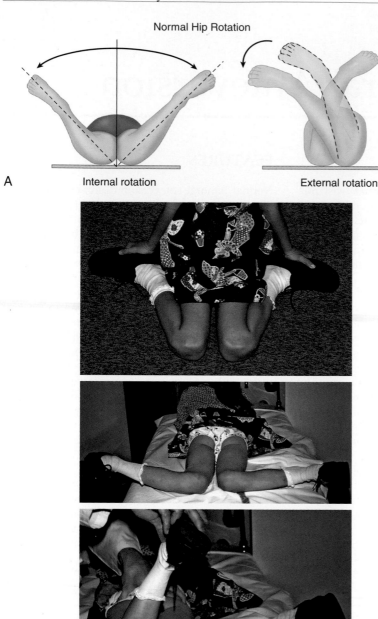

Normal Hip Rotation

A

Internal rotation          External rotation

B

FIGURE 9-1. **A**, Normal internal and external hip rotation. **B**, Accentuating her excessive femoral anteversion, this moderately affected child prefers to sit in the W or reversed tailor position. Hip rotation is measured by having the child lie prone on the examination table with the knees flexed 90 degrees and allowing the legs to fall inward and outward by gravity alone. The amount of internal and external rotation of the hip should be similar, inscribing a total arc of about 90 degrees. Internal rotation in excess of 70 degrees suggests excessive femoral anteversion. With mildly excessive femoral anteversion, there are 70 to 80 degrees of internal rotation and 10 to 20 degrees of external rotation. With severe femoral anteversion, there is no external rotation and internal rotation is greater than 90 degrees.

(Courtesy of Saul Bernstein, Cedar Sinai Medical Center, Los Angeles, Calif.)

90 degrees. Tibial rotation is determined by measuring the thigh-foot angle, which is the angular difference between the axis of the foot and the axis of the thigh when the patient is in the prone position with the knees flexed 90 degrees and the foot in neutral position. A negative value means the tibia is rotated internally (internal tibial torsion),

and a positive value means the tibia is rotated externally (external tibial torsion). An infant normally has a negative thigh-foot angle that becomes progressively positive with age, resulting in a mean thigh-foot angle during childhood of +10 to +15 degrees (normal range, −5 to +30 degrees). As the child with excessive femoral anteversion ages, compensatory external rotation of the tibia may develop, giving rise to a torsional malalignment syndrome that leads to patellofemoral joint instability and anterior knee pain. Quantification of rotational abnormalities is usually done by physical examination, and imaging is used only when a significant rotational abnormality does not resolve with time. Pelvic radiographs may be taken to rule out hip dysplasia as a cause of femoral anteversion, but tibial radiographs are not helpful in assessing tibial torsion.

## MANAGEMENT, PROGNOSIS, AND COUNSEL

Management is seldom required, and spontaneous resolution occurs by late childhood in more than 80% of cases.[1-8] After release from the constraining intrauterine position, progressive straightening of the legs tends to occur. The same preventive measures for sleeping posture as were mentioned for metatarsus adductus and tibial torsion may be used. In a patient with a family history of rotational anomalies that persist into adulthood, it is less likely that such rotational anomalies will resolve spontaneously. Treatment for femoral anteversion is controversial, with no effective nonsurgical treatment identified and with significant risks for major complications associated with derotational osteotomies. Children with cerebral palsy have an increased incidence of excessive femoral anteversion, which seldom improves with time in these children. In children with hemiplegia, there is increased femoral anteversion on the hemiplegic side. Physical therapy can be helpful in treating excessive femoral anteversion in children with cerebral palsy.[9] There is no evidence that intoeing causes osteoarthritis or back pain, and the use of shoe modifications or night splints is not indicated.[6]

## DIFFERENTIAL DIAGNOSIS

Three causes of intoeing affect otherwise normal children: metatarsus adductus, internal tibial torsion, and excessive femoral anteversion. Rotational anomalies, even if severe, are not painful; therefore, any history of pain should prompt a search for another cause. Surgery is usually only contemplated in skeletally mature individuals with insufficient spontaneous correction. Tibial torsion occurs because the tibia is medially rotated on its long axis at birth, but this may not be noticed until the child begins to walk, and the lower legs may be more bowed than usual because of a variety of generalized neuromuscular or skeletal disorders, many of which require surgical management. Associated short stature may suggest the presence of a skeletal dysplasia or metabolic bone disease. An abnormal neurologic examination should prompt consideration of mild cerebral palsy, spinal dysraphism, hydrocephalus, or hereditary motor-sensory neuropathies.

## References

1. Staheli LT, Corbett M, Wyss G, et al: Lower extremity rotational problems in children, *J Bone Joint Surg Am* 67:39–47, 1985.
2. Staheli LT: Rotational problems in children, *J Bone Joint Surg Am* 75:939–949, 1993.
3. Heirich SD, Sharps CH: Lower extremity torsional deformities in children: a prospective comparison of two treatment modalities, *Orthopedics* 14:655–659, 1991.
4. Bruce RW Jr: Torsional and angular deformities, *Pediatr Clin North Am* 43:867–881, 1996.
5. Guidera KJ, Ganey TM, Keneally CR, et al: The embryology of lower-extremity torsion, *Clin Orthoped Relat Res* 302:17–21, 1994.
6. Li YH, Leong JCY: Intoeing gait in children, *Hong Kong Med J* 5:360–366, 1999.
7. Sass P, Hassan G: Lower extremity abnormalities in children, *Am Fam Physician* 68:461–468, 2003.
8. Lincoln TL, Suen PW: Common rotational variations in children, *J Am Acad Orthop Surg* 11:312–320, 2003.
9. Cibulka MT: Determination and significance of femoral neck anteversion, *Phys Ther* 84:550–558, 2004.

# Joint Dislocations

# 10 Joint Dislocation

## GENERAL

Joints normally develop secondarily within the condensed mesenchyme that will form the bones (Fig. 10-1). Hence, a dislocated joint represents a displacement of the bone from the original site of the joint. Once a joint has been dislocated, the joint capsule becomes stretched into an unusual form, and ligamentous attachments become elongated and deformed. If the dislocation is of sufficient duration, the aberrant forces will alter the form of the original joint socket. The occurrence of dislocation is dependent on at least three factors:

1. Biomechanical forces affecting the alignment of bones within the joint
2. Laxity of ligaments that hold the joint together
3. Mesenchymal boney precursors within the joint itself (Fig. 10-2)

The joint that is most liable to dislocation is the hip joint because of the major forces that may be brought to bear on it by such situations as breech presentation in later fetal life and because of the sloping angulation of the acetabulum. The second most common dislocation is of the proximal head of the radius, and the third most common dislocation is at the knee, yielding a genu recurvatum. Because of the relative importance and frequency of dislocation of the hip, it will be given more extensive coverage in this text.

When multiple joint dislocations are present, it usually suggests the presence of a genetic malformation syndrome, such as Larsen syndrome, or a genetic connective tissue dysplasia, such as one of the many different types of Ehlers-Danlos syndrome that lead to ligamentous laxity. Larsen syndrome results in multiple joint dislocations because of joint malformation.[1,2] This syndrome is caused by autosomal dominant mutations in Filamen B *(FLNB)*, a cytoplasmic protein expressed in growth plate chondrocytes and in vertebral bodies that serves to regulate the structure and activity of the cytoskeleton by cross-linking actin into three-dimensional networks.[1] Ehlers-Danlos syndrome is a heritable group of connective tissue disorders characterized by joint hypermobility, skin extensibility, and tissue fragility.[2] Skin extensibility is evaluated on the volar surface of the forearm by pulling skin until resistance is felt (this is difficult in young children due to subcutaneous fat). Joint hypermobility is confirmed by a score of 5 or more points out of 9 on the Beighton scale:

1. Dorsiflexion of the fifth finger more than 90 degrees (1 point for each hand).
2. Apposition of the thumb to flexor aspect of forearm (1 point for each hand).
3. Hyperextension of the elbow beyond 10 degrees (1 point for each elbow).
4. Hyperextension of the knee beyond 10 degrees (1 point for each knee).
5. Forward flexion of the trunk with knees extended so that palms lie flat on the floor (1 point).

Tissue fragility manifests as easy bruising with spontaneous recurrent ecchymoses, causing brownish discoloration and dystrophic scars with

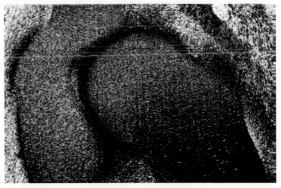

FIGURE 10-1. Normal fetal hip joint developing secondarily within the condensed mesenchyme, which will form the head of the femur and pelvic acetabulum.

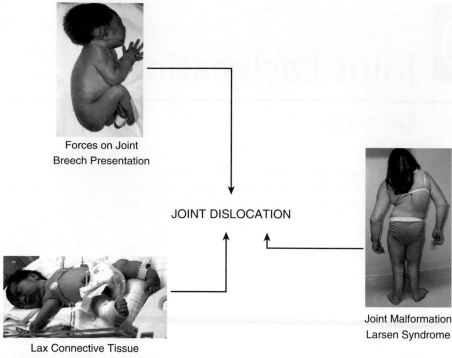

Forces on Joint
Breech Presentation

JOINT DISLOCATION

Joint Malformation
Larsen Syndrome

Lax Connective Tissue
Ehlers–Danlos Syndrome VIIA

FIGURE 10-2. Factors that interact in the genesis of joint dislocation, with examples relating to altered forces due to extrinsic deformation (e.g., breech deformation sequence), ligamentous laxity (e.g., Ehlers-Danlos syndrome, Type VIIA due to an autosomal dominant alteration in protease cleavage site from skipping of Exon 6 in COL1A1), and joint malformation (e.g., Larsen syndrome due to an autosomal dominant mutation in FLNB). In the latter two examples, the presence of multiple joint dislocations suggests a genetic disorder involving connective tissue or skeletal development.

a thin, atrophic papyraceous appearance, occurring mostly over pressure points.[2] In addition to the Ehlers-Danlos syndromes and Larsen syndrome, numerous other syndromes result in multiple joint dislocations, such as pseudodiastrophic dysplasia (autosomal recessive), Desbuquois dysplasia (autosomal recessive), and various types of arthrogryposis.

## References

1. Krakow D, Robertson SP, King LM, et al: Mutations in the gene encoding filamen B disrupt vertebral segmentation, joint formation and skeletogenesis, *Nat Genet* 36:405–410, 2004.
2. Beighton P, De Paepe A, Steinmann B, et al: Ehlers-Danlos syndromes: revised nosology, Vellefranche, 1997, Ehlers-Danlos National Foundation (USA) and Ehlers-Danlos Support Group (UK), *Am J Med Genet* 77:31–37, 1998.

# 11 Developmental Dysplasia of the Hip (Congenital Dislocation of the Hip)

## GENESIS

The definition of developmental dysplasia of the hip (DDH), formerly termed "congenital dislocation of the hip" (CDH), remains complex and controversial, making precise determination of incidence figures difficult. Fig. 10-2 depicts some of the interacting factors that relate to the genesis of DDH. When hip dislocation develops as a consequence of genetic connective tissue dysplasia, it may not become evident until after birth. Under such circumstances, use of the term *congenital hip dislocation* is inappropriate. Laxity of connective tissue is an important factor, and the 4:1 to 5:1 female-to-male predilection toward the occurrence of DDH is considered a consequence of the female fetus being more lax than the male. This might be due to a lack of testosterone effect in the female fetus.[1] Testosterone in the male fetus may result in tighter muscles and tougher connective tissue, as has been demonstrated in the hip capsule of young rodents.[2] Pelvic ligaments are also more relaxed in infant girls, possibly due to differential receptor responses to relaxing hormones in late gestation. Dunn[3] has shown the excess of dislocation of the hip in the female to be as high as 13:1 when it is an isolated deformation; however, when there is breech presentation and/or the presence of multiple deformations, the sex ratio is closer to equal. Carter and Wilkinson[4] noted laxity of three or more joints in 7% of individuals in the general population compared with an incidence of 22% among first-degree relatives with sporadic cases of dislocation of the hip. This suggests a possible heritable tendency toward increased joint laxity in association with congenital hip dislocation. When there were multiple cases of dislocation of the hip in a family, 65% of first-degree relatives had undue joint laxity.[4]

The same forces that tend to thrust the head of the femur out of the acetabulum also cause stretching of the joint capsule and ligamentum teres (Fig. 11-1). These forces are most commonly the result of constraint in late fetal life and thus are more likely to affect the first-born offspring. Certain presentations during late gestation are particularly likely to cause dislocation of the hip, and breech presentation is notorious in this respect. About 50% of patients with hip dislocation had been in breech presentation at birth.[3] Among breech term births (about 3.5% of all births), the frequency of dislocation of the hip is 17%, and for breech births with extended legs in utero (frank breech), the incidence is 25%.[3] When 224 term breech singleton infants were compared with 3107 term vertex singleton infants, congenital dislocation of the hip occurred 15 times more frequently among the infants in breech presentation (0.9%) compared with infants in vertex presentation (0.06%).[5] Breech presentation, with the fetal buttocks located in the maternal pelvis and the hips tightly flexed against the abdomen, tends to displace the femoral heads out of the acetabulum, especially when the legs are extended and "caught" between the fetal abdomen and the maternal uterine wall.

The fact that the fetus more commonly lies with the left side toward the mother's spine may explain why the left hip is more commonly dislocated than the right.[3] Left-sided hip dislocation is noted four times more frequently than right-sided hip dislocation. Constraint of the fetus due to oligohydramnios deformation sequence is associated with an increased frequency of hip dislocation, partly due to the increased frequency of breech presentation with oligohydramnios. Dunn noted that hip dysplasia is more common when other postural deformations are present, particularly congenital muscular torticollis, talipes equinovarus, metatarsus adductus, and hyperextension or dislocation of the knee (usually all resulting from the same deforming posture in late gestation).[3]

The position of the infant after birth is also important in the genesis of DDH. The hip joint may be lax at birth and usually becomes tighter

69

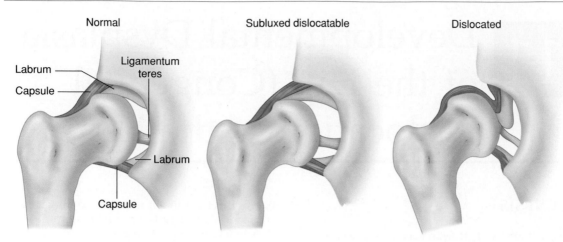

FIGURE 11-1. The normal hip, the moderately stretched capsule and ligaments of the dislocatable hip, and the overstretched capsule and ligaments of the dislocated hip. (From Clarren S, Smith DW: Congenital deformities, *Pediatr Clin North Am* 24:665–677, 1977.)

after birth, hence hips rarely become dislocated postnatally unless some type of developmental dysplasia of the hip is present. Undue leg extension in early infancy, at a time when the femoral head is not yet perfectly round, can be a factor in the postnatal genesis of DDH.[4] Thus, the hip that has been flexed, with a relatively contracted psoas muscle in utero, is more likely to be thrust out of its socket by forced extension of the leg. The increased frequency of DDH in both American Indians and Lapps has been at least partially attributed to their practice of swaddling young infants with their legs extended. On the other hand, the relatively low incidence of hip dislocation among the Hong Kong Chinese population has been attributed to the custom of carrying the infant on the mother's lower back, with the infant's hips flexed and partially abducted (which mechanically favors maintenance of the femoral head in the acetabulum).[6] In dogs, canine hip dysplasia is the most common developmental defect, and the risk in very large-sized breeds is 20 to 50 times greater, respectively, than that in small and medium breeds, with no apparent difference evident between sexes.[7]

Therefore, certain risk factors warrant close surveillance for congenital hip dislocation: family history of DDH, breech presentation, first-born children, female sex, accompanying postural deformations (particularly congenital muscular torticollis, which also manifests a left-sided predominance), and certain postnatal positioning practices (papoose or swaddling with the hips fully extended).[3-6] All gradations of dislocation, from a partially stretched, dislocatable hip to a fully dislocated hip, occur with an overall frequency of about 1%.[3] Considering the full spectrum, Barlow[8] observed that 60% of these dislocatable hips are stable in the normal location by 1 week of age, and 88% are stable by 2 months of age. The remaining 12% represents frank dislocation of the hip that was evident at birth or during early infancy, suggesting a frequency of 1.2 per 1000.

Additional controversy regarding the incidence of DDH results from differences in criteria for defining a genuinely pathologic neonatal hip. Prior to the introduction of routine clinical screening programs for neonatal detection of DDH (c. 1920–1950), diagnostic criteria were so varied that incidence figures ranged from 0 to 200 per 1000 children.[9] After routine clinical neonatal screening was introduced (c. 1950–1980), data on the incidence of DDH were based mainly on clinical findings that denoted neonatal hip instability, leading to some overdiagnosis and overtreatment, with an incidence of 0.41 to 168.6 per 1000.[9] After ultrasonography began to be used in neonatal screening for DDH, higher sensitivity resulted in higher incidence figures (71.5 to 518.5 per 1000), but sonographic diagnoses did not always correlate with clinical diagnoses.[9] In an effort to correlate this data with Barlow's clinical findings (which suggested that 88% of unstable hips eventually become normal without treatment), Bialik et al[9] tried to correlate neonatal ultrasound screening with clinical findings and treatment to determine the true incidence of DDH. They screened 9030 neonates at 1 to 3 days of life; any infants found to have sonographic abnormalities were reexamined at 2 to 6 weeks, depending on the severity of their findings. Only hips that had not improved or had deteriorated were treated; all others were examined periodically until age 12 months. Sonographically abnormal hips had an incidence of 55.1 per 1000 hips, while the true incidence of DDH requiring treatment was 5 per 1000 hips, with all others evolving into normal hips and no new instances of DDH at 12 months.[9]

## FEATURES

The usual direction for hip dislocation is posterior. The major problem with DDH is that it is seldom readily evident on gross inspection of the newborn and may not become apparent until early postnatal life. Thus, the diagnosis of congenital hip dislocation involves a directed physical examination (Figs. 11-2 to 11-4), searching for signs of the whole dislocation spectrum, from the lax dislocatable hip, to the dislocated hip that can still be relocated into the acetabulum, to the dislocated hip that cannot be relocated. The following hip examinations are warranted for all infants. In newborns, positive Ortolani and Barlow tests (see Figs. 11-3 and 11-4) continue to be effective clinical screening tests for unstable hips. From these tests, the examiner should be able to determine whether the hip is actually dislocated or subluxable.

It is of utmost importance that the infant is relaxed during the hip examination, and use of a

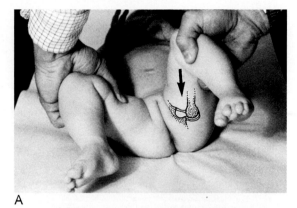

A

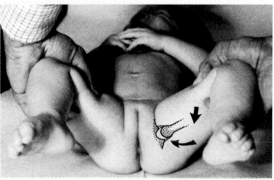

B

FIGURE 11-3. Technique for the Ortolani maneuver, which assists in the detection of the dislocated hip that can be repositioned into the acetabulum. **A,** Downward pressure further dislocates the hip; **B,** inward rotation of the hip will force the femoral head over the acetabular rim, leading to a noticeable "clunk."

(Courtesy of Lynn Staheli, Dept. of Pediatric Orthopedics, Children's Orthopedic Hospital, Seattle, Wash.)

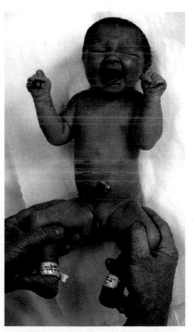

FIGURE 11-2. The usual position of an infant for neonatal hip examination.

pacifier or bottle may be of value in this regard. For the Ortolani test, the infant is placed in the supine position with the hips and knees flexed to 90 degrees and mildly abducted. The examiner, who is facing the baby's buttocks, grasps each thigh. The thumb of each hand is placed on the medial part of the upper thigh, and the index and third fingers are placed over the lateral aspect of the upper thigh at the level of the greater trochanter. The first maneuver is to lift up and out quite gently on the thigh and, at the same time, push the upper thigh toward the groin with the third finger. If the hip is dislocated posteriorly (the usual direction for dislocation) and can be relocated into the acetabulum, the examiner will feel a noticeable "clunk" as the femoral head slips over the acetabular shelf and into the acetabular socket. This is considered a positive Ortolani sign (see Fig. 11-3). If the result of this test is negative, then a Barlow test is performed by pulling out gently on the thigh while at the same time pushing the

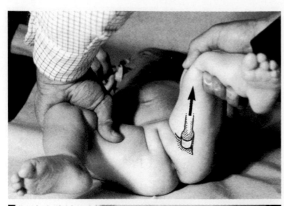

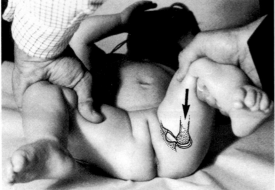

FIGURE 11-4. Technique for the Barlow maneuver, which assists in detecting the unstable dislocatable hip that is in the acetabulum. The leg is forcibly pulled up during the maneuver. Passage over the rim usually yields a noticeable "clunk."

(Courtesy of Lynn Staheli, Dept. of Pediatric Orthopedics, Children's Orthopedic Hospital, Seattle, Wash.)

upper thigh away from the groin with the thumb. Barlow's test (see Fig. 11-4) is a provocative test to determine whether the hip is dislocatable, implying a shallow socket with hip instability. If Barlow's test results in a noticeable (palpable) "clunk" as the femoral head is forced over the acetabular rim into a posteriorly dislocated position, the hip may be referred to as *dislocatable* or *unstable*. Minor clicks may be noted in about one third of examinations and do not appear to be of any consequence. Rather, it is the palpable "clunk" or "thunk" that is relevant. If either test is positive, referral to a pediatric orthopedist is indicated within the first 2 weeks of life; if equivocal, clinical reevaluation is indicated in 2 weeks. If suspicion still exists after 4 weeks, then hip ultrasonography and referral to an orthopedist are indicated. Ultrasound is the appropriate imaging modality for infants from birth to 4 to 6 months of age; radiography is used after the femoral heads begin to ossify.

It is important to understand that neither maneuver will be positive in an older infant whose hip is dislocated and cannot be manually relocated; thus, the Barlow and Ortolani maneuvers are reserved for infants younger than 3 or 4 months. In older infants with DDH, the hip will usually show a limitation in abduction, the greater trochanter may be felt to be posteriorly and superiorly displaced, and the upper leg may appear relatively short (Fig. 11-5, *A*). When the dislocation is unilateral or asymmetric in degree, then the relative length of the legs may be asymmetric,

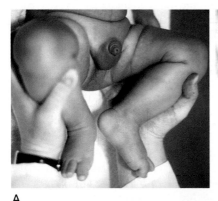

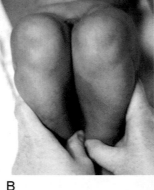

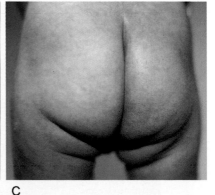

A                          B                          C

FIGURE 11-5. Developmental dysplasia of the hip in an older infant with rigid spine myopathy. Aberrantly increased muscular forces resulted in postnatal hip dislocation, evident as tight hips with limited abduction (**A**), upper leg length discrepancy with uneven knee height (**B**), and asymmetric thigh creases (**C**).

although the lower legs and feet will be the same length. Thus, when the infant is placed in supine position with the hips and knees flexed and the feet flat on the examination table, if one knee is noticeably lower than the other knee (Galeazzi's sign), DDH is suggested (Fig. 11-5. *B*). An obvious discrepancy may also be observed in the creases of the thigh folds between the two sides (Fig. 11-5, *C*).

The Ortolani and Barlow maneuvers are only indicated during the first 4 months of life. After this time, the soft tissues around the hip joint tighten and the dislocated hip cannot be replaced within the hip socket. As a result, the adductor muscles appear relatively tight on the involved side, resulting in limited abduction. It is paramount to understand that not all dislocation of the hip can be detected in the newborn nursery, and continued surveillance throughout the first 12 months is merited. To check for DDH in infants older than 4 months, flex both hips and both knees to 90 degrees with the infant lying supine on the exam table, bringing each knee toward the chest and checking for limited abduction by moving each leg sideways back toward the exam table. Older children with DDH or neuromuscular disease may have a positive Trendelenburg sign, which is tested by having the child stand on one foot and then the other. Normally, the hip opposite the weight-bearing leg elevates because the hip on the weight-bearing side abducts. With a positive Trendelenburg sign, the opposite hip drops because the weight-bearing hip does not abduct. This also affects the gait, resulting in a Trendelenburg gait (also called an *abductor lurch*) due to weakness of the abductor muscles. The child with this gait leans the upper trunk over the affected side to maintain his or her center of gravity while walking.

Radiography is of little value in the newborn because of incomplete ossification of the acetabulum and lack of ossification in the femoral head, but it becomes more valuable after 6 months of age. To detect evidence of dislocation when such a problem is clinically suspected, a plain anteroposterior radiograph of the pelvis in the frogleg position is useful. Ultrasonography should be used prior to this time and in the immediate neonatal period, particularly when the other risk factors mentioned previously are present. A number of associated aberrations in morphogenesis may occur secondary to dislocation of the hip (Fig. 11-6), depending on the age of development and the duration and extent of the dislocation. These aberrations include deformation of the femoral head; imperfect articular cartilage; adher-

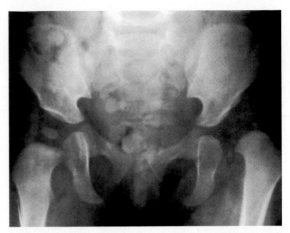

FIGURE 11-6. Secondary changes in acetabulum and neck of femur, as well as the unseen hourglass elongation of the hip capsule, elongated ligamentum teres, and foreshortened muscle attachments relating to long-term dislocation of the hip.
(Courtesy of Lynn Staheli, Dept. of Pediatric Orthopedics, Children's Orthopedic Hospital, Seattle, Wash.)

ence between the articular surface of the femoral head and the capsular tissues; short psoas, adductor, and hamstring muscles; anteversion of the hip; development of a false acetabulum; and elongation of the ligamentum teres with a stretched joint capsule. When such changes are profound, it may be difficult or even impossible to accomplish a closed reduction of the femoral head into its original acetabulum.

## MANAGEMENT, PROGNOSIS, AND COUNSEL

If either Ortolani's sign or Barlow's test is positive during the first few months of life, referral to an orthopedist is indicated. Likewise, limited abduction, leg length discrepancy, or asymmetry of skin folds on the leg in addition to ultrasound or radiographs revealing abnormal findings in the hip should also prompt a referral. Early, simple, conservative management of DDH will usually result in a normal hip by the age of walking. If DDH is discovered after 1 year of age, the condition usually requires prolonged, complicated management and may result in varying degrees of lifelong disability (Fig. 11-7). Hence, early diagnosis, as emphasized previously, is key to successful management.

The most common hip diagnosis at birth is the dislocatable or unstable hip. In a study of 1,059,479 newborns born between 1970 and 1988 in Norway, the overall prevalence of clinically

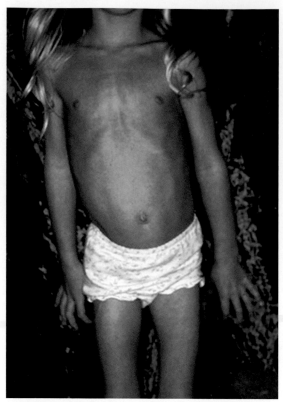

FIGURE 11-7. This girl was born with hip dislocation in breech presentation from a maternal bicornuate uterus. Late diagnosis and treatment resulted in an uneven pelvis and altered gait.

detected neonatal hip instability at birth was 0.9% (0.6% in males and 1.4% in females).[10] With breech presentation, the rate was 4.4% compared with 0.9% with vertex presentation; the incidence was also higher in first-borns. In female infants, the rate of neonatal hip instability increased with the duration of pregnancy, particularly with breech presentation, but this was not seen in males.[10] Family history was important, with the risk of DDH in males increasing from 4.1 per 100 to 9.4 per 1000 with a positive family history. Risks were even greater in females, increasing from 19 per 1000 to 44 per 1000 with a positive family history. These data support the hypothesis that mechanical factors in combination with familial and hormonal factors (primarily relaxing female hormones) play an important role in causing neonatal hip instability.

Despite the introduction of clinical screening for early detection of DDH in Norway and many other Western countries, the incidence of late DDH appeared to increase, so in 1987 one hospital compared ultrasound and clinical examination prospectively and noted a low incidence of late DDH during the 9-month study period (0.9 per 1000 vs 3.5 per 1000 with clinical screening from 1982 to 1985).[11] This same group subsequently showed that the major impact of general ultrasound screening (a combination of clinical screening plus ultrasound screening of all infants) versus clinical screening alone was a higher treatment rate of early DDH using a Frejka pillow splint (3.4% vs 1.8%) and a lower rate of late DDH, usually requiring hospitalization and surgery (0.3 per 1000 vs 1.3 per 1000).[12] Selective screening (clinical screening plus ultrasound screening of all female infants and those male infants with known risk factors for DDH) resulted in intermediate figures.[12] When overall costs for these programs were compared, they were similar for all three groups, but the costs of late treatment accounted for only 22% of the general screening group versus 65% in the other two groups.[13] These studies demonstrate the effectiveness of a national program of screening linked to treatment, but concerns have been raised about the efficacy of clinical screening alone in lowering the rate of late detection of DDH in the United Kingdom.[14-16] Using current diagnostic techniques, the late presentation of DDH can be minimized but not eliminated, and approximately 15% of DDH cases at birth are not detectable, even by experienced examiners or ultrasonographers.[17]

If the hips are unstable even though the femoral head is in a normal position at birth, it is considered best to provide prophylactic splinting of the dislocatable hip to prevent the very real possibility of insidious hip dislocation during early infancy. Such splinting is continued until the hip is held firmly in place by its own connective tissues, which may have become stretched prior to birth. The aim of splinting is to maintain the femoral head in the acetabulum with reliable but not excessive constraint. The recommended position is with the hips flexed about 90 degrees and abducted about 25 to 30 degrees. The full frogleg position has been discouraged because the constant and possibly excessive forcing of the femoral head into the acetabulum may occasionally result in avascular necrosis in the head of the immobilized femur. Various types of splints have been used (Fig. 11-8), but the Pavlik splint is generally preferred. For the dislocatable hip, a period of 4 to 6 weeks of splinting is usually adequate to yield a "tight" hip.

The dislocated hip that can be relocated into the acetabulum should be splinted, with assurance that the femoral head remains in the acetabulum. For this type of dislocated hip, the Pavlik splint

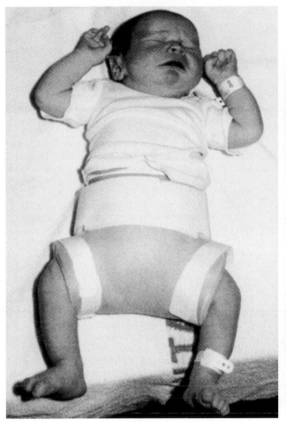
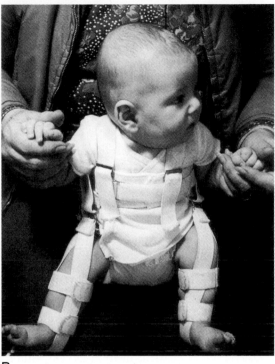

A                                                      B

FIGURE 11-8. **A,** Plastizote splint used for the dislocatable hip in early infancy. **B,** Pavlik splint used for maintaining the repositioned dislocated hip in early infancy.

(see Fig. 11-8, *B*) may be preferable. Ultrasound has been found to be valuable for assessment and monitoring of treatment in the Pavlik harness, which resulted in a reduction success rate of >95% in a study of 370 ultrasonographically abnormal hips in 221 infants detected through ultrasound screening (treatment rate, 5.1 per 1000 live births), with a low (0.4%) rate of avascular necrosis and a low rate of late presentation (0.26 per 1000 live births).[18] The duration of splinting varies with the severity of the problem and the age at diagnosis. When detected at birth to 1 month of age, the mean duration of splinting is 3.6 months, but detection at 1 to 3 months requires 7 months of splinting. If the dislocation was not detected until 3 to 6 months, the mean duration of splinting is 9.3 months.[9] Use of ultrasound to monitor treatment in the Pavlik harness makes it possible to distinguish between recalcitrant and gradually improving subluxation, and it also appears to lower the rate of avascular necrosis as well as the rate of late or persistent dysplasia.[18]

If it is not possible to manually reduce the dislocation, leg traction may be used in an effort to lengthen the contracted muscles and (ideally) allow for a closed reduction. If this is not possible, then surgical correction is merited. Surgery may include lengthening or detachment of contracted muscles and reconstruction of the distorted joint capsule. Surgery is often postponed until the infant is about 1 year old because of the risk of ischemic necrosis following hip surgery at an earlier age. Uncorrected dislocation of the hip will adversely affect walking (see Fig. 11-7), resulting in the development of a limp and osteoarthritis during late adulthood. Although a dislocated hip will usually not become painful until after age 40, a subluxated hip (acetabular dysplasia) becomes painful in late adolescence. In children with untreated DDH who are older than 3 years, it is unclear whether preoperative traction lowers the rate of avascular necrosis, and some surgeons believe that femoral shortening is preferable to traction for the late reduction of DDH.[19] Magnetic resonance imaging can be useful to evaluate the position of the femoral head after operative reduction because this positioning is critical to the success of the procedure and to the prevention of avascular necrosis.[20]

The recurrence risk of the more common type of dislocation of the hip is in the range of 3% to 6% and is higher when a male is affected.[4] If both the parent and child are affected, the recurrence risk may be as high as 30%.

## DIFFERENTIAL DIAGNOSIS

Certain malformations that enhance the likelihood of breech positioning, such as spina bifida, and genitourinary malformations leading to oligohydramnios (and thereby resulting in both constraint and breech positioning) are associated with an increased frequency of dislocation of the hip secondary to these more primary malformation problems. A number of neurologic disorders may lead to dislocation of the hip, presumably on the basis of diminished muscle strength while holding the femoral head in the acetabulum and/or muscular imbalance. Thus dislocation of the hip may be secondary to meningomyelocele and may occur in certain types of cerebral palsy or neuromuscular diseases, especially when there is flexion and/or adduction spasm at the hip. In some forms of arthrogryposis (multiple joint contractures), especially amyoplasia congenita, the hip may be dislocated. Additionally, dislocation of the hip occurs as a frequent or occasional defect in a number of syndromes. One of the most striking examples is Larsen syndrome, in which there tend to be multiple joint dislocations, an unusually low nasal bridge, and spatulate thumbs. Treatment of these dislocations is not the same as for DDH in an otherwise normal child because this type of joint dislocation is due to malformation of the joints themselves (see Fig. 10-2).

One other entity that warrants mention is voluntary habitual hip dislocation in a child.[21,22] This rare condition is six times more frequent in females than in males and is not associated with underlying joint laxity or a history of trauma. It consists of voluntary recurrent popping of one hip (more commonly the right hip) with no associated pain, with visualization of a radiographic or sonographic vacuum phenomenon within the hip capsule. Surgery is not needed, and behavioral management halts the behavior with no long-term sequellae.[21,22]

## References

1. Fernando J, Arena P, Smith DW: Sex liability to single structural defects, *Am J Dis Child* 132:970–972, 1978.
2. Hama H, Yamamuro T, Titkeda T: Experimental studies on connective tissue of the capsular ligament, *Acta Orthop Scand* 47:473–479, 1976.
3. Dunn PM: Perinatal observations on the etiology of congenital dislocation of the hip, *Clin Orthop* 119:11–22, 1976.
4. Carter CO, Wilkinson JA: Genetic and environmental factors in the etiology of congenital dislocation of the hip, *Clin Orthop Rel Res* 33:119–128, 1964.
5. Hsieh Y-Y, Tsai F-J, Lin C-C, et al: Breech deformation complex in neonates, *J Reprod Med* 45:933–935, 2000.
6. Chan A, McCaul KA, Cundy PJ, et al: Perinatal risk factors for developmental dysplasia of the hip, *Arch Dis Child Fetal Neonatal Ed* 76:94F–100F, 1997.
7. Priester WA, Mulvihill JJ: Canine hip dysplasia: relative risk by sex, size, and breed, and comparative aspects, *J Am Vet Assoc* 160:735–739, 1972.
8. Barlow TG: Early diagnosis and treatment of congenital dislocation of the hip, *J Bone Joint Surg* 44B:292–301, 1962.
9. Bialik V, Bialik G, Blazer S, et al: Developmental dysplasia of the hip: a new approach to incidence, *Pediatrics* 103:93–99, 1999.
10. Hinderaker T, Daltveit AK, Irgens LM, et al: The impact of intra-uterine factors on neonatal hip instability: an analysis of 1,059,479 children in Norway, *Acta Orthop Scand* 65:239–242, 1994.
11. Rosendahl K, Markestad T, Lie RT: Congenital dislocation of the hip: a prospective study comparing ultrasound and clinical examination, *Acta Paediatr* 81:177–181, 1992.
12. Rosendahl K, Markestad T, Lie RT: Ultrasound screening for congenital dislocation of the hip in the neonate: the effect on treatment rate and incidence of late cases, *Pediatrics* 94:47–52, 1994.
13. Rosendahl K, Markestad T, Lie RT, et al: Cost-effectiveness of alternative screening strategies for developmental dysplasia of the hip, *Arch Pediatr Adolesc Med* 149:643–648, 1995.
14. Godward S, Dezateux C: Surgery for congenital dislocation of the hip in the UK as a measure of outcome of screening, *Lancet* 351:1149–1152, 1998.
15. Dunn P: Screening for congenital dislocation of the hip, *Lancet* 352:317, 1998.
16. Jones D: Neonatal detection of developmental dysplasia of the hip (DDH), *J Bone Joint Surg Br* 80B:943–945, 1998.
17. Cady RB: Developmental dysplasia of the hip: definition, recognition, and prevention of late sequelae, *Pediatr Ann* 35:92–101, 2006.
18. Taylor GR, Clarke NMP: Monitoring the treatment of developmental dysplasia of the hip with the Pavlik harness: the role of ultrasound, *J Bone Joint Surg Br* 79B:719–723, 1997.
19. Ryan MG, Johnson LO, Quanbeck DS, et al: One-stage treatment of congenital dislocation of the hip in children three to ten years old: functional and radiographic results, *J Bone Joint Surg Am* 80A:336–344, 1998.
20. McNally EG, Tasker A, Benson MK: MRI after operative reduction for developmental dysplasia of the hip, *J Bone Joint Surg Br* 79B:724–726, 1997.
21. Walker J, Rang M: Habitual hip dislocation in a child, *Clin Pediatr* 31:562–563, 1992.
22. Chan YL, Cheng JCY, Tang APY: Voluntary habitual dislocation of the hip: sonographic diagnosis, *Pediatr Radiol* 23:147–148, 1993.

# 12 Knee Dislocation (Genu Recurvatum)

## GENESIS

Hyperextension of the leg with dislocation at the knee may result from the legs being in an extended posture with breech presentation, oligohydramnios, or other unusual late gestational constraint due to uterine myomas or structural defects. It can also occur in various genetic connective tissue disorders, such as Ehlers-Danlos syndrome, atelosteogenesis types 1 and 3, Larsen syndrome, or (occasionally) arthrogryposis. Dislocation of the hips is frequently associated with congenital knee dislocation and is much more common in females, especially when there is no associated syndrome.[1] This condition is relatively rare, occurring in roughly 1 in 10,000 live births. It is frequently associated with other musculoskeletal problems, especially dislocation of the hip and clubfoot.[2]

## FEATURES

Curvature of the knee is "backward" with an unstable and sometimes dislocated knee. Subclas-

sification (Fig. 12-1) depends on the radiographic relationship between the tibia and the femur: (1) simple hyperextension (or severe genu recurvatum); (2) anterior subluxation; or (3) anterior dislocation. If the tibia is displaced anterior to the long axis of the femur, the knee is considered *dislocated*, but if longitudinal contact is at least partially maintained, it is *subluxed*. Simple hyperextension exists when there is no displacement of the joint surfaces.[2] The quadriceps muscle tends to be short, and the distal quadriceps may be relatively fibrotic; these findings have been noted as early as 19.5 weeks of gestation in a fetus with bilateral, congenitally dislocated knees. When compared with age-matched controls, there was also absence of a suprapatellar pouch and incomplete patellofemoral joint cavitation.[3] Neither altered muscle/joint pathology nor intrauterine factors explain all cases, and this condition appears to be multifactorial. The patella, a sesamoid bone that normally forms in the quadriceps tendon in response to stress, may be small or absent, possibly because of the lack of tension on the quadriceps tendon.

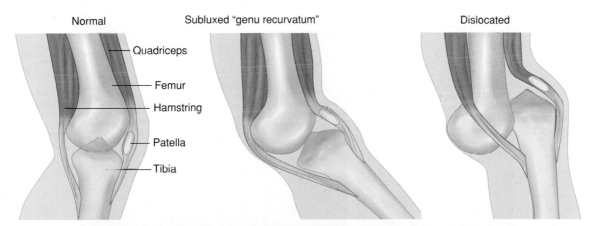

FIGURE 12-1. Normal knee with tissues stretched to the point of being subluxed, also termed *genu recurvatum* (most commonly occurring in prolonged frank breech presentation), and with a dislocated knee. The patella develops as a sesamoid bone in the tendon of the quadriceps muscle. With less tension, the sesamoid bone may be small to absent. (From Clarren SK, Smith DW: Congenital deformities, *Pediatr Clin North Am* 24:665–677, 1977.)

## MANAGEMENT, PROGNOSIS, AND COUNSEL

Treatment depends on the severity of the knee dislocation and the age when treatment begins, with most authors recommending early conservative treatment. Early traction, manipulation, splinting, and/or serial casting in a corrected position to increase knee flexion may suffice to bring about a correction by age 8 weeks in about 50% of cases, but prompt early treatment is often critical to the success of these measures. For patients with no associated syndromes who are seen within the first 2 days after birth (when high levels of maternal relaxing hormones are still circulating in the neonate and softening the connective tissues),

reduction may sometimes be achieved with gentle traction to align the tibia and femur, followed by serial splinting or casting every 2 weeks for 6 to 8 weeks. After the first 2 days, passive stretching of the quadriceps and anterior knee capsule, combined with serial splinting and casting, may still be successful.[2] If these initial measures are not successful, then traction in the prone position for 1 to 2 weeks may permit closed reduction with or without anesthesia; however, recalcitrant cases usually require quadriceps lengthening with surgical correction of the stretched knee joint capsule and its attachments, with the goal of achieving 90 degrees of flexion intraoperatively.[2]

Among 19 neonates with congenital dislocation of the knee, in 6 cases (all females with no asso-

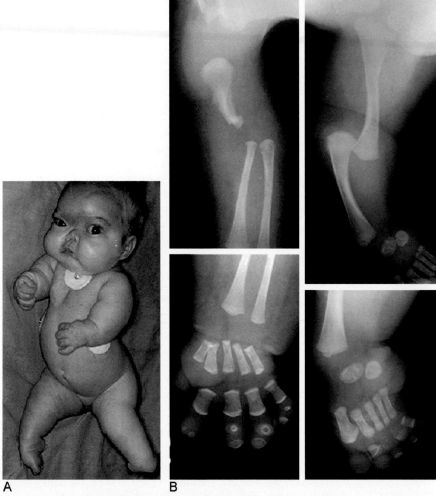

A                    B

FIGURE 12-2. **A,** Dislocated knees and elbows in an infant with atelosteogenesis type 3 and a mutation in the gene *FLNB*. **B,** Radiographs demonstrating dislocations with tapered distal humeri and characteristic hand and foot changes.

ciated anomalies) spontaneous reduction was achieved with application of a simple posterior splint with a fixed degree of knee flexion for a short duration. In four of these patients, there were either associated deformations (hip dislocation, foot deformation, or elbow contracture) or fetal constraint due to oligohydramnios, uterine myomas,

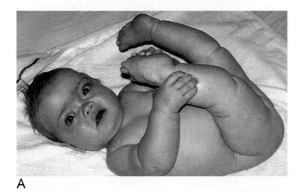

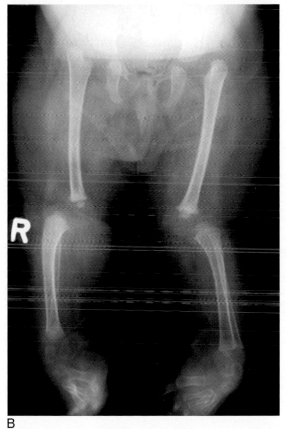

A

B

FIGURE 12-3. **A–B,** Multiple dislocations in a patient with Larsen syndrome. Multiple joint dislocations in a patient with Larsen syndrome and a mutation in *FLNB*.

or coiling of the umbilical cord around the affected limb.[1] Cases associated with clubfoot, arthrogryposis, or Larsen syndrome were resistant to such conservative treatment and sometimes required surgery for persistent knee instability. Among 17 patients seen and treated conservatively over a 7-year period, in 5 cases there was immediate reduction within 20 hours of birth; 7 patients seen within 2 days of birth responded to passive stretching of the quadriceps and anterior knee capsule, followed by splinting and/or casting; and 5 patients required traction for as long as 26 days, with or without anesthesia, to achieve reduction.[2] The pathoanatomies of congenital knee and hip dislocation are very similar, with soft tissue contractures becoming more severe if the dislocation is not reduced early; therefore, the subluxed or dislocated knee should be treated as early as possible.

Cases with signs of late gestational constraint that reduce spontaneously or with minimal treatment may represent a type of congenital postural deformity produced by abnormal intrauterine posture in late gestation.[1] Because congenital hip

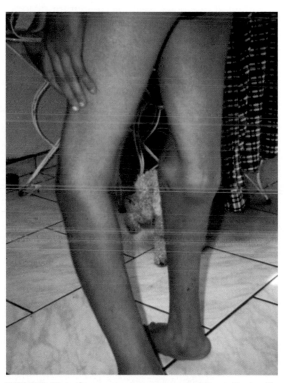

FIGURE 12-4. Genu recurvatum in an older patient with Larsen syndrome.

dislocation is frequently associated with congenital knee dislocation in more than 50% of cases, it is important to evaluate the hips sonographically, because the dislocated knee needs to be reduced before the hip dislocation is treated. Concurrent treatment of both the knee and hip dislocations with a Pavlik harness has also been successful.[2] Long leg casting has been used to treat concurrent knee and foot deformation after the knee has been reduced. When progressive genu valgus deformity occurs with global instability of the knee due to an underlying genetic connective tissue disorder, reconstruction of the medial knee structures with prolonged bracing can provide good results.[2] Recurrence risk is related to whether there is an underlying genetic connective tissue disorder; most cases occur sporadically and with no prior family history.[4] Because cervical spine instability and/or kyphosis in Larsen syndrome can result in quadriplegia with traction during vaginal delivery, it is recommended that fetuses who are diagnosed prenatally with congenital knee dislocation be delivered by cesarean section.

# DIFFERENTIAL DIAGNOSIS

Differential diagnosis is similar to that for dislocation of the hip, but knee dislocation is less likely to occur with neurologic disorders and is especially common in certain genetic connective tissue disorders. The differential diagnosis includes atelosteogenesis (Fig. 12-2), Larsen syndrome (Figs. 12-3 and 12-4), Ehlers-Danlos syndrome (Fig. 12-5), or arthrogryposis.[4]

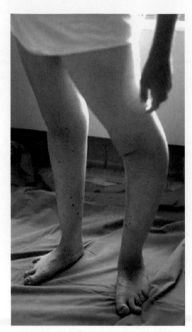

FIGURE 12-5. Genu recurvatum in a patient with Ehlers-Danlos syndrome.

## References

1. Haga N, Nakamura S, Sakaguchi R, et al: Congenital dislocation of the knee reduced spontaneously or with minimal treatment, *J Pediatr Orthop* 17:59–62, 1997.
2. Ko J-Y, Shih C-H, Wenger DR: Congenital dislocation of the knee, *J Pediatr Orthop* 19:252–259, 1999.
3. Uthoff HK, Ogata S: Early intrauterine presence of congenital dislocation of the knee, *J Pediatr Orthoped* 14:254–257, 1994.
4. Elchalal U, Itzhak IB, Ben-Meir G, et al: Antenatal diagnosis of congenital dislocation of the knee: a case report, *Am J Perinatol* 10:194–196, 1993.

# 13 Dislocation of the Radial Head

## GENESIS

Dislocation of the radial head is the most common congenital anomaly of the elbow, but it is relatively rare, accounting for 0.15% to 0.2% of outpatient orthopedic visits.[1-3] It can occur as an isolated abnormality or as part of a number of different syndromes. The presence of associated anomalies and bilateral involvement suggest a congenital joint dislocation syndrome. Some authors believe that many unilateral cases might be attributed to low-energy greenstick fractures, which may result in transient mild symptoms that are unnoticed by parents.[4] It is difficult to distinguish radiographically between congenital dislocation and late post-traumatic cases,[5] so the genesis of many isolated cases is seldom understood.

Radial head dislocation can be associated with radioulnar synostosis, antecubital pterygia, distal hand and limb anomalies, congenital hip dislocation, extra sex chromosomes, arthrogryposis, Larsen syndrome, Ehlers-Danlos syndrome, occipital horn syndrome (X-linked cutis laxa), multiple exostosis, nail-patella syndrome, cleidocranial dysplasia, surviving camptomelic dysplasia, atelosteogenesis, small patella syndrome, and craniofacial dysostosis.[1,3,6,7] Bilateral congenital posterior dislocation of the radial heads without other anomalies can also be inherited as an autosomal dominant trait.[8] Vertical transmission within one consanguineous family was interpreted as possibly being due to autosomal recessive inheritance,[9] but most isolated hereditary cases appear to manifest autosomal dominant inheritance. The dislocation of the proximal head of the radius toward the posterolateral results in the inability to fully supinate at the elbow and some limitation in extension (Fig. 13-1). It generally gives rise to little disability and is seldom treated.

## FEATURES

The direction of bowing of the ulna depends on the type of dislocation of the radial head, and if an abnormal position is initiated by one of the bones of the forearm, the other bone will bend accordingly as it grows (see Fig. 13-1). Therefore, in unreduced congenital anterior dislocation of the radial head, the ulna bends forward. In posterior dislocation, it bends backward, and in lateral dislocation, the ulna bends laterally.[5] Radiographic criteria suggesting congenital anterior dislocation include hypoplastic or absent capitellum, dome-shaped radial head with a long neck, and long radius in relation to ulna.[8] Additional findings that suggest a congenital etiology include bilateral involvement, presence of associated anomalies, familial occurrence, no history of trauma, and dislocation noted at birth.[2] Progression from subluxation to dislocation has been observed, and most patients have no pain and minimal functional limitations during childhood.

## MANAGEMENT, PROGNOSIS, AND COUNSEL

Some untreated patients experience pain, progressive limitation in movement, and prominence of the radial head during adulthood (see Fig. 13-1, B and C), in which case radial head excision can alleviate pain and improve appearance but seldom increases movement.[2] Many syndromic cases and those with isolated bilateral involvement are inherited in an autosomal dominant fashion. When radial head dislocation occurs in association with congenital hip dislocation, marked joint hypermobility, and lax redundant skin in a male, the diagnosis of X-linked cutis laxa (occipital horn syndrome) should be considered. When radial head dislocation occurs with patellar hypoplasia and decreased pubic ossification, surviving camptomelic dysplasia or small patella syndrome should be considered. When there are multiple joint dislocations at birth in addition to a flat midface, cleft palate, and broad thumbs with cylindrical fingers, Larsen syndrome should be considered (see Fig. 13-1).

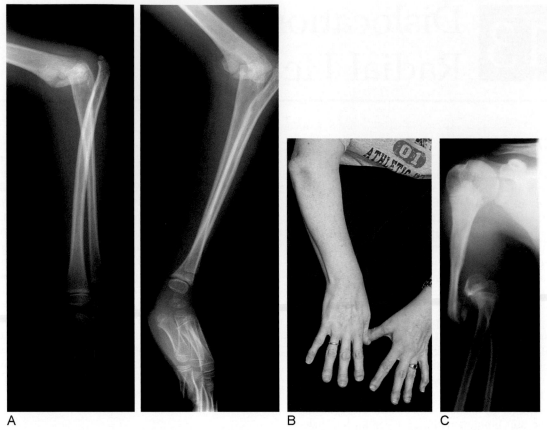

A                                    B                                    C

FIGURE 13-1. **A,** Dislocated radial heads in a child with Larsen syndrome. **B** and **C,** Dislocated radial heads in an adult with Larsen syndrome and a mutation in *FLNB*. Note the protrusion of the radial head with long cylindric fingers and broad thumbs.

## DIFFERENTIAL DIAGNOSIS

Radial head dislocation, which is associated with congenital synostosis of the upper end of the radius, should be considered part of radioulnar synostosis and not a true dislocation. Congenital radioulnar synostosis is due to defective longitudinal segmentation that results in persistent interzonal mesenchyme between the proximal radius and ulna, which later becomes ossified, resulting in marked limitation of pronation, supination, and extension. Some cases of Erb's palsy result in subluxation of the radial head as a result of muscle imbalance, and this is not true dislocation.[10]

### References

1. Almquist EE, Gordon LH, Blue AI: Congenital dislocation of the head of the radius, *J Bone Joint Surg Am* 51:1118–1127, 1969.
2. Mardam-Bey T, Ger E: Congenital radial head dislocation, *J Hand Surg* 4:316–320, 1979.
3. Agnew DK, Davis RJ: Congenital unilateral dislocation of the radial head, *J Pediatr Orthoped* 13:526–528, 1993.
4. Lloyd-Roberts GC, Bucknill TM: Anterior dislocation of the radial head in children, *J Bone Joint Surg Br* 59:402–407, 1977.
5. Caravias DE: Some observations on congenital dislocation of the head of the radius, *J Bone Joint Surg Br* 39:86–90, 1957.
6. Bongers EM, Van Bokhoven H, Van Thienen MN, et al: The small patella syndrome: description of five cases from three families and examination of possible allelism with familial patella aplasia–hypoplasia and nail-patella syndrome, *J Med Genet* 38:209–213, 2001.
7. Mansour S, Offiah AC, McDowall S, et al: The phenotype of survivors of camptomelic dysplasia, *J Med Genet* 39:597–602, 2002.
8. Reichenbach H, Hormann D, Theile H: Hereditary congenital posterior dislocation of radial heads, *Am J Med Genet* 55:101–104, 1995.
9. Gunn DR, Pillay VK: Congenital dislocation of the head of the radius, *Clin Orthop* 34:108–113, 1964.
10. McFarland B: Congenital dislocation of the head of the radius, *Br J Surg* 24:41–49, 1936.

# Neurapraxias (Palsies)

# 14 Facial Palsy

## GENESIS

Prolonged compression or stretching of a peripheral nerve may lead to compression palsy, apparently on the basis of neural ischemia. The frequency of congenital facial palsy is 0.71 to 1.4 per 1000.[1] The mechanism of injury is usually either direct trauma from forceps or compression of the side of the face and nerve against the sacral promontory, with the side of the injured facial nerve usually corresponding with the side of the fetal face that was lying against the maternal sacrum during delivery. The facial nerve exits the skull through the stylomastoid foramen behind the ear, where it is protected by the mastoid bone, and then travels to the parotid gland, where it divides and sends branches to all the muscles of the face. Direct forceps injury may occur behind the ear or over the parotid region, although both the maternal sacral promontory and fetal shoulder can also cause intrauterine nerve compression. Traumatic cases are usually unilateral and present with weakness of the frontalis, orbicularis oculi, buccinator, orbicularis oris, and platysma. There may be a history of prolonged or difficult labor or forceps delivery or evidence of periauricular ecchymoses or hemotympanum. Traumatic facial nerve palsy is associated with birth weight >3500 g, forceps-assisted deliveries, and prematurity.[2,3]

Congenital facial nerve paralysis is generally considered to be of either developmental or traumatic origin. When facial nerve paralysis is of developmental origin, it may be part of a broader pattern of altered morphogenesis, such as Möbius syndrome (Fig. 14-1), oculoauriculovertebral (OAV) sequence (hemifacial microsomia) (Fig. 14-2), or CHARGE syndrome (coloboma, heart disease, atresia choanae, retarded growth and development and/or central nervous system anomalies, genital hypoplasia, and ear anomalies and/or deafness) (Fig. 14-3).[4,5] In OAV sequence, there is unilateral microtia with conductive deafness and varying degrees of jaw hypoplasia, ocular dermoids, and cervical vertebral abnormalities.[4] In CHARGE syndrome, there is ocular colobomata, choanal

atresia, dysplastic ears with sensorineural deafness, hypoplasia of the cochlea and semicircular canals, heart defects, and hypogonadotropic hypogonadism.[5] Facial paralysis with associated distal limb deficiency has been seen after early chorion villus sampling, failed dilation and curettage, maternal use of either thalidomide or misoprostol after the first trimester, and maternal hyperthermia during the first trimester, suggesting it may be a manifestation of brainstem disturbances during the first trimester.[6–8] Congenital facial paralysis of traumatic etiology in otherwise normal children accounts for 8% to 25% of all facial nerve palsies occurring in the pediatric population, and it requires a systematic evaluation to exclude other associated anomalies, particularly those affecting vision and hearing.[9]

## FEATURES

Facial nerve palsy is usually unilateral, and decreased movement on the side of the palsy occurs

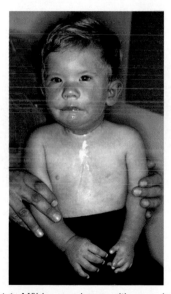

FIGURE 14-1. Möbius syndrome with associated absent left pectoralis muscle and hypoplastic left hand in a child whose mother had prolonged high fever toward the end of the first trimester.

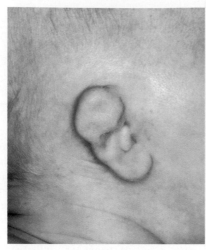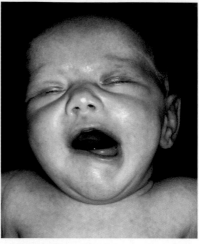

FIGURE 14-2. Right facial nerve palsies in a child with OAV sequence.

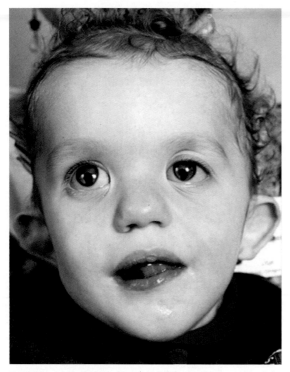

FIGURE 14-3. Child with CHARGE syndrome with right facial weakness, dysplastic ears, and bilateral iris colobomata.

with facial animation (Fig. 14-4). At rest, the affected side has decreased forehead wrinkling, increased eye opening (resulting in the inability to close the eye, with resultant corneal drying and irritation), a decreased nasolabial fold, and flattening of the corner of the mouth.

## MANAGEMENT AND PROGNOSIS

Immediate management of facial palsy is usually not necessary, although a careful clinical evaluation should be performed to search for other anomalies. Periauricular bruising or lacerations should heighten the suspicion of facial nerve trauma. Electrophysiologic testing (electroneuronography, or ENOG), whereby the facial nerve is stimulated transdermally near the stylomastoid foramen, can help provide objective assessment of facial nerve function.[9] The quantity of nerve deficit parallels the muscle deficit in developmental paralysis, whereas in traumatic cases, the nerve may be injured although the muscle is spared. Nontraumatic bilateral facial nerve weakness without ocular muscle weakness has been reported as an autosomal dominant trait with two defined loci, and facial weakness with impaired ocular abduction due to abducens weakness (Möbius syndrome) has been attributed to both teratogenic and genetic developmental abnormalities of rhombencephalic development.[10] When associated limb defects are present, a teratogenic etiology is more likely than a genetic defect. In developmental cases, temporal bone computed tomography and brainstem auditory evoked-response testing can evaluate the middle ear, inner ear, and semicircular canals for associated anatomic and functional problems, particularly in the case of CHARGE syndrome and OAV sequence. When facial nerve compression has occurred in late gestation or during delivery, there is usually a full return of function within a matter of days to weeks because the injury does

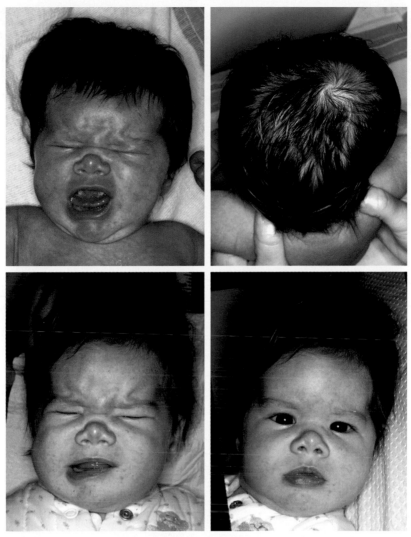

FIGURE 14-4. Child with right lower facial nerve palsy with right facial droop and associated traumatic right parietal cephalohematoma.

not usually disrupt the axon. Spontaneous recovery occurs within 4 weeks in 90% of traumatic congenital facial paralysis cases.[11] Adequate eye care to prevent exposure keratitis is important and consists of taping the eyelid shut and frequently applying artificial tears until the nerve recovers. With developmental facial palsy, the eyelid may need to be partially closed surgically. The surgical treatment of facial paralysis consists of staged techniques using autologous muscle or tendon transplantation to the paralyzed side of the face or reanimation procedures using regional muscle transfers and nerve crossovers.[9] These operations are generally not done until early school age, when the child can actively participate in and understand the necessary postoperative physical therapy exercises.

## References

1. Painter MJ, Bergman I: Obstetrical trauma to the neonatal central and peripheral nervous system, *Sem Perinatol* 6:89–104, 1982.
2. Falco NA, Ericksson E: Facial nerve palsy in the newborn: incidence and outcome, *Plast Reconstr Surg* 85:1–4, 1986.
3. Towner D, Castro MA, Eby-Wilkens E, et al: Effect of mode of delivery in nulliparous women on neonatal intracranial injury, *N Engl J Med* 341:1709–1714, 1999.
4. Carvalho GJ, Song CS, Vargervik K, et al: Auditory and facial nerve dysfunction in patients with hemifacial microsomia, *Arch Otolaryngol Head Neck Surg* 125:209–212, 1999.
5. Graham JM Jr: A recognizable syndrome within CHARGE association: Hall-Hittner syndrome [editorial comment], *Am J Med Genet* 99:120–123, 2001.
6. Pastuszak AL, Schuler L, Speck-Martins CE, et al: Use of misoprostol during pregnancy and Möbius syndrome in infants, *N Engl J Med* 338:1881–1885, 1998.

7. Grundfast KM, Guarisco JL, Thornsen JR, et al: Diverse etiologies of facial paralysis in children, *Int J Pediatr Otorhinolaryngol* 19:223–229, 1990.

8. Graham JM  Jr, Edwards MJ, Edwards MJ: Teratogen update: gestational effects of maternal hyperthermia due to febrile illnesses and resultant patterns of defects in humans, *Teratology* 58:209–221, 1998.

9. Shapiro NL, Cunningham MJ, Parikh SR, et al: Congenital unilateral facial paralysis, *Pediatrics* 97:261–264, 1996.

10. Verzijl H, van der Zwaam B, Cruysberg JRM, et al: Möbius syndrome redefined: a syndrome of rhombencephalic maldevelopment, *Neurology* 61:327–333, 2003.

11. Smith JD, Crumley RL, Lee AH: Facial paralysis in the newborn, *Otolaryngol Head Neck Surg* 89:1021–1024, 1981.

# 15 Brachial Plexus Palsy

## ERB'S PALSY, KLUMPKE'S PALSY, OBSTETRIC PALSY

## GENESIS

The frequency of brachial plexus palsy has been decreasing with improved obstetric management and is currently 0.37 to 1.89 per 1000 newborns.[1,2] Supraclavicular traction or stretching of the brachial plexus during delivery can injure nerve fibers; hence this injury is sometimes termed *obstetric palsy*. The fibers that originate from the fifth and sixth cervical segments are usually the most commonly and severely affected. Occasionally fibers from C7, C8, and T1 can also be affected. Lesions that affect the upper segments (C5–C7) result in Erb's palsy, whereas lesions that affect the lower spinal segments (C7–T1) result in Klumpke's palsy. There may be associated injuries suggesting a difficult delivery, such as fracture of the clavicle or humerus (9%–21% of cases), diaphragmatic paralysis (5%–9%), or facial palsy (5%–14%).[3,4] The position at delivery is related to the risk of brachial plexus injury, and infants delivered vaginally from an occipitoposterior position have a higher incidence of Erb's palsy and facial palsy than those delivered from the occipitoanterior position.[5]

Traction to the plexus, especially the upper plexus, occurs during delivery when the angle between the neck and shoulder is suddenly and forcibly increased, with the arms in an adducted position. This can occur during vertex deliveries when traction is placed on the head to deliver the after-coming shoulder, particularly when the shoulders are caught against the pelvic brim in shoulder dystocia, as forceful contractions push the head and trunk forward. Brachial plexus palsy can also occur during breech deliveries when the adducted arm is pulled forcefully downward to free the after-coming head (accounting for 24% of brachial plexus palsies) or during other malpresentations when the head is rotated to achieve an occipitoanterior presentation.[3] The lower plexus is most susceptible to injury when traction is exerted on an abducted arm, such as occurs in vertex deliveries when traction

is applied to an abducted prolapsed arm, or during breech deliveries when traction is applied to the trunk or legs while the after-coming arm is fixed in abduction.[3] Spinal nerves are attached to the vertebral transverse process distal to the intervertebral foramen, encased in funnel-shaped dural sleeves, and enmeshed in a network of rami, cords, and trunks to form the brachial plexus; these factors serve to protect the plexus from traction injury. When traction is excessively rapid and forceful, then diffuse multifocal injury occurs, including avulsion of the roots from the cord in the most severe injuries. Risk factors include technically difficult (57%) or breech (9%) deliveries, fetal macrosomia (weight >4 kg) (55%), shoulder dystocia, multiparous mothers, prolonged labor, or fetal hypotonia leading to loss of the normal cushioning effect of intact muscle tone.[3-6] There are also reports of prenatal-onset brachial plexus injuries in which denervation was demonstrated by electromyography (EMG) shortly after birth. One child demonstrated left brachial plexus injury, left Horner's syndrome, left phrenic nerve injury, and hypoplasia of the left hand in addition to distortion of the first four ribs due to pressure on the left side of the neck and shoulder from the septum of a bicornuate uterus.[7]

The advent of microsurgical techniques and neuroelectrodiagnostic techniques has fostered development of new neurosurgical techniques to repair brachial plexus injuries, although most infants recover spontaneously by age 4 months and only 10% to 20% of cases require surgery.[8] Severe lateral flexion of the infant's neck at delivery makes avulsion of the lower brachial plexus nerve roots four times more common than avulsion of the upper plexus.[8] Among 91 infants observed through age 2 years who sustained a brachial plexus birth injury and were treated with only physical and occupational therapy, 63 children with an upper or middle plexus injury recovered good to excellent shoulder and hand function.[9] Of the remaining 28 infants, 12 sustained global injury, resulting in a useless arm, and 16 infants showed inadequate recovery of deltoid and biceps function by age 6 months. These authors concluded that children with global injury would clearly benefit from early nerve reconstruction. By age 6 months, careful examination of the infant in the seated position (in order to evaluate shoulder function) demonstrated the potential for almost full recovery in most infants. Recovery of motor and sensory nerve function is attributed to axonal regeneration with re-innervations of original target muscle tissue, and functional improvement may continue for 5 years or longer.[10] This longer period of recovery mirrors adaptational mechanisms at the spinal and supraspinal level, which overcome initial motor neuron loss.[10,11] After perinatal upper brachial plexus injury to spinal roots C5 and C6, spinal root C7 contributes to biceps and deltoid innervations, but this does not occur in the adult.[11,12]

## FEATURES

Lesions that affect the upper segments (C5, C6, and sometimes C7) result in Erb's palsy, paralyzing the abductors, external rotators, and extensors of the shoulder as well as injuring the flexors and supinators of the forearm (Fig. 15-1). The infant's arm tends to hang limply adducted and internally rotated at the shoulder, with pronation and extension at the elbow, absent biceps and brachioradialis tendon jerks, and absent Moro response on the side of the lesion.[3,4] If C7 is also involved, then a wrist drop will be noted, with the hand flexed in a

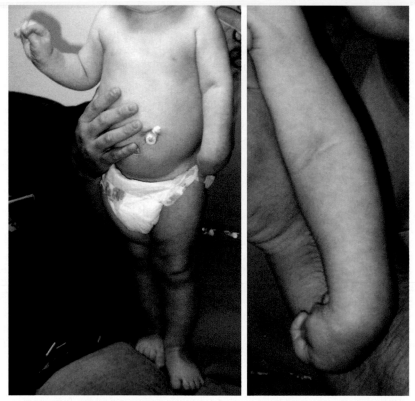

FIGURE 15-1. This large-for-gestational-age infant experienced shoulder dystocia, resulting in a traumatic delivery that damaged his left brachial plexus, affecting C5, C6, and C7 and resulting in Erb's palsy. This injury paralyzed the abductors, external rotators, and extensors of his left shoulder and injured the flexors and supinators of his forearm. His arm hangs limply adducted and internally rotated at the shoulder, with pronation and extension at the elbow, absent biceps and brachioradialis tendon jerks, and absent Moro response on the side of the lesion. Due to involvement of C7, he manifests wrist drop, with the hand flexed in a "waiter's tip" position and with an absent triceps jerk.

"waiter's tip" position and with an absent triceps jerk. Upper plexus injuries (Erb's palsy) may be present without lower plexus injuries; however, lower plexus injury is usually accompanied by some degree of upper plexus damage. Lesions that affect only lower spinal segments (C7, C8, and T2) are much less common, and loss of C7 results in paralysis of the elbow, wrist, and finger extensors, causing wrist drop. Loss of C8 and T1 causes loss of wrist and finger flexors as well as intrinsic hand muscles causing extension of the metacarpal-phalangeal joints and flexion at the proximal and distal interphalangeal joints (Klumpke's palsy).[3,4] The infant manifests a flexed arm with the shoulder in a normal position with flexed wrist and fingers, absent grasp reflex, sensory loss, and loss of sweating on the arm and hand. Injury to T1 at the root level can affect sympathetic fibers to the face, resulting in ipsilateral Horner's syndrome (ptosis, miosis, anhydrosis, facial flushing, and failure of iris pigmentation). Lesions that affect C5 and C6 are most common and account for 58% to 72% of brachial plexus palsies, followed by those affecting C5, C6, and C7 (18%) and those affecting the entire brachial plexus (C5–T1) (10%). Most cases are unilateral (56% right-sided, 41% left-sided), with only 3% affecting both arms.[3,6]

## MANAGEMENT AND PROGNOSIS

Diagnosis is based on clinical features of lower motor neuron weakness. Additional studies may help determine prognosis, such as motor conduction velocities in the median and ulnar nerves; assessment of sensory action potentials in the median, ulnar, and radial nerves; EMG of affected muscles; radiographs; and magnetic resonance imaging (MRI) or myelography with contrast when avulsion of roots is suspected. Although the mainstay of treatment is physical therapy with range-of-motion exercises, no treatment is advised during the first 7 to 10 days after birth because traumatic neuritis makes arm movement painful.[3] Physical therapy should then be promptly initiated because contractures can develop quickly in this condition. For upper plexus injuries, range-of-motion exercises should be initiated for the shoulder and elbow, along with abduction of the arm with the scapula fixed by one hand in order to prevent the development of scapulohumeral adhesions.[3] For middle and lower plexus injuries, the paralyzed hand and wrist require range-of-motion exercises as well as a long opponens splint to maintain the hand and wrist in a position

of function, with the wrist slightly extended and the phalanges slightly flexed.[3]

Complete recovery occurs in 70% to 92% of cases; in most of the remaining cases, recovery is partial. Recovery usually begins distally, with all cases of complete recovery evident by age 5 months. Although some improvement may continue through age 18 months, no improvement has been noted after age 24 months. Children with residual deficits usually manifest shoulder muscle weakness (especially in the external rotators), with associated muscular atrophy and contractures. Infants with lower plexus injuries are less likely to make a complete recovery than those with upper plexus injuries. Associated elevation of the hemidiaphragm on chest radiograph, Horner's syndrome, inability to retract or shrug the shoulders, or scapular winging may indicate damage to nerve fibers that originate from spinal roots close to the cord, thereby signifying avulsion, which is an irreversible injury. The most useful prognostic indicator is recovery that begins within 2 weeks after delivery.[3] The "towel test" has been advocated as a clinical tool to assess shoulder and elbow flexion/extension, biceps contraction, and finger flexion/extension because absence of biceps recovery by age 3 months is an indication to consider surgical reconstruction.[13] The infant's face is covered with a towel, and the infant is then observed to see if he or she can remove the towel with either arm. Among 21 infants with brachial plexus palsy, none of the infants could remove the towel with either arm at 2 to 3 months; at 6 and 9 months, all infants could remove the towel with the normal arm, but 11 of 21 could not remove it with the affected arm.[13]

Surgery may be indicated if there is little improvement by 4 to 6 months, with early neural repair resulting in improvement in 90% of cases, and repair after 6 months resulting in improvement in only 50% to 70% of cases.[8] Older children with brachial plexus injuries (>3 years after injury) require tendon and muscle transfers to achieve functional improvement. Neuromas involving ruptured nerve roots of C5 and C6 are the most common lesions (found in 95% of plexi explored). If EMG conduction post-neuroma decreases by more than 50% compared with pre-neuroma, the lesion is excised with grafting of the proximal and distal nerve roots, which usually involves interpositional sural nerve grafts to guide the proximal sprouting neural bulb to the severed ends.[8] Pseudomeningoceles due to nerve root avulsions are thought to be predictive of significant injury to the brachial plexus and can be visualized by MRI.[14]

Some children in whom complete neurologic recovery is apparent may develop a shoulder contracture or subluxation during growth; therefore, ongoing monitoring and intervention is recommended to minimize functional problems.[9] Glenoid dysplasia and posterior shoulder subluxation with resultant shoulder stiffness is a well-recognized complication in infants with neonatal brachial plexus palsy. It is attributed to slowly progressive glenohumeral deformation due to muscle imbalance and/or physeal trauma. Clinical signs include asymmetric axillary skin folds, asymmetric humeral shortening, asymmetric fullness in the posterior shoulder region, and/or a palpable click during shoulder manipulation (thereby resembling the clinical signs of congenital hip dislocation).[15] Among 134 infants with neonatal brachial plexus palsy who were followed monthly, 11 (8%) had posterior shoulder dislocation diagnosed at a mean age of 6 months, as evidenced by a rapid loss of passive external rotation between monthly examinations and confirmed by ultrasound.[15]

## DIFFERENTIAL DIAGNOSIS

Arthrogryposis and neonatal muscular dystrophy should be easily distinguished by the presence of joint stiffness or ankylosis and the absence of associated features suggesting birth trauma. Sometimes pseudoparalysis may occur after a humeral fracture.

### References

1. Leffert RD: *Brachial plexus injuries*, New York, 1985, Churchill Livingstone, pp 91–120.
2. Towner D, Castro MA, Eby-Wilkens E, et al: Effect of mode of delivery in nulliparous women on neonatal intracranial injury, *N Engl J Med* 341:1709–1714, 1999.
3. Painter MJ, Bergman I: Obstetrical trauma to the neonatal central and peripheral nervous system, *Semin Perinatol* 6:89–104, 1982.
4. Al-Rajeh S, Corea JR, Al-Sibai MH, et al: Congenital brachial palsy in the eastern province of Saudi Arabia, *J Child Neurol* 5:35–37, 1990.
5. Pearl ML, Roberts JM, Laros RK, et al: Vaginal delivery from the persistent occiput posterior position: influence on maternal and neonatal morbidity, *J Reprod Med* 38:955–961, 1993.
6. Boo NY, Lye MS, Kanchanamala M, et al: Brachial plexus injuries in Malaysian neonates: incidence and associated risk factors, *J Trop Pediatr* 37:327–330, 1991.
7. Dunn DW, Engle WA: Brachial plexus palsy: intrauterine onset, *Pediatr Neurol* 1:367–369, 1985.
8. Laurent JP: Neurosurgical intervention for birth-related brachial plexus injuries, *Neurosurg Quart* 7:69–75, 1997.
9. DiTaranto P, Campagna L, Price AE, et al: Outcome following nonoperative treatment of brachial plexus injuries, *J Child Neurol* 19:87–90, 2004.
10. Birch R: Obstetrical brachial plexus palsy, *J Hand Surg Br* 27:3–8, 2002.
11. Vredeveld JW, Blaauw G, Slooff BA, et al: The findings in paediatric obstetric brachial palsy differ from those in older patients: a suggested explanation, *Dev Med Child Neurol* 42:158–161, 2000.
12. Korak KJ, Tam SL, Gordon T, et al: Changes in spinal cord architecture after brachial plexus injury in the newborn, *Brain* 127:1488–1495, 2004.
13. Bertelli JA, Ghizoni MF: The towel test: a useful technique for the clinical and electromyographic evaluation of obstetric brachial plexus palsy, *J Hand Surg Br* 29:155–158, 2004.
14. Abbott R, Abbott M, Alzate J, et al: Magnetic resonance imaging of obstetrical brachial plexus injuries, *Childs Nerv Syst* 20:720–725, 2004.
15. Moukoko D, Ezaki M, Wilkes D, et al: Posterior shoulder dislocation in infants with neonatal brachial plexus palsy, *J Bone Joint Surg Am* 86:787–793, 2004.

# 16 Diaphragmatic Paralysis

## GENESIS

Approximately 5% to 9% of children with brachial plexus palsies also have diaphragmatic paralysis, which has a similar etiology in that the cervical roots forming the phrenic nerve (C4 and C5) lie immediately superior to those forming the brachial plexus.[1] Traction to the phrenic nerve during difficult deliveries or vaginal breech deliveries can occur, and 75% of diaphragmatic paralysis caused by birth injury has associated brachial plexus palsy.[1,2] Thoracic surgery for cardiovascular or tracheoesophageal fistula repair may also injure the phrenic nerve and result in diaphragmatic paralysis.

## FEATURES

Symptoms of diaphragmatic paralysis are relatively nonspecific and can include respiratory distress and recurrent atelectasis and/or pneumonia, with chest radiographs demonstrating elevation of the diaphragm on one side as the infant is breathing spontaneously (Fig. 16-1). If bilateral paralysis is present or if the infant is being ventilated, chest radiographs are not diagnostic, and chest fluoroscopy to demonstrate an immobile diaphragm or one with paradoxical motion (i.e., elevation during inspiration) may be required.[1,2]

## MANAGEMENT AND PROGNOSIS

Neonates are less able to tolerate diaphragmatic paralysis than are older children or adults; hence, they often require prolonged ventilatory support with supplemental oxygen. Most authors state that if early recovery of diaphragmatic function is going to occur, it will do so during the first 2 weeks after birth, during which time ventilatory support is usually necessary. After that time, diaphragmatic plication may be indicated in infants with persistent paralysis. Plication prevents paradoxical

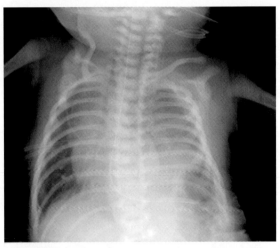

FIGURE 16-1. This infant was delivered from an obese mother and had shoulder dystocia, Erb's palsy and a left diaphragmatic paralysis that resulted in respiratory distress during the first 3 weeks and then resolved. Note the elevated left hemidiaphragm and stomach bubble. This hemidiaphragm did not move on fluoroscopy.

inspiratory shifting of abdominal contents into the ipsilateral thoracic cavity.[1] Eventual recovery of diaphragmatic function occurs in 50% to 60% of cases.[1,2] Treatment depends on the degree of respiratory compromise, with mild cases requiring little more than chest physical therapy and use of antibiotics for any associated pneumonia.

## DIFFERENTIAL DIAGNOSIS

Arthrogryposis and neonatal muscular dystrophy should be easily distinguished by the presence of joint stiffness or ankylosis and the absence of associated features suggestive of birth trauma.

### References
1. Painter MJ, Bergman I: Obstetrical trauma to the neonatal central and peripheral nervous system, *Semin Perinatol* 6:89–104, 1982.
2. Green WL, L'Heureux P, Hunt CE: Paralysis of the diaphragm, *Am J Dis Child* 129:1402–1405, 1975.

# 17 Other Peripheral Nerve Palsies

## GENESIS AND FEATURES

Radial nerve compression along the humerus due to fetal crowding in late gestation may lead to wrist drop (Fig. 17-1) as a function of radial nerve palsy.[1,2] Wrist drop may also result from compression of the posterior interosseous nerve, when prolonged intrauterine palmar flexion results in traction on the posterior interosseous nerve over a fixed point at the origin of the nerve in the supinator muscle.[3] Constricting amniotic bands can also lead to distal nerve dysfuction.[4]

Sciatic compression may cause weakness in one or both legs. In infants with prolonged breech presentation and extended legs, traction on the sciatic nerve may exert a selective effect on the peroneal nerve due to relative fixation of the nerve at the neck of the fibula. This results in foot drop.[3] Prolonged extreme abduction, flexion, and external rotation of the leg at the hip can result in traction on the obturator nerve as it is stretched between fixation points at the pubic ramus and knee joint. This results in limitation of active internal rotation and adduction of the thigh and limitation of knee extension.[3,5]

## MANAGEMENT AND PROGNOSIS

Diagnosis is based on clinical features of lower motor neuron weakness. Additional studies such as motor conduction velocities, sensory action potentials, and electromyography of affected muscles may help determine prognosis. Although the mainstay of treatment is physical therapy with range-of-motion exercises, no treatment is advised for the first 7 to 10 days of life because traumatic neuritis makes limb movement painful.[1] Physical therapy should then be promptly initiated because contractures may develop quickly in this condition. The paralyzed hand and wrist requires range-of-motion exercises in addition to splinting to maintain the hand and wrist in a position of function, with the wrist slightly extended and the phalanges slightly flexed.[1] Complete recovery occurs in most cases; patients who do not completely recover usually show some degree of improvement. Complete recovery is usually evident by age 5 months, but significant improvement may continue for another 12 months. No improvement has been noted in any series after age 24 months. The most useful prognostic indicator is recovery that begins within 2 weeks of delivery.[1]

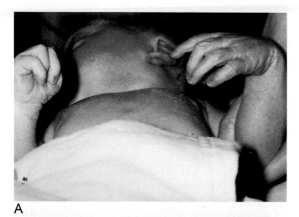

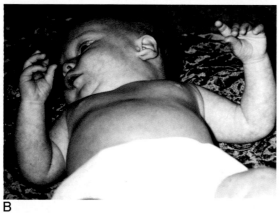

FIGURE 17-1. Unilateral radial palsy from compression at birth **(A)** and 12 weeks later **(B),** by which time wrist function was normal. The compression in this case was due to prolonged engagement in a restricted birth canal for 5 weeks prior to delivery.

## References

1. Painter MJ, Bergman I: Obstetrical trauma to the neonatal central and peripheral nervous system, *Semin Perinatol* 6:89–104, 1982.
2. Feldman GV: Radial nerve palsies in the newborn, *Arch Dis Child* 32:469–471, 1957.
3. Craig WS, Clark JMP: Of peripheral nerve palsies in the newly born, *J Obstet Gynaecol Br Emp* 65:229–237, 1958.
4. Weeks PM: Radial, median, and ulnar nerve dysfunction associated with a congenital constricting band of the arm, *Plast Reconst Surg* 69:333–336, 1982.
5. Craig WS, Clark JMP: Obturator palsy in the newly born, *Arch Dis Child* 37:661–662, 1962.

# 18 Lung Hypoplasia

## GENESIS

Lung hypoplasia implies an abnormal reduction in the weight and/or volume of the lung without the absence of any of its lobes; this condition is different than agenesis or aplasia of the lungs. Lung hypoplasia can result from various phenomena. During the fourth week of gestation, the laryngotracheal groove forms in the esophageal portion of the endotracheal tube, and shortly thereafter lung development begins with the evagination of two buds from the ventral surface of this groove. Between 6 and 16 weeks of gestation, these buds invade the thoracic mesenchyme by dichotomous branching so that the conducting airway system is complete by the end of the 16th week. Formation of the acini begins proximally and proceeds distally in the lung, and alveoli appear as early as 32 weeks and continue to develop throughout childhood.[1]

Decreased lung weight and volume can result from a decreased number of bronchial branches, reduced numbers of alveoli, decreased alveolar size, or any combination of these phenomena.[1] Bilateral pulmonary hypoplasia can be associated with various types of problems: oligohydramnios, thoracic wall abnormalities, lung compression by abdominal contents, central nervous system abnormalities, or a group of miscellaneous conditions including fetal hydrops, extralobar seques tration, or cloacal dysgenesis.[1,2] Restriction of thoracic cage expansion by a small uterine cavity can be associated with lung hypoplasia. Certain lethal skeletal dysplasias that result in rib shortening and a small thorax (e.g., thanatophoric dysplasia or asphyxiating thoracic dysplasia [Figs. 18-1 and 18-2]) can have the same impact. Fetal akinesia that results in diaphragmatic paralysis and failure to swallow amniotic fluid is associated with polyhydramnios and leads to lack of lung expansion (e.g., Pena-Shokeir syndrome) and pulmonary hypoplasia. Prolonged oligohydramnios due to either renal agenesis or prolonged rupture of membranes can lead to pulmonary hypoplasia. Thus distension of the lung with lung liquid and

fetal lung movements are both needed for normal lung growth.[3]

Restrained thoracic growth was initially hypothesized to cause the lungs to remain small and underdeveloped in oligohydramnios sequence,[4] but it is the inhibition of breathing movements (essential for lung growth) and/or abnormal fluid dynamics within the lung that result in decreased intraluminal fluid pressures and cause poor lung growth.[5] The gestational age at the time of premature rupture of membranes relates to the histologic development of the lungs, which can be divided into three stages. During the pseudoglandular stage (from 5 to 17 weeks of gestation), all major lung elements are formed except those related to gas exchange. During the canalicular stage (16 to 25 weeks), terminal bronchioles give rise to respiratory bronchioles and then to thin-walled terminal sacs. During the terminal sac stage (24 weeks to birth), the number of terminal sacs rapidly increases, which increases the total gas exchange area. If oligohydramnios is limited to

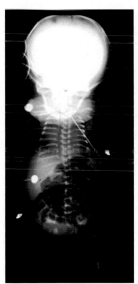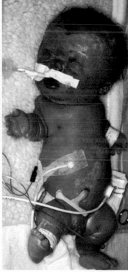

FIGURE 18-1. Thanatophoric dysplasia is caused by mutations in *FGFR3* and results in short-limbed dwarfism with short ribs, a small thorax, and markedly hypoplastic lungs.

99

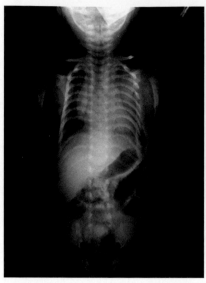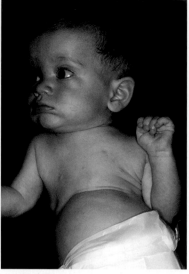

FIGURE 18-2. Radiographic and clinical appearance of a patient with asphyxiating thoracic dystrophy, showing less severely reduced thoracic volume.

the terminal sac stage, it does not affect lung growth, but when oligohydramnios is induced during the canalicular stage, it results in a cumulative reduction in lung size.[7] Thus, the risk for pulmonary hypoplasia diminishes when oligohydramnios occurs after 24 weeks of gestation.[5-8] The duration of severe oligohydramnios and the gestational age at which oligohydramnios had its onset are independent risk factors, and severe oligohydramnios lasting more than 14 days with rupture of membranes before 25 weeks results in a mortality rate greater than 90%.[8]

## FEATURES

Lung hypoplasia is best defined by the ratio of lung weight to body weight; hence, it is usually defined by the pathologist during postmortem examination. This ratio is 0.012 for infants older than 28 weeks of gestation and 0.015 for younger fetuses.[9] Another method of detecting lung hypoplasia involves the radial alveolar count, which is the number of alveolar septae traversed by a perpendicular line drawn from the center of a respiratory bronchiole to the nearest connective tissue septum. As the lung matures, bronchioles extend peripherally, so pathologists often take the most peripheral bronchiole in the section and count the number of alveoli to the pleural surface. The radial count is standardized for gestational age. At 18 weeks of gestation the count averages 1.5 alveolar spaces, whereas at term it averages

5 alveolar spaces.[10] Pulmonary hypoplasia with limited alveolar development leads to respiratory insufficiency.

## MANAGEMENT AND PROGNOSIS

Premature rupture of membranes occurs in approximately 10% of all pregnancies, and pulmonary hypoplasia occurs in 13% to 21% of cases with midtrimester premature rupture of membranes.[11] The duration of severe oligohydramnios (amniotic pocket less than 1 cm and lasting more than 14 days) and gestational age (fetus younger than 25 weeks of gestation) are independent risk factors for lethal pulmonary hypoplasia.[11,12] Lethality usually results in a 25-week fetus with more than 3 days of oligohydramnios, but when chronic leakage of amniotic fluid occurs after 27 weeks of gestation, every measure toward providing adequate oxygenation should be taken in the hope of maintaining survival until lung development can become adequate for normal respiration. The lungs in thanatophoric dysplasia (see Fig. 18-1) and Pena-Shokeir syndrome are invariably too hypoplastic to allow for survival, and extended respiratory support is generally futile. In disorders such as asphyxiating thoracic dystrophy (see Fig. 18-2), spondylothoracic dysplasia (Fig. 18-3, *A*), or spondylocostal dysostosis (Fig. 18-3, *B*), the prognosis is extremely variable, which leaves little tolerance for additional insults such as respiratory syncytial

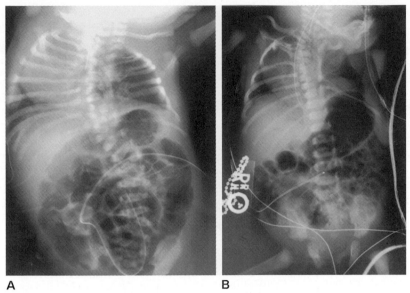

**A**                                  **B**

FIGURE 18-3. Radiographs of neonates with spondylothoracic dysplasia **(A)** and spondylocostal dysostosis **(B)**.

virus (RSV) infection. Spondylocostal dysostosis is an autosomal recessive disorder that has been linked to mutations of the Notch signaling gene *DLL3* at 19q13.1.[13-15] Spondylothoracic dysplasia (Jarcho-Levin syndrome) is an autosomal recessive disorder linked to 2q32.1, with high prevalence in the Puerto Rican population. It is characterized by a fan-like configuration of the ribs (crab-like chest) due to fusion of the ribs at the costovertebral junction without intrinsic costal anomalies.[16] Early mortality due to respiratory insufficiency occurs within the first 6 months in 44% of patients, but surgical enlargement of the chest may lead to increased survival in some cases.[17] Bilateral renal agenesis leads to complete absence of urine production, termed *Potter syndrome*, which is associated with extremely hypoplastic lungs (Figs 18-4 and 18-5).

## DIFFERENTIAL DIAGNOSIS

Oligohydramnios may be the result of inadequate urine flow into the amniotic space (e.g., bilateral renal agenesis, polycystic kidney disease, or cystic dysplastic kidneys), in which case the prognosis is usually poor. Instillation of fluid has been used successfully in some cases of oligohydramnios, and fetal bladder catheterization has been used in some cases of bladder outlet obstruction. (See Chapter 46

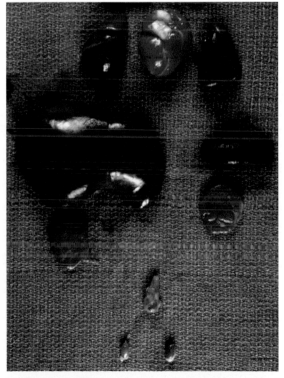

FIGURE 18-4. Relative organ size in an infant with bilateral renal agenesis, resulting in prolonged oligohydramnios due to complete failure of urine flow. Note the extremely small size of both lungs and the discoid appearance of both adrenal glands when both kidneys are absent.

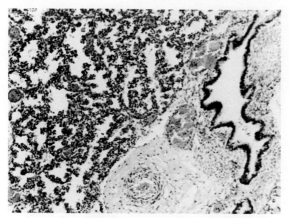

FIGURE 18-5. Histology in hypoplastic lungs due to prolonged oligohydramnios.

for a more complete discussion of the oligohydramnios deformation sequence.) Diaphragmatic hernia not only limits lung development on the side of the hernia but also shifts the mediastinal contents toward the opposite side, thereby limiting lung growth on that side as well. Hence infants with this condition may die from respiratory insufficiency due to lung hypoplasia unless fetal surgery is attempted to correct the diaphragmatic hernia. Several skeletal dysplasias have a profound impact on thoracic cage growth, thereby resulting in lung hypoplasia and associated respiratory insufficiency. One such disorder is thanatophoric dwarfism. The word *thanatophoric* means "death dealing", and death in this condition is usually the consequence of respiratory insufficiency.

## References

1. Askin F: Respiratory tract disorders in the fetus and neonate. In Wigglesworth JS, Singer DB, eds: *Textbook of fetal and perinatal pathology*, Boston, 1991, Blackwell Scientific, pp 643–688.
2. Gilbert-Barness E: *Potter's pathology of the fetus and infant*, St Louis, 1997, Mosby, pp 733–734.
3. Wigglesworth JS, Desai R: Is fetal respiratory function a major determinant of perinatal survival? *Lancet* 1:264–267, 1982.
4. Thomas IT, Smith DW: Oligohydramnios, cause of the non-renal features of Potter's syndrome, including pulmonary hypoplasia, *J Pediatr* 84:811–814, 1974.
5. Richards DS: Complications of prolonged PROM and oligohydramnios, *Clin Obstet Gynecol* 41:817–826, 1998.
6. Nimrod C, Varela-Gittins F, Machin G, et al: The effect of very prolonged membrane rupture on fetal development, *Am J Obstet Gynecol* 148:540–543, 1984.
7. Moessinger AC, Collins MH, Blanc WA, et al: Oligohydramnios-induced lung hypoplasia: the influence of timing and duration in gestation, *Pediatr Res* 20:951–954, 1986.
8. Kilbride HW, Yeast J, Thiebault DW: Defining limits of survival: lethal pulmonary hypoplasia after midtrimester premature rupture of membranes, *Am J Obstet Gynecol* 175:675–681, 1996.
9. Wigglesworth JS, Desai R, Guerrini P: Lung hypoplasia: biochemical and structural variations and their possible significance, *Arch Dis Child* 56:606–615, 1981.
10. Cooney TP, Thurlbeck WM: The radial alveolar count method of Emery and Mithal: a reappraisal. 2. Intrauterine and early postnatal lung growth, *Thorax* 37:580–583, 1982.
11. Rotschild A, Ling EW, Poterman ML, et al: Neonatal outcome after prolonged preterm rupture of the membranes, *Am J Obstet Gynecol* 162:46–52, 1990.
12. Suzuki K: Respiratory characteristics of infants with pulmonary hypoplasia syndrome following preterm rupture of membranes: a preliminary study for establishing clinical diagnostic criteria, *Early Hum Dev* 79:31–40, 2004.
13. Turnpenny PD, Whittock N, Duncan J, et al: Novel mutations in *DLL3*, a somatogenesis gene encoding a ligand for Notch signaling pathway, cause a consistent pattern of abnormal segmentation in spondylocostal dysostosis, *J Med Genet* 40:333–339, 2003.
14. Bonafe L, Giunta C, Gassner M, et al: A cluster of autosomal recessive spondylocostal dysostosis caused by three newly identified *DLL3* mutations segregating in a small village, *Clin Genet* 64:28–35, 2003.
15. Whittock NV, Ellard S, Duncan J, et al: Pseudodominant inheritance of spondylocostal dysostosis type 1 caused by two familial delta-like 3 mutations, *Clin Genet* 66:67–72, 2004.
16. Cornier AS, Ramirez N, Arroyo S, et al: Phenotype characterization and natural history of spondylothoracic dysplasia syndrome: a series of 27 new cases, *Am J Med Genet* 128A:120–126, 2004.
17. Campbell RM Jr, Smith JT: Correspondence: response to "spondylothoracic dysplasia syndrome: a series of 27 new cases" by Cornier et al, *Am J Med Genet* 128A:132, 2004.

# 19 Pectus Excavatum and Pectus Carinatum

## GENESIS

Pectus excavatum is common, with a reported frequency of 1 in 300. There is a positive family history in 37% to 43% of cases, and it occurs more often in males (5:1).[1,2] This deformity is often due to overgrowth of costal cartilages, which becomes more apparent during the period of rapid skeletal growth in early adolescence. Pectus carinatum is less common than pectus excavatum, with an estimated frequency of 1 in 1500, and it also progresses during adolescence. Pectus carinatum is caused by abnormal growth of costal cartilages with precocious fusion of sternal growth plates, resulting in anterior bowing of the superior costal cartilages and consequent protrusion of the superior portion of the sternum. Growth of costal cartilages alone is solely responsible for pectus excavatum.[3] A positive family history was found in 27% of pectus carinatum cases.[4] Intrauterine pressure may distort the shape of the thoracic cage and result in depression or protrusion of the sternum; hence, the association with urethral obstruction malformation sequence, resulting in marked abdominal distension and oligohydramnios. Prolonged partial airway obstruction also contributes to the occurrence of pectus deformities, which explains the association with Robin sequence and Jeune syndrome. Abnormal skeletal growth in a variety of skeletal dysplasias and genetic connective tissue disorders can result in pectus deformities, which are especially frequent in patients with Marfan syndrome (Fig. 19-1). Because of these associated genetic connective tissue disorders, mitral valve prolapse and scoliosis are common associated defects and are found in approximately 20% of patients with pectus deformities. In addition, open thoracotomy for repair of cardiovascular defects during early childhood sometimes affects the growth of costal cartilages, leading to pectus deformities with secondary associated scoliosis. Pectus excavatum has also been reported in Noonan syndrome and Van Den Ende-Gupta syndrome (Fig. 19-2).

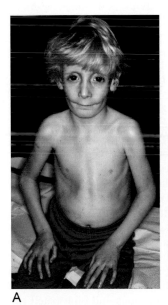
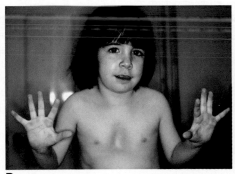
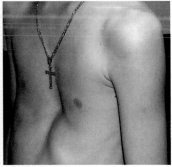

A          B

FIGURE 19-1. Pectus carinatum **(A)** and pectus excavatum **(B)** in unrelated children with Marfan syndrome, an autosomal dominant connective tissue disorder that results in laxity of connective tissues due to mutations in fibrillin-1.

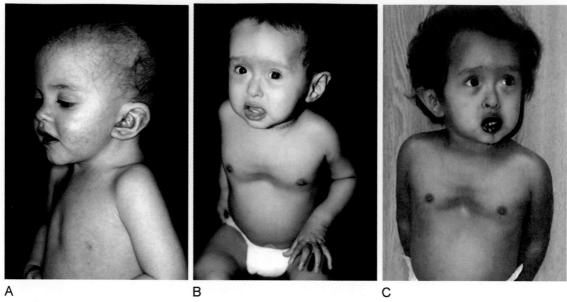

A                                    B                                    C

FIGURE 19-2. Early pectus excavatum in a 10-month-old girl with Noonan syndrome **(A)** and progression of pectus excavatum between ages 2 and 4 years in a boy with Van Den Ende-Gupta syndrome **(B** and **C).**

## FEATURES

Pectus excavatum results in a central anterior chest depression (inward sternum), whereas pectus carinatum results in sternal protrusion (prominent sternum). Frequently the sternum faces to the right in pectus excavatum, and the deepest depression is usually near the xyphoid. Deep inspiration commonly accentuates the pectus depression, and the heart is often displaced into the left chest, interfering with right atrial filling and limiting pulmonary expansion on inspiration. Respiration during exercise often requires deeper diaphragmatic excursions to compensate for diminished chest wall expansion, and younger adolescents may become easily fatigued during exercise, with decreased stamina and endurance.[5] Some patients experience exercise-induced asthma and/or low anterior chest pain as well as bronchiectasis, and spontaneous regression of pectus excavatum or pectus carinatum rarely occurs. About 20% to 25% of patients have associated mild to moderate scoliosis, and body-building exercises may result in worsening of the cosmetic appearance.[5] Severe pectus excavatum deformities are usually repaired during childhood because this deformity tends to worsen during the adolescent growth spurt. With improved surgical techniques, surgery yields improvements in respiratory symptoms and exercise tolerance with excellent cosmetic results and short hospital stays.[5]

## MANAGEMENT AND PROGNOSIS

In mild cases, no management is necessary, but because most cases progress with growth, surgical intervention merits early consideration. A pectus severity index has been developed to assist in making such determinations.[6] The pectus severity index is determined by dividing the inner width of the chest at the widest point (on a chest computed tomography scan or radiograph) by the distance between the posterior surface of the sternum and the anterior surface of the spine. The mean pectus severity index of normal adults is 2.56, and the mean of 23 operated symptomatic adults was 5.3 in one series[5] and 4.42 in another.[6] If the index is greater than 3.25, surgery should be considered. Because the deformity is progressive and results in secondary rib abnormalities that cannot be corrected surgically, the ideal age for correction is 4 to 6 years, before these rib changes develop.[6] In previous surgical procedures, the chest and abdominal muscles were reflected laterally and inferiorly, the sternum was fractured and elevated to the desired position, and a stainless-steel strut was used to support the tip of the sternum for 6 to 10 months and then subsequently removed (various versions of the Ravitch procedure).[7-9] Recent modifications that have minimized incisions and eliminated the need for a second operation include use of bioabsorbable strut materials and development of a

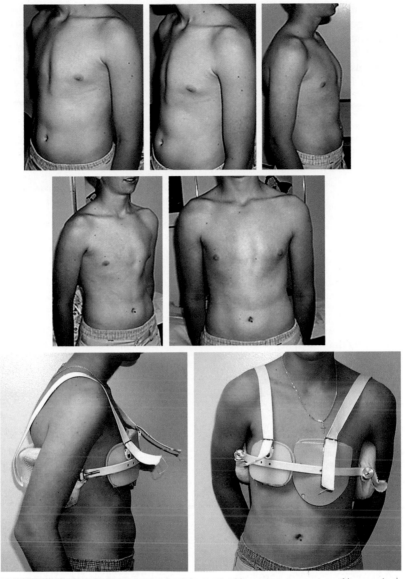

FIGURE 19-3. An otherwise normal adolescent with pectus excavatum. Nonsurgical correction of pectus excavatum was attempted via orthotic bracing.

sternal turnover technique.[10,11] Innovative miniature access techniques (Nuss procedure), open repairs with minimal cartilage resection, and endoscopic techniques have also been developed.[12–15] Similar surgical techniques have been used for pectus carinatum, but good results have also been reported with prolonged use of an orthotic sternal brace prior to and during the early adolescent growth spurt (see Figs. 19-1 to 19-3).[16–19] Operations performed too early (i.e., before the age of 4 years), especially those in which five or more costal cartilages are removed, can result in limited chest wall growth with marked limitation in ventilatory function.[20]

## DIFFERENTIAL DIAGNOSIS

Pectus deformities may occur concomitantly with abdominal muscle weakness in a number of neurologic disorders, and they also occur with certain genetic connective tissue disorders and skeletal dysplasias (e.g., Jeune syndrome [see Fig. 18-2]) as well as other conditions (e.g., Poland sequence,

Robin sequence, and urethral obstruction malformation sequence). About two thirds of patients with Marfan syndrome have pectus excavatum, which may manifest later in childhood than in other patients, who usually present before age 2 years. Patients with Marfan syndrome are also much more likely to experience recurrence if sternal support bars are not used postoperatively, and they may benefit from pectus repair performed before aortic replacement is necessary.[20] Pectus excavatum can be inherited as an isolated autosomal dominant trait without any associated syndrome.[21]

## References

1. Ellis DG: Chest wall deformities, *Pediatr Rev* 11:147–151, 1989.
2. Shamberger RC, Welch KJ: Surgical repair of pectus excavatum, *J Pediatr Surg* 23:615–622, 1988.
3. Haje SJ, Harcke HT, Bowen JR: Growth disturbance of the sternum and pectus deformities: imaging studies and clinical correlation, *Pediatr Radiol* 29:334–341, 1999.
4. Shamberger RC, Welch KJ: Surgical correction of pectus carinatum, *J Pediatr Surg* 22:48–53, 1987.
5. Fonkalsrud EW, Bustorff-Silva J: Repair of pectus excavatum and carinatum in adults, *Am J Surg* 177:121–124, 1999.
6. Haller JA Jr, Kramer SS, Lietman SA: Use of CT scans in selections of patients for pectus excavatum surgery: a preliminary report, *J Pediatr Surg* 22:904–906, 1987.
7. Haller JA Jr, Scherer LR, Turner CS, et al: Evolving management of pectus excavatum based on a single institutional experience of 664 patients, *Ann Surg* 209:578–583, 1989.
8. Fonkalsrud EW, Salman T, Guo W, et al: Repair of pectus deformities with sternal support, *J Thorac Cardiovasc Surg* 107:37–42, 1994.
9. Nakajima H, Chang H: A new method of reconstruction for pectus excavatum that preserves blood supply and costal cartilage, *Plast Reconstr Surg* 103:1661–1666, 1999.
10. Lane-Smith DM, Gillis DA, Roy PD: Repair of pectus excavatum using a Dacron vascular graft strut, *J Pediatr Surg* 29:1179–1182, 1994.
11. Matsui T, Kitano M, Nakamura T, et al: Bioabsorbable struts made from poly-l-lactide and their application for treatment of chest deformity, *J Thorac Cardiovasc Surg* 108:162–168, 1994.
12. Fonkalsrud EW: Open repair of pectus excavatum with minimal cartilage resection, *Ann Surg* 240:231–235, 2004.
13. Kim YI, Choe JW, Park YW: Minimally invasive concomitant cardiac procedures and repair of pectus excavatum: case report, *Heart Surg Forum* 7:E216–E217, 2004.
14. Zallen GS, Glick PL: Miniature access pectus excavatum repair: lessons we have learned, *J Pediatr Surg* 39:685–689, 2004.
15. Seiichiro K, Yoza S, Komoro Y, et al: Correction of pectus excavatum and pectus carinatum by the endoscope, *Plast Reconstr Surg* 99:1037–1045, 1997.
16. Haje SA, Bowen RJ: Preliminary results of orthotic treatment of pectus deformities in children and adolescents, *J Pediatr Orthop* 12:795–800, 1992.
17. Haje SA: Pectus deformities from an orthopedic standpoint. Orthopedic Transactions, *J Bone Joint Surg* 17:977–978, 1993/94.
18. Mielke CH, Winter RB: Pectus carinatum successfully treated with bracing: a case report, *Int Orthop* 17:350–352, 1993.
19. Haller JA Jr, Colombani PM, Humphries CT, et al: Chest wall constriction after too extensive and too early operations for pectus excavatum, *Ann Thorac Surg* 61:1618–1625, 1996.
20. Scherer LR, Arn PH, Dressel DA, et al: Surgical management of children and young adults with Marfan syndrome and pectus excavatum, *J Pediatr Surg* 23:1169–1172, 1988.
21. Leung AKC, Hoo JH: Familial congenital funnel chest, *Am J Med Genet* 26:887–890, 1987.

# 20 Scoliosis

## GENESIS

The development and progression of spinal deformities can be explained in biologic and mechanical terms. External fetal constraint rarely causes persistent scoliosis but can result in infantile idiopathic scoliosis that responds to physical therapy (Fig. 20-1). Infantile idiopathic scoliosis has been associated with a history of breech presentation,[1] and Lloyd-Roberts and Pilcher[2] studied the natural history of 100 infants with no associated malformations or radiologic defects who presented with a lateral curve of the thoracic spine that did not disappear on suspension (67% male predilection); convexity to the left was noted in 85% of cases, with similar sex and sidedness predilections as noted for torticollis. The mean angle of curvature was 15 degrees (range, 5–40 degrees), and the affected infants were observed for an average of 3 years until complete resolution (92%) or obvious progression (5%), with secondary structural scoliosis (double primary curves) noted in 3%.[2] Because of the high rate of associated torticollis-plagiocephaly deformation sequence (83%), with rib prominence on the convex side (50%) and pelvic tilting that followed the curve of the trunk,

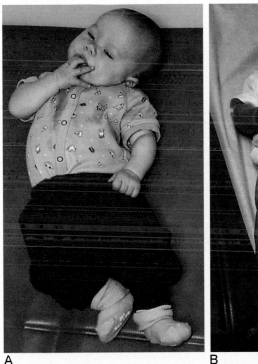 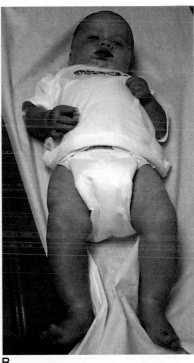

A           B

FIGURE 20-1. Idiopathic infantile scoliosis before (A) and after (B) physical therapy in an infant with late fetal constraint due to an abnormal fetal lie. At age 3 months, he presented with scoliosis and left torticollis-plagiocephaly deformation sequence. His mother wore an elastic maternity girdle during the final 2 weeks of her pregnancy to keep her fetus in vertex presentation after undergoing version for a transverse lie.

these researchers interpreted these defects as being secondary to fetal constraint and used the term *molded baby syndrome*.

Spontaneous resolution during infancy occurred in most cases of infantile idiopathic scoliosis but curves with an initial rib-vertebra angle difference greater than 20 degrees that failed to improve in 3 months, or those that developed compensatory curves above and/or below the primary curve, tended to relentlessly progress, compromising cardiorespiratory function.[2-4] In a study of causative factors of infantile idiopathic scoliosis, Wynne-Davies[5] noted an excess of males, with most curves convex to the left, as well as postnatal development of forehead flattening on the same side as the convexity and accompanied by contralateral occipital flattening. She noted an excess of breech presentation (17.6%), with only 3% of such infants sleeping in prone position (which she compared with the markedly reduced incidence of infantile idiopathic scoliosis among prone-sleeping North American infants). Among infants with idiopathic scoliosis, 64% were born between July and December, and they developed curves between October and March, suggesting that limitation to free movement due to being heavily wrapped during cold weather played a role.[5] Infantile idiopathic scoliosis differs from adolescent-onset idiopathic scoliosis in that it frequently resolves spontaneously, is more common in males, and shows a marked predilection for left thoracic curves, whereas most adolescent-onset cases progress and occur more commonly in females and on the right side. The occurrence of resolving infantile idiopathic scoliosis in Edinburgh (Scotland) was markedly reduced, from 42% of all patients with idiopathic scoliosis in 1968–1971 to 4% in 1980–1982, when infant sleep positioning changed from supine to prone and centralized heating became more available.[6] Because the current infant sleeping practice has switched back to supine sleep positioning, the incidence of infantile idiopathic scoliosis may increase once again but this can easily be treated with physical therapy.[7]

Progressive scoliosis has also been noted after chest wall resection in children who undergo surgical repair of esophageal atresia or congenital heart defects. The degree of curvature is related to the number of ribs resected, with posterior rib resection leading to scoliosis much more readily than anterior rib resection (which seldom leads to significant scoliosis).[8] Scoliosis may also result from plural tethering following tumors, irradiation, or empyema. In the past, paralytic scoliosis after poliomyelitis was a cause of scoliosis, and there is progressive neuromuscular scoliosis in spinal muscular atrophy as well as in severe spastic cerebral palsy.[9,10] Patients with anterior chest wall deformities manifest associated scoliosis in more than 20% of cases, and 18% and 14% of patients with pectus excavatum and pectus carinatum, respectively, require therapeutic intervention for scoliosis via bracing or surgery.[11]

## FEATURES

Constraint-related infantile scoliosis is not associated with vertebral anomalies or underlying neuromuscular disease, and there is usually a history of fetal constraint and/or abnormal fetal lie, supported by an unusual position of comfort shortly after birth (see Fig. 20-1). Congenital scoliosis can be caused by abnormal development of the vertebral bodies during the sixth week of gestation, resulting in unilateral bar, block vertebrae, hemivertebrae, wedge vertebrae, and other complex forms due to multiple vertebral anomalies.[12] It is usually progressive, with the degree and rate of progression dependent on the type and location of the spinal defects. Bracing is ineffective, and operative intervention with posterior spinal fusions, with or without instrumentation, combined with anterior and posterior arthrodeses is necessary in about 50% of such cases to preserve respiratory function and stabilize progressive curvature. Therefore in such cases, surgery is usually done early, and any associated spinal dysraphism or tethering of the cord must be identified prior to surgery.[12]

Adolescent idiopathic scoliosis is characterized by a lateral bending of the spine and an associated rotation of vertebral bodies over 5 to 10 segments of the spine. It is the most common spinal deformity that affects adolescents 10 to 16 years of age. Its etiology remains unknown, but genetic factors appear to play a role because family history is positive in 27% to 30% of cases.[13,14] There is a much stronger family history of scoliosis among girls with adolescent idiopathic scoliosis, suggesting dominant inheritance.[13]

## MANAGEMENT AND PROGNOSIS

Physical therapy is merited for infantile scoliosis due to fetal constraint, with manipulative stretching exercises performed by caretakers and careful follow-up to determine whether full correction will occur after initiation of physical therapy. Most pediatric orthopedists believe that the probability of progression is low if the scoliotic curve is 15 degrees or less and growth is complete. For patients who are skeletally immature with curves between 20 and 25 degrees, observation and follow-up are indicated. For curves between 25 and 45 degrees with a high probability of progression, treatment usually consists of underarm bracing with a thoracolumbosacral orthosis worn under the clothing during the day and at night. Occasionally, a nighttime brace is used to hold the spine in an overcorrected position. Surgery is usually recommended for mature adolescents with curves of 40 to 50 degrees that are likely to progress during adulthood.[14] Surgery is intended to diminish the scoliotic curve and maintain spinal correction during the next 6 months while fusion and healing occur. Spinal instrumentation prevents the need for postoperative immobilization in a cast or brace, and there are usually few long-term limitations.[14]

## DIFFERENTIAL DIAGNOSIS

Vertebral anomalies can result in congenital scoliosis (see Fig. 18-3), as can neurologic problems that alter muscle tone (Fig. 20-2). Some genetic connective tissue disorders such as Marfan syndrome or Ehlers-Danlos syndrome (Figs. 20-3 and 20-4)

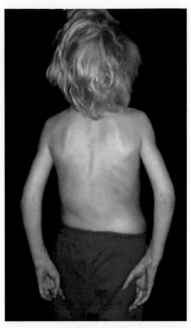

FIGURE 20-3. Scoliosis is associated with laxity of connective tissues in Marfan syndrome, an autosomal dominant genetic connective tissue disorder that results from mutations in the *FBN1* gene.

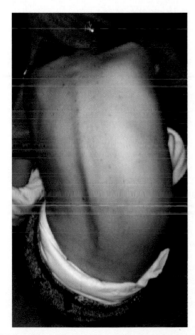

FIGURE 20-2. Neuromuscular scoliosis is associated with increased muscle tone in a young woman with Rett syndrome, an X-linked dominant disorder that is lethal in males and is due to mutations in *MECP2*, a gene involved in the process of silencing other genes.

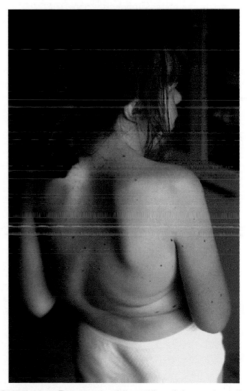

FIGURE 20-4. Progressive idiopathic adolescent scoliosis in a young woman with classic Ehlers-Danlos syndrome.

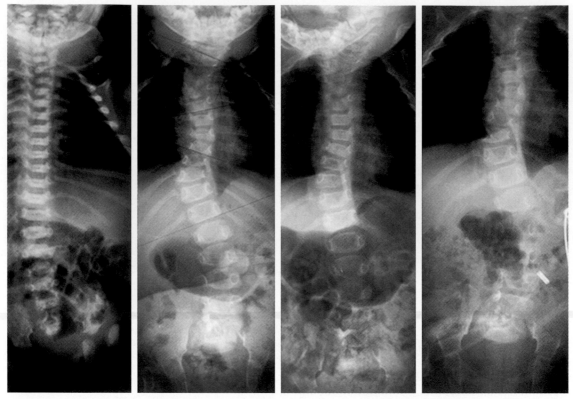

FIGURE 20-5. Progressive scoliosis occurs in diastrophic dysplasia, an autosomal recessive skeletal dysplasia, because of mutations in a sulfate transporter gene *(SLC 26A2)*. This condition typically results in abnormal connective tissues with fixed equinovarus foot deformities, phalangeal synostosis, and proximally placed thumbs and halluces. The changes in spinal curvature shown in this patient occurred over the course of the first 18 months of her life.

can lead to scoliosis, as can certain skeletal dysplasias such as camptomelic dysplasia or diastrophic dysplasia (Fig. 20-5).

## References

1. Wynne-Davies R, Littlejohn A, Gormley J: Aetiology and relationship of some common skeletal deformities (talipes equinovarus and calcaneovalgus, metatarsus varus, congenital dislocation of the hip, and infantile idiopathic scoliosis), *J Med Genet* 19:321–328, 1982.
2. Lloyd-Roberts GC, Pilcher MF: Structural idiopathic scoliosis in infancy: a study of the natural history of 100 patients, *J Bone Joint Surg Br* 47:520–523, 1965.
3. Ferreira JH, James JIP: Progressive and resolving infantile idiopathic scoliosis, *J Bone Joint Surg Br* 54:648–655, 1972.
4. Thompson SK, Bentley G: Prognosis in infantile idiopathic scoliosis, *J Bone Joint Surg Br* 62:151–154, 1980.
5. Wynne-Davies R: Infantile idiopathic scoliosis: causative factors, particularly in the first six months of life, *J Bone Joint Surg Br* 57:138–141, 1975.
6. McMaster MJ: Infantile idiopathic scoliosis: can it be prevented? *J Bone Joint Surg Br* 65:612–617, 1983.
7. Philippi H, Faldum A, Bergmann H, et al: Idiopathic infantile asymmetry, proposal of a measurement scale, *Early Hum Dev* 80:79–90, 2004.
8. DeRosa GP: Progressive scoliosis following chest wall resection in children, *Spine* 10:618–622, 1985.
9. Rodillo E, Marini ML, Heckmatt JZ, et al: Scoliosis in spinal muscular atrophy: review of 63 cases, *J Child Neurol* 4:118–123, 1989.
10. Saito N, Ebara S, Ohotsuka K, et al: Natural history of scoliosis in spastic cerebral palsy, *Lancet* 351:1687–1692, 1998.
11. Waters P, Welch K, Micheli LJ, et al: Scoliosis in children with pectus excavatum and pectus carinatum, *J Pediatr Orthop* 9:551–561, 1989.
12. Lopez-Sosa F, Guille JT, Bowen JR: Rotation of the spine in congenital scoliosis, *J Pediatr Orthop* 15:528–534, 1995.
13. Wynne-Davies R: Familial (idiopathic) scoliosis: a family survey, *J Bone Joint Surg Br* 50:24–30, 1968.
14. Killian JT, Mayberry S, Wilkinson L: Current concepts in adolescent scoliosis, *Pediatr Ann* 28:755–762, 1999.

# Head and Neck Deformations

# 21 Nose Deformation

## GENESIS

A small nose may result from limitation of nasal growth in a face presentation or transverse lie or from compression due to a small uterine cavity. A compressed nose is also a feature of oligohydramnios and severe crowding, such as can occur in a bicornuate uterus (Fig. 21-1). Infants born to mothers with a bicornuate uterus have about a fourfold greater risk of congenital defects, and nasal hypoplasia and limb deficiencies occur more frequently in infants born to mothers with a bicornuate uterus.[1] Nasal deformities consisting of columellar necrosis, flaring of nostrils, and snubbing of the nose have been reported in very-low-birth-weight infants after prolonged application of flow-driver nasal prongs for continuous positive airway pressure.[2] Midfacial hypoplasia has also been reported in preterm infants with bronchopulmonary dysplasia who were subjected to prolonged nasotracheal intubation for 68 to 243 days.[3]

Nasal septal deviations (Fig. 21-2) occur in as many as 17% to 22% of newborns examined immediately after vaginal delivery but occur less frequently in infants delivered by cesarean section; therefore nasal septal deviations are thought to be related to passage through the birth canal.[4,5] Among 273 newborns examined at 12-hour intervals, the septum straightened spontaneously during

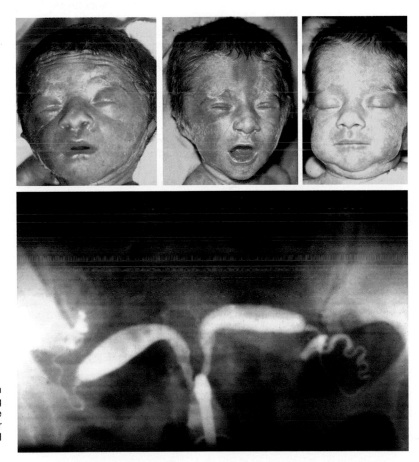

FIGURE 21-1. Nasal compression can occur with severe crowding due to a maternal bicornuate uterus, with gradual recovery over the first few weeks of postnatal life, as shown.

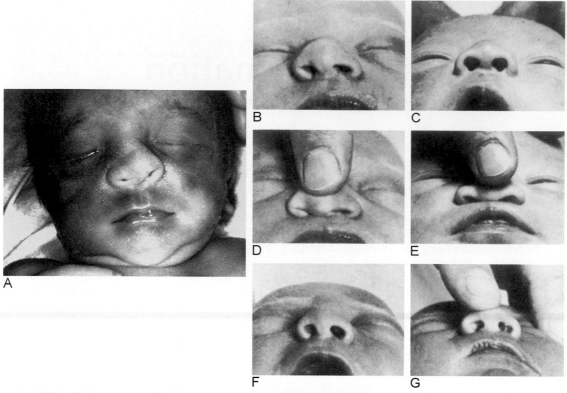

FIGURE 21-2. **A,** Nasal deviation due to mechanical pressure during vaginal delivery from a right occiput transverse position. **B** and **C,** Deviated nasal septum **(B)** versus normal **(C)**. The compression test is positive when dislocation of the lower edge of the nasal cartilage has occurred **(D)** and the nasal cartilage is unable to return to its former slot in the vomerine ridge **(E)**. The normal response to compression is shown on the right. After reduction of the dislocation of the cartilaginous septum, there is still slight asymmetry **(F),** but the compression test **(G)** shows that the cartilage is relocated into its slot in the vomerine ridge.

(From Stoksted P, Schønsted-Madsen U: Traumatology of the newborn's nose. *Rhinology* 17:77–82, 1979.)

the first 3 days of life.[5] Newborns delivered from a left occipitoanterior (LOA) presentation were more prone to anterior nasal septal deviations to the right, whereas newborns delivered from a right occipitoanterior presentation (ROA) had deviations directed to the left. During LOA presentation, the head turns in a clockwise direction and the nasal cartilage moves to the right as the nasal tip is directed to the left; the reverse is true for infants delivered from ROA presentation.[4,5] Gray is generally credited with attributing anterior nasal septum deviations to deformation from maxillary pressure during pregnancy or birth,[6] but others have suggested that posterior septal deformities and one type of anterior septal deformation might be inherited.[7] More severe deviation of the nasal septum can result in frank nasal septum dislocation. About 2% to 4% of neonates have an anterior dislocation of the nasal septum, and about 17% to 22% of neonates have some type of septum deformation.[8]

## FEATURES

A deviated nose is not rare and appears to be secondary to mechanical force during normal vaginal delivery. The lower edge of the nasal cartilage may be dislocated from its usual placement on the vomerine ridge, which results in an asymmetric nose with slanting of the columella and a smaller nasal aperture on the side toward which the cartilaginous septum is dislocated (see Fig. 21-2).

## MANAGEMENT AND PROGNOSIS

Nasal compression and nasal septum deviation generally resolve spontaneously, but most authors believe that nasal septum dislocation should be treated by manual reduction in the newborn nursery (see Figs. 21-2 and 21-3).[8,9] An unresolved

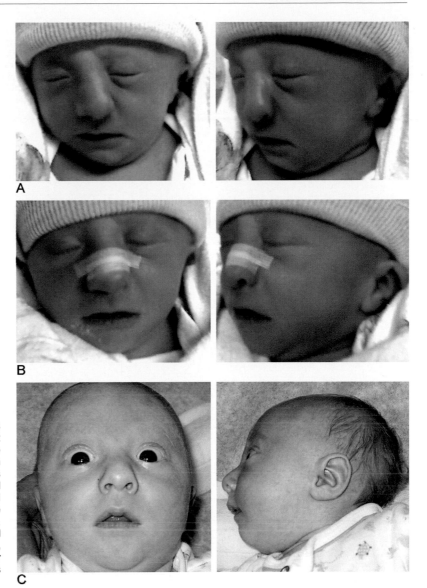

FIGURE 21-3. **A,** This infant was delivered by cesarean section at 37 weeks from a prolonged face presentation with a nasal septum dislocation to the left side. **B,** His nasal septum was relocated shortly after birth, and external taping was used to maintain the correction. **C,** At age 2 months, his nose appeared fully corrected with symmetric nares. (**A** and **B,** Courtesy of Dr. Gene Liu, Cedar Sinai Medical Center, Los Angeles, Calif.)

dislocated nasal septum should be treated by the third day after birth by repositioning the septal cartilage into the anatomic groove in the floor of the nose. The cartilaginous part of the nose should be grasped (with gauze) between the thumb and forefingers and then lifted forward while a probe or elevator is inserted into the nares below the free edge of the dislocated septum, forcing it into its normal location.[8,9] A slight nasal asymmetry may persist for several weeks after relocation before the normal form is fully reestablished. Regarding the deformed septum that is not dislocated, there is no known contraindication to manipulation in an effort to restore the nasal septum to a normal alignment.

## DIFFERENTIAL DIAGNOSIS

A small nose may be a distinguishing feature of a number of specific disorders.

### References

1. Martinez-Frias ML, Bermejo E, Rodriquez-Pinilla E, et al: Congenital anomalies in the offspring of mothers with a bicornuate uterus, *Pediatrics* 101:e10, 1998.
2. Robertson NJ, McCarthy LS, Hamilton PA, et al: Nasal deformities resulting from flow driver continuous positive airway pressure, *Arch Dis Child* 75:F209–F212, 1996.
3. Rotschild A, Dison PJ, Chitayat D, et al: Midfacial hypoplasia associated with long-term intubation for bronchopulmonary dysplasia, *Am J Dis Child* 144:1302–1306, 1990.

4. Korantzis A, Cardamakis E, Chelidonis E, et al: Nasal septum deformity in the newborn infant during labor, *Eur J Obstet Gynecol Reprod Funct* 44:41–46, 1992.

5. Kawalski H, Spiewak P: How septum deformations in newborns occur, *Int J Pediatr Otorhinolaryngol* 44:23–30, 1998.

6. Gray LP: Septal and associated cranial birth deformities (types, incidence and treatment), *Med J Aust* 1:557–563, 1974.

7. Mladina R, Subaric M: Are some types of septal deformities inherited? Type 6 revisited, *Int J Pediatr Otorhinolaryngol* 67:1291–1294, 2003.

8. Podoshin L, Gertner R, Fradis M, et al: Incidence and treatment of deviation of nasal septum in newborns, *Ear Nose Throat J* 70:485–487, 1991.

9. Stoksted P, Schønsted-Madsen U: Traumatology of the newborn's nose, *Rhinology* 17:77–82, 1979.

# 22 External Ears

## GENESIS

Overfolding of the upper helix and/or other parts of the cartilaginous auricle are common constraint-related deformations, as is flattening of the ear against the head (Figs. 22-1 and 22-2). Prolonged constraint of the external ear may also result in asymmetric overgrowth of the ear.[1] Ear enlargement is commonly observed on the side opposite the muscular torticollis in torticollis-plagiocephaly deformation sequence (Fig. 22-3). On the side of the tightened sternocleidomastoid muscle, the ear is usually measurably smaller,

with an uplifted lobe due to pressure from the shoulder. In nonsynostotic deformational posterior plagiocephaly, the position of the ear is also displaced anteriorly on the side toward which the head is turned (as the occiput on that side becomes flattened with persistent supine positioning). Such ear malposition usually corrects with timely and appropriate treatment of the torticollis-plagiocephaly deformation sequence. Similarly, the vertical position of the ear can be lowered with unilateral coronal or lambdoidal craniosynostosis, and it also corrects with timely and appropriate surgical correction (Fig. 22-4).

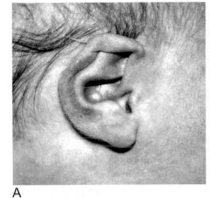
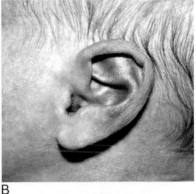

FIGURE 22-1. Constraint-induced overfolding of the scapha holix (**A**) and partial crumpling of the concha (**B**). In a more severe example of abdominal pregnancy with prolonged oligohydramnios, the right ear is markedly enlarged due to compression, while the left ear is markedly crumpled. Respiratory insufficiency associated with oligohydramnios led to death shortly after birth.

A                           B

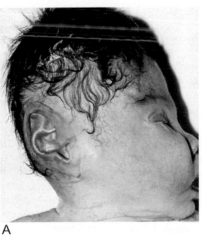
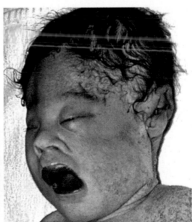

FIGURE 22-2. **A** and **B,** Crumpling of the helix as the result of late gestational constraint due to prolonged oligohydramnios associated with an ectopic abdominal pregnancy.

(Courtesy of Will Cochran, Beth Israel Hospital and Harvard Medical School, Boston, Mass.)

A                           B

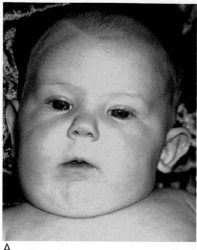
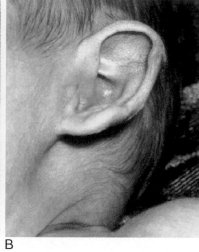

FIGURE 22-3. **A,** Uplifted left ear lobe caused by an oblique skewed head position in utero, with the left auricle between the head and left shoulder and the right ear compressed against the calvarium. **B,** Note the asymmetric overgrowth of the right ear and the prominent sulcus under the left mandible due to compression against the left shoulder.

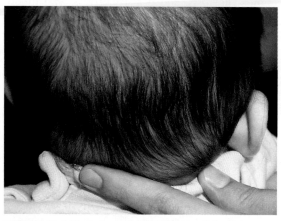

FIGURE 22-4. Posterior bony prominence of the right mastoid region with downward displacement of the right ear due to right lambdoid synostosis.

The incidence of ear deformation varies with age and the degree of attentiveness of the observer. Matsuo studied the ears of 1000 neonates over time and noted that more than 50% of the neonates had external ear shape abnormalities, most of which self-corrected during the first few months.[2] Extrinsic and intrinsic ear muscles play a role in shaping ears and may overcome the impact of fetal head constraint in many instances.[2,3] For example, Stahl's ear (third crus) was noted in 47% of neonates but only seen in 7% of the same infants at 1 year of age. On the other hand, protruding ears were only seen in 0.4% of neonates, but 5.5% of the same infants

had protruding ears at 1 year of age, usually due to persistently turning the head toward one side while being maintained in a supine sleeping position.[2] These researchers noted that when constriction was accompanied by a lop ear deformity, it was unlikely to correct spontaneously over time.

Inactivity of the posterior auricular muscles with associated loss of facial nerve function in Möbius syndrome leads to prominent ears, which suggests that some ear deformities result from aberrant neuromuscular function.[2] Maternal relaxing hormones that circulate prior to parturition can soften the cartilages of the fetus and neonate, making the auricles more susceptible to deforming external forces.[2] Based on this pliability of ear cartilage in the first few days after birth, many ear shape abnormalities can be corrected by splinting the ear into a normal shape with custom molds fashioned from polymer dental compound, thermoplastic materials, or flexible wire splints encased in plastic tubing and taped in place for the first few weeks.[2,4-7] Such splinting is much less effective and generally requires longer treatment periods when initiated in older children.[7] The elasticity of ear cartilages affects successful treatment more than does age, and ear cartilages tend to lose elasticity with age. Many types of congenital auricular deformities are caused by abnormalities in intrinsic and extrinsic ear muscles, with shortened muscles increasing the prominence of cartilages. Thus, shortened muscles can be corrected by mechanical stretching with a splint, but stretched muscles are more difficult to shorten by splinting.[8]

## FEATURES

Ears are often crumpled and distorted by late gestational forces, and their folded forms reflect the impact of these deforming forces. If an ear can be straightened out beneath a plate of clear glass or plastic so that all of its normal cartilaginous landmarks can be identified, this suggests the presence of deformations rather than malformations. Some minor ear shape abnormalities can be inherited in an autosomal dominant pattern, which is readily ascertained by inspection of the parents' ears. Other ear shape anomalies and malformations should prompt a search for other anomalies that might suggest the presence of a recognizable syndrome, such as oculoauriculovertebral sequence, branchiootorenal syndrome, Treacher-Collins syndrome, or CHARGE (*colo-oloboma, *h*eart defect, *a*tresia choanae, *r*etarded growth and development and/or central nervous system abnormalities, *g*enital hypoplasia, and *e*ar anomalies and/or deafness) syndrome.[9,10] In a recent series of 1000 patients with branchial arch malformations resulting in microtia, 36.5% had obvious soft tissue and bony abnormalities suggesting hemifacial microsomia, 15.2% had facial nerve weakness, 2.5% had macrostomia, 4.3% had cleft lip and/or palate, 4% had urogenital defects, 2.5% had cardiovascular abnormalities, and 1.7% had other anomalies such as cervical vertebral abnormalities.[11] Microtia occurs in 1:5000 live births and is more frequently right-sided (58.2%) than left-sided (32.4%) or bilateral (9.4%), and it is found more frequently in males (63.1%).[11]

## MANAGEMENT AND PROGNOSIS

A return to normal auricular form within the first few postnatal days tends to confirm the deformational origin of such ear defects, which usually require no management. When the ear is abnormally crumpled into a form that is unlikely to resolve within the first day or so, wax molds or thermoplastic splints can be individually fashioned and taped in place (Figs. 22-5 to 22-7). This is most effective if done in the first few days of life, while the ear cartilage is still relatively soft and pliable as a consequence of maternal relaxing hormones still circulating in the neonatal bloodstream.[2,4-8] When a child's ear was protruded laterally because of torticollis-plagiocephaly deformation sequence, one parent with an engineering background designed a modification for the child's cranial orthotic device that compressed

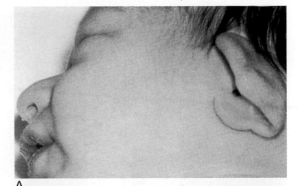

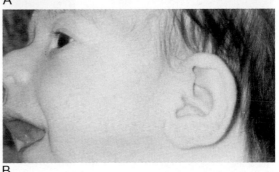

FIGURE 22-5. **A,** Overfolded auricle secondary to constraint during an asymmetric breech presentation in a septate uterus. **B,** Twelve weeks later, the auricle has largely returned to normal form. Taping the ear may accelerate the process of reformation.

the protruding auricles against the adjacent cranium (Fig. 22-8). Microtia requires surgical correction (Fig. 22-9), which is usually done around 6 years of age before correction of any associated canal atresia or mandibular asymmetry is attempted.[5,11] It is extremely important to assess a child with auricular malformations for the possibility of associated hearing loss.[9,10] This can be done safely and effectively in young infants through otoacoustic emission evaluations, which can detect malfunction of cochlear hair cells at hearing thresholds >35 decibels, or by auditory brainstem responses, which can detect neurologic hearing losses >80 decibels.[12] Early amplification is extremely important for the normal development of speech, and cochlear implantation in early childhood is indicated for children with severe or profound cochlear deafness.[12]

## DIFFERENTIAL DIAGNOSIS

Aberrations of ear form caused by defects in the development and/or function of intrinsic or

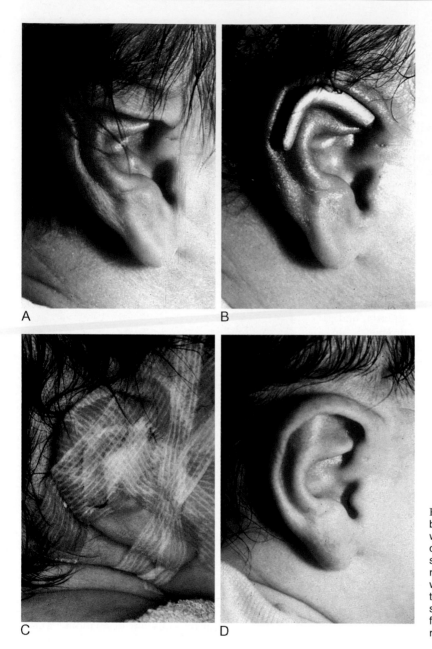

A

B

C

D

FIGURE 22-6. Crumpled ears can be re-formed with the aid of dental wax molds. **A,** Initial Stahl's ear deformity that had also been present in the infant's mother, who required surgical correction. Dental wax molds were applied to reshape the ear **(B)** and were taped securely in place **(C)**. **D,** The ear form remained normal after removal of taping and wax molds.

extrinsic auricular ear muscles, such as protruding auricle or lop ear, usually do not improve after birth. Ear malformations that result from deficient cartilaginous support seldom improve and may be associated with a significant risk for hearing loss and renal anomalies.[9,10] A truly low-set ear is a very rare malformation, but vertical or anterior displacement is quite common and usually is a consequence of associated cranial abnormalities such as deformational plagiocephaly or lambdoid craniosynostosis. Some types of ear deformities spontaneously resolve on their own without treatment, such as the characteristic ear swelling seen in diastrophic dysplasia (Fig. 22-10).

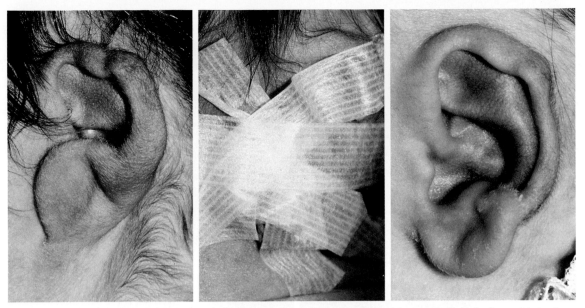

FIGURE 22-7. This crumpled ear in an infant with Turner's syndrome was corrected nonsurgically by taping molds in place to correct the abnormally folded ears.

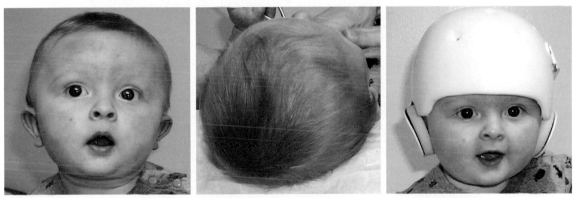

FIGURE 22-8. When his infant's ear protruded laterally because of brachycephaly with a head turn to the right, a parent with an engineering background designed a modification for the cranial orthotic device, which compressed the protruding auricle against the adjacent cranium.

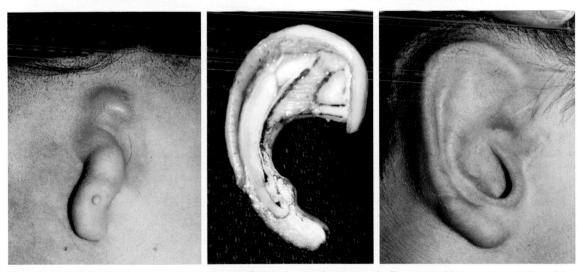

FIGURE 22-9. This microtic ear in a child with hemifacial microsomia was surgically corrected by carving a portion of the child's rib cartilage into a normal auricular form, sliding this form under the skin, and using the ear tag to help form an ear lobe. (Courtesy of Dr. Robert Ruder, Cedar-Sinai Medical Center.)

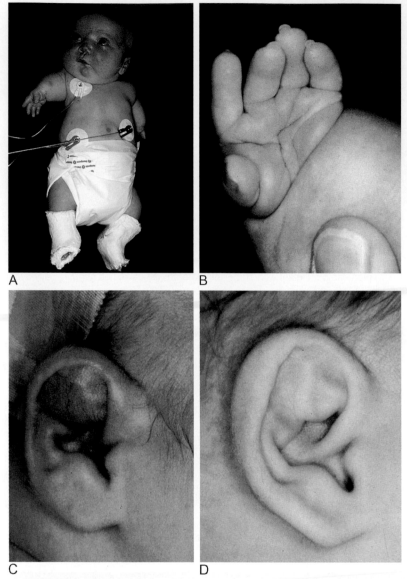

FIGURE 22-10. This child with diastrophic dysplasia (**A** and **B**) developed character-istic ear swellings shortly after birth **(C)**, which gradually resolved over the first few months without treatment **(D)**.

## References

1. Aase JM: Structural defects as a consequence of late intrauterine constraint: craniotabes, loose skin, and asymmetric ear size, *Semin Perinatol* 7:270–273, 1983.
2. Matsuo K, Hayashi R, Kiyono M, et al: Nonsurgical correction of congenital auricular deformities, *Clin Plast Surg* 17:383–395, 1990.
3. Smith DW, Takashima H: Ear muscles and ear form, *Birth Defects Orig Artic Ser* 16:299–302, 1980.
4. Brown FE, Cohen LB, Addante RR, et al: Correction of congenital auricular deformities by splinting in the neonatal period, *Pediatrics* 78:406–411, 1986.
5. Ruder RO, Graham JM Jr: Evaluation and treatment of the deformed and malformed auricle, *Clin Pediatr* 35:461–465, 1996.
6. Yotsuyanagi T, Yokoi K, Urushidate S, et al: Nonsurgical correction of congenital auricular deformities in children older than early neonates, *Plast Reconstr Surg* 101:907–914, 1998.
7. Furnas DW: Nonsurgical treatment of auricular deformities in neonates and infants, *Pediatr Ann* 28:387–390, 1999.
8. Yotsuyanagi T: Nonsurgical correction of congenital auricular deformities in children older than early neonates, *Plast Reconstr Surg* 114:190–191, 2004.

9. Wang R, Earl DL, Ruder RO, et al: Syndromic ear anomalies and renal ultrasounds, *Pediatrics* 108:E32, 2001.

10. Wang R, Martinez-Frias ML, Graham JM Jr: Infants of diabetic mothers are at increased risk for the oculo-auriculo-vertebral sequence: a case-based and case-control approach, *J Pediatr* 141:611–617, 2002.

11. Brent B: The pediatrician's role in caring for patients with congenital microtia and atresia, *Pediatr Ann* 28:374–383, 1999.

12. Slattery WH, Fayad JN: Cochlear implants in children with sensorineural inner ear hearing loss, *Pediatr Ann* 28:359–363, 1999.

# 23 Mandibular Deformation

## GENESIS

Compression of the chin against the chest or intrauterine structures may limit the growth of the jaw prior to birth, and when asymmetric, jaw retrusion is more commonly left-sided (Fig. 23-1). If the compression is of prolonged duration, there may be pressure indentation or skin necrosis on the upper thoracic surface. As shown in Fig. 23-1, one deformational cause of asymmetric mandibular growth deficiency is prolonged oligohydramnios. Asymmetric mandibular growth deficiency with a laterally tilted mandible is most commonly the result of head rotation with one side of the mandible compressed against the shoulder or chest, and it is commonly associated with muscular

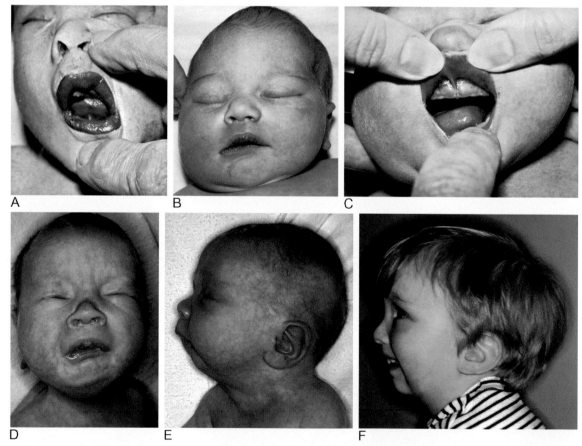

FIGURE 23-1. **A,** This infant was delivered abdominally from an extrauterine location behind the uterus with marked distortion of the face and jaw. Respiratory insufficiency associated with oligohydramnios led to death shortly after birth. **B** and **C,** This infant was also an abdominal pregnancy; her head was under the mother's stomach, and her feet were under the gallbladder. **D** to **F,** This infant experienced prolonged oligohydramnios with transverse lie due to premature rupture of amnion at 26 weeks, with delivery at 36 weeks. **D** and **E,** There is striking mandibular growth restriction with necrotic neck folds. **F,** At age 30 months, mandibular growth deficiency persisted. (**A–C,** Courtesy of Will Cochran, Beth Israel Hospital and Harvard Medical School, Boston, Mass.)

torticollis on the same side as the deficient mandible (Fig. 23-2). Such asymmetric mandibular growth deficiency is often the first indication that an infant might have associated congenital muscular torticollis.

If the ear on the side of the small jaw is dysplastic or microtic, or if there are associated ear tags or epibulbar dermoids, the diagnosis of oculoauriculovertebral sequence (OAVS) should be considered (Fig. 23-3). OAVS is etiologically

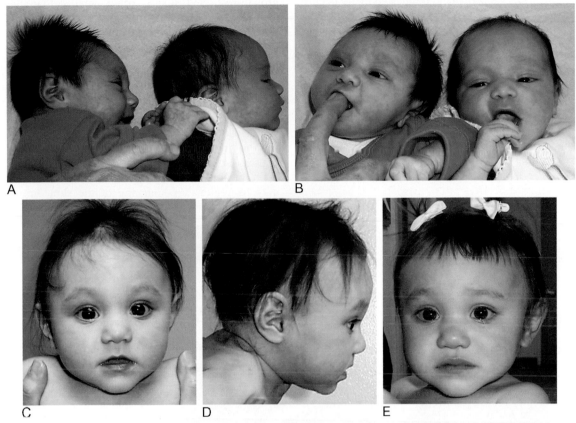

A   B

C   D   E

FIGURE 23-2. These twins were born at term to a primigravida woman; the left twin was carried in a prolonged vertex presentation low in the uterus. This twin had severe congenital left muscular torticollis at birth **(A, B),** which responded well to neck physical therapy, although mild jaw asymmetry was still evident at age 7 months **(C–E).**

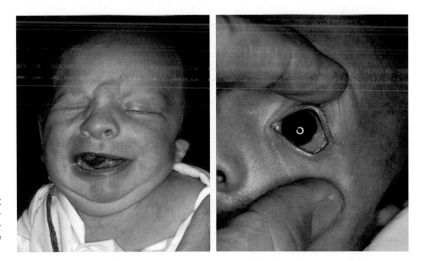

FIGURE 23-3. This infant has left hemifacial microsomia with mandibular growth deficiency, epibulbar dermoid, and microtia on the left.

heterogeneous, and a careful family and gestational history, renal ultrasound, and cervical vertebral radiographs may help evaluate the possibility of an associated syndrome (Figs. 23-4 to 23-6).[1,2] Muscular torticollis with mandibular asymmetry results from late gestational fetal constraint, whereas OAVS with mandibular asymmetry occurs in early gestation as part of a malformation syndrome. Symmetric undergrowth of the jaw occurs with Pierre Robin malformation sequence with associated posterior cleft palate and glossoptosis (Fig. 23-7), which can also be etiologically heterogeneous. Skin redundancy under the chin suggests pressure-induced growth restriction of the jaw, especially when there is no associated cleft posterior palate (Fig. 23-8), whereas unilateral mandibular growth deficiency with an associated sulcus that corresponds with compression by the shoulder suggests congenital muscular torticollis (see Fig. 22-3, A).

## FEATURES

In constraint-related mandibular growth restriction associated with torticollis, the head is often tilted toward the growth-restricted mandible while the chin points toward the other side. The ear on the growth-restricted side is often smaller than the other ear, and there may be a prominent mandibular sulcus, with an upward cant to the mandible on that same side (see Figs. 23-1 and 23-2). Neck rotation is often restricted. These features warrant early neck physical therapy once concerns about any possible structural cervical spine anomalies have been resolved through careful physical examination and radiographs, if necessary. With symmetric jaw deficiency due to a face presentation or transverse lie, retroflexion of the head with a prominent occipital shelf may be noted. With prolonged compression of the jaw, there may be regional redundancy of the skin due to

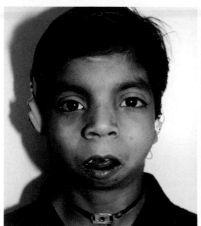
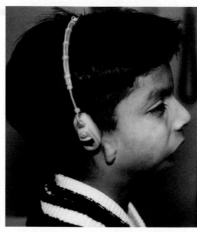

FIGURE 23-4. This boy has branchiootorenal syndrome with deafness, bilateral mandibular deficiency, microtia, conjunctival dermoids, and branchial cleft cysts; he was initially diagnosed with familial Goldenhar's syndrome.

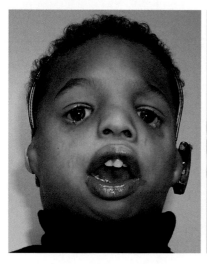
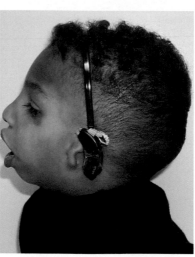

FIGURE 23-5. This child has Treacher Collins syndrome with microtia, deafness, malar clefts, down-slanting palpebral fissures, mandibular growth deficiency, and cleft palate.

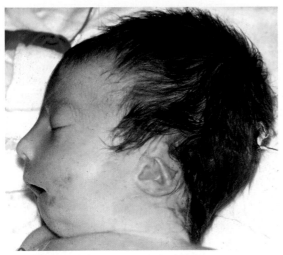

FIGURE 23-6. This child has CHARGE syndrome with characteristic dysplastic ears lacking lobes, sensorineural deafness, bilateral choanal atresia, micrognathia, cleft palate, DiGeorge sequence, genital hypoplasia, and tetralogy of Fallot.

constraint-induced overgrowth of the skin in that region (Fig. 23-9). This skin redundancy is usually not present if the mandibular growth deficiency is due to an underlying syndrome. If there are associated ear malformations or if the neck is wide and short with limited mobility, the possibility of cervical spine anomalies should be considered.

## MANAGEMENT AND PROGNOSIS

If there is associated congenital muscular torticollis, early neck physical therapy with frequent variation of the infant's sleeping position should be initiated to prevent the development of secondary deformational posterior plagiocephaly.[3,4] Because the infant's neck does not begin to extend vertically until the second half of the first year, asymmetric mandibular growth restriction may be difficult to detect in young infants, but parents may note that the eye on the side of the

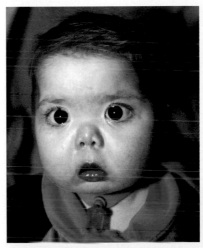
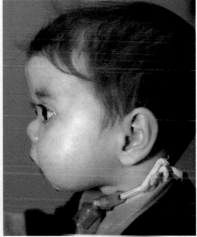

FIGURE 23-7. This child has Stickler syndrome with deafness, Pierre Robin malformation sequence, flat nasal bridge, and severe myopia.

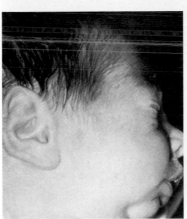
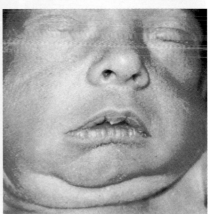

FIGURE 23-8. This infant has mandibular growth deficiency due to jaw compression. Note the redundancy of skin secondary to constraint-induced overgrowth of skin.

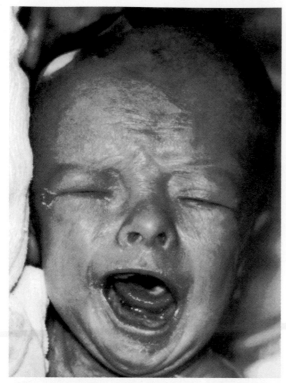

FIGURE 23-9. This neonate has marked jaw asymmetry due to unilateral shoulder compression in utero.

growth-restricted mandible appears to open less widely due to vertical displacement of the soft tissues of the cheek when the mandible is compressed against the chest on that side. Failure to treat muscular torticollis appropriately can result in marked, persistent mandibular asymmetry, facial

scoliosis, and rotatory cervical spine subluxation.[5-7] With effective treatment of the torticollis, most of the associated jaw asymmetry usually resolves by the end of the second year (Fig. 23-10). There is also an association between hemifacial microsomia and craniofaciocervical scoliosis when associated underlying cervical vertebral anomalies are present.[8,9] Infants with cervical vertebral anomalies resulting in torticollis benefit from early cranial orthotic therapy in an effort to prevent or at least minimize craniofacial deformation. Such orthotic molding should begin during the first few months and continue through the second year. When mandibular growth deficiency is symmetric and a consequence of abnormal fetal presentation, it may resolve with little more than gentle mandibular massage, but if compression has been prolonged and severe, mandibular growth deficiency may persist (see Fig. 23-1).

## DIFFERENTIAL DIAGNOSIS

Micrognathia is an associated feature in a number of malformation syndromes (see Figs. 23-3 to 23-7). Mandibular asymmetry may occur with OAVS. Striking mandibular growth deficiency can be associated with a posterior cleft palate and glossoptosis in the Pierre Robin malformation sequence, which is etiologically heterogeneous.[10,11] Among 117 patients with Pierre Robin malformation sequence, 31% had an underlying syndrome; Stickler syndrome, Treacher Collins syndrome, velocardiofacial syndrome, chromosomal disorders, and teratogenic disorders accounted for about half of these

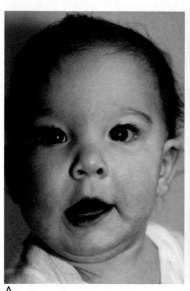

A

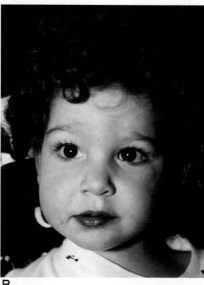

B

FIGURE 23-10. This child was born with left congenital muscular torticollis and had asymmetric mandibular deficiency on the side of the torticollis (A), which resolved by age 2 years (B).

syndromes. Another 20% had associated malformations affecting the skeleton, heart, eye, and central nervous system, which resulted in mental retardation in 67% of these cases, whereas 49% were isolated.[11] Thus, a careful search for associated anomalies often reveals the presence of other anomalies that might lead to the diagnosis of an associated syndrome.

## References

1. Wang R, Earl DL, Ruder RO, et al: Syndromic ear anomalies and renal ultrasounds, *Pediatrics* 108:E32, 2001.
2. Wang R, Martinez-Frias ML, Graham JM Jr: Infants of diabetic mothers are at increased risk for the oculo-auriculo-vertebral sequence: a case-based and case-control approach, *J Pediatr* 141:611–617, 2002.
3. Persing J, James H, Swanson J, et al: Prevention and management of positional skull deformities in infants, *Pediatrics* 112:199–202, 2003 [Letters to the editor. *Pediatrics* 13:422–424, 2003].
4. Graham JM Jr, Gomez M, Halberg A, et al: Management of deformational plagiocephaly: repositioning versus orthotic therapy, *J Pediatr* 146:258–262, 2005.
5. Kane AA, Lo L-J, Vannier MW, et al: Mandibular dysmorphology in unicoronal synostosis and plagiocephaly without synostosis, *Cleft Palate Craniofac J* 33:418–423, 1996.
6. Putnam GG, Postlethwaite KR, Chate RA, et al: Facial scoliosis—a diagnostic dilemma, *Int J Oral Maxillofac Surg* 22:324–327, 1993.
7. Slate RK, Posnick JC, Armstrong DC, et al: Cervical spine subluxation associated with congenital muscular scoliosis and craniofacial asymmetry, *Plast Reconstr Surg* 91:1187–1195, 1993.
8. Poole MD, Briggs M: The cranio-facio-cervical scoliosis complex, *Br J Plast Surg* 43:670–675, 1990.
9. Padwa BL, Bruneteau RJ, Mulliken JB: Association between plagiocephaly and hemifacial microsomia, *Am J Med Genet* 47:1202–1207, 1993.
10. Cohen MM Jr: Robin sequences and complexes: causal heterogeneity and pathogenetic/phenotypic variability, *Am J Med Genet* 84:311–315, 1999.
11. Holder-Espinasse M, Abadie V, Cormier-Daire V, et al: Pierre Robin sequence: analysis of 117 consecutive cases, *J Pediatr* 139:588–590, 2001.

# 24 Congenital Muscular Torticollis

## GENESIS

The term *torticollis* is derived from the Latin terms *torus*, meaning "twisted," and *collum*, meaning "neck," and it refers to the posture that results from the head being twisted and turned to one side. This is most often due to a congenital asymmetry in the length and/or strength of the sternocleidomastoid (SCM) muscles on each side of the neck, which must be distinguished from acquired torticollis and from structural torticollis due to cervical vertebral anomalies. Prenatally acquired congenital muscular torticollis (CMT) is the most common type of torticollis, and when it remains partly or completely untreated, it results in facial asymmetry and plagiocephaly (see Chapter 25), which may be a presenting feature for CMT. According to Dunn, these conditions occurred together once in every 300 live births prior to 1974,[1] when infants were positioned on their stomachs for sleep and with their heads turned toward one side or the other. Since the "Back to Sleep" campaign was initiated in 1992 for the prevention of sudden infant death syndrome (SIDS), the frequency of deformational posterior plagiocephaly has increased. The reported incidence of torticollis among live births has varied from 0.3% in the United Kingdom to 1.9% in Japan, possibly reflecting differences in classification, methodology, and infant sleeping position.[1,2] Cheng and colleagues reported a 1.3% incidence of torticollis among Chinese children and studied outcomes in 1086 children with CMT who were classified into three groups according to severity (from most severe to least severe): 42.7% with a sternomastoid tumor, 30.6% with sternocleidomastoid tightness but no tumor, and 22.1% with postural torticollis who presented with congenital torticollis but no demonstrable tightness or tumor.[2]

CMT may occur as a consequence of early fetal head descent or an abnormal fetal position with the head tilted and turned, thereby resulting in muscle imbalance, with occasional associated deformations involving the back, hips, and feet (the intrauterine theory). More severe shortening and fibrosis of the muscle may be caused by venous occlusion from persistent lateral flexion and rotation of the neck (the vascular etiology) and/or trauma to the muscle during difficult deliveries (the birth trauma theory).[1] Many clinical studies have demonstrated that infants with CMT are more commonly first-born and have an increased incidence of other deformations, such as metatarsus adductus, developmental dysplasia of the hip, and talipes equinovarus.[3] Histology of affected muscles has demonstrated replacement of muscle by dense fibrous tissue, and when magnetic resonance imaging (MRI) was used to study the affected muscle, altered signal characteristics suggested that CMT might be caused by sequelae of an intrauterine or perinatal sternomastoid compartment syndrome.[3] In cadaver studies, flexion with lateral bending and rotation of the head and neck caused the ipsilateral sternomastoid muscle to kink on itself, resulting in ischemia and edema within the sternomastoid muscle compartment. When birth histories were compared with MRI findings, the side of birth presentation correlated with the side of the torticollis.[3]

The intrauterine theory concerning the etiology of CMT (which does not exclude the compartment theory) is based on epidemiologic data and emphasizes the concept that CMT is one of a group of associated deformations arising from malposition of the fetus during the third trimester.[1] This theory relies on the association between unilateral hip dislocation, CMT, infantile idiopathic scoliosis, and plagiocephaly (see Chapter 20 for a discussion of scoliosis and the molded baby syndrome). It is suggested that the ipsilateral coexistence of a *t*urned head, *a*dduction contracture of the hip, and truncal *c*urvature (TAC syndrome) indicates a specific intrauterine asymmetric posture of the fetus (see Figs. 20-1 and 24-1).[4] Based on a study of 108 infants born with the clinical triad of TAC syndrome, this condition occurs in 5.8 per 1000 live births with a preponderance of females, first-born children, winter births, low birth weights, children born to mothers with small abdominal circumference, and first-born children of mothers of advanced maternal age. The frequency of change of position in utero was significantly reduced from that in normal fetuses, and the side of fetal position

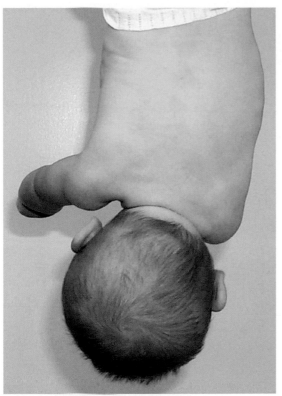

FIGURE 24-1. When a young infant is suspended upside down by holding the feet and ankles securely above an examination table, any generalized tightness of the neck or trunk musculature will cause the infant's neck and body to curve toward the tight side. This infant suspension test can be used to monitor the course of physical therapy, and it will often show differences between multiple gestation infants according to the degree of gestational constraint each fetus experienced. Normally, an infant with no muscular asymmetry should hang straight down like a plumb bob. This infant has left CMT with associated curvature of the trunk (idiopathic infantile scoliosis) and mild deformational posterior plagiocephaly. The coexistence of TAC syndrome suggests the specific intrauterine asymmetric posture of this infant as a fetus. He responded well to physical therapy with repositioning.

correlated with the side of the TAC syndrome. When the left side of the fetus in vertex presentation was against the mother's spine, with the back on the left, the hip adduction contracture and torticollis were also on the left; the reverse was true when the back of the fetus was on the mother's right side.[4]

Interstitial fibrosis of the muscle is sometimes palpable as a fusiform fibrous mass or "tumor" that becomes evident within the first 3 weeks after birth and reaches maximum size by age 1 month.[5] This mass is composed of myoblasts, fibroblasts, myofibroblasts, and mesenchyme-like cells that usually mature and differentiate, resulting in disappearance of the mass over the first 4 to 8 months of life with variable sequelae.[6] Such

masses usually involve the lower two thirds of the muscle, and their evolution can be followed by ultrasound,[7] which also allows for simultaneous ultrasound screening for hip dysplasia.[8] Hip dysplasia occurred in 17% of 47 infants confirmed to have CMT by ultrasound, although only 8.5% of these infants required treatment with a Pavlik harness or surgery.[8] If myoblasts in the mass differentiate in a normal way, the mass will disappear and conservative treatment with neck physical therapy will have a high likelihood of success; however, if the myoblasts degenerate and the remaining fibroblasts produce excess collagen, the result may be a scar-like band that is visible by ultrasound and causes muscular contracture. Myoblasts can be mechanically stimulated to undergo hypertrophy and hyperplasia in vitro by intermittent stretching and relaxation, and the proper orientation of skeletal fibers during myogenesis is maintained by rhythmic contractions.[9-11] Thus, there is good physiologic justification for the early initiation of neck physical therapy to prevent muscle fibrosis.

A number of associated features suggest that CMT is related to late gestational constraint. The laterality of the birth head position usually matches the laterality of the torticollis.[3,4,12] In most series, there is a slight excess of males and of left-sided involvement, possibly reflecting the predilection for most fetuses to be in the left occiput transverse presentation.[2,13-18] If combinations of CMT with hip dysplasia are considered, there is a slight excess of females. Females may be protected from torticollis for the same reasons that make them more susceptible to developmental dysplasia of the hip. The female fetus is more lax than the male, possibly due to the lack of testosterone effect in the female fetus, or it may be that ligaments are more relaxed in females than males due to differential receptor responses to relaxing hormones in late gestation. CMT is also more common with multiple gestation.[12,18] Without treatment, the shortened muscle tends to maintain the aberrant posture of the head and neck, with the head tilted toward the affected side and the chin rotated toward the opposite side. This results in deformational posterior plagiocephaly with a rhomboid head shape that can progress in severity if the infant's head remains turned toward one side. Early physical therapy, frequent "tummy time" when the infant is awake and under adult observation, and head repositioning onto the more prominent occiput can prevent many of these secondary positional craniofacial effects. Eventually, uncorrected torticollis has the potential to result in permanent craniofacial asymmetry, but surgical correction of torticollis need not be attempted until after at least 6 months of neck physical therapy has failed to correct the torticollis or the muscle has clearly become fibrotic.

## FEATURES

Characteristically, the infant manifests lateral head and neck flexion toward one shoulder, with the ear lobule on that side uplifted and the jaw canted upward due to compression against the shoulder or chest (see Figs. 22-3 and 23-2). The head is tilted toward the tighter, shorter SCM muscle, with the chin turned away. CMT can be difficult to diagnose at birth because of the normal shortness of the neck in a neonate, but it becomes more evident as the neck lengthens during the second 6 months of life. Jaw asymmetry may be the first indication that CMT is present, and some mothers note that the infant has difficulty turning the head to nurse equally from both breasts or that one eye appears to be more closed than the other due to upward displacement of cheek soft tissues as the jaw rests against the chest on the side of the torticollis (see Figs. 23-2 and 24-2). The ear is usually noticeably smaller on the side of the torticollis, having been relatively protected by the shoulder from the uterine compression experienced by the other ear. When the infant is held in suspension with the head down (see Fig. 24-1), the neck and trunk often flex toward the tight side, as mentioned previously in the discussion of idiopathic infantile scoliosis (see Chapter 20). SCM muscle imbalance is part of a spectrum of CMT that includes muscle length/ strength asymmetry at one end and muscle shortening and fibrosis at the other end. With consistent supine positioning, the occiput on the side toward which the head is turned becomes progressively flattened, displacing the ear and forehead forward on the side opposite the torticollis (Fig. 24-2). When infants customarily slept in prone position, the natural tendency to turn the head toward each side helped correct many cases of postural torticollis, and many torticollis treatment programs emphasize a prone sleeping position with the head turned toward the side of the torticollis to help maintain the corrected posture.[2,13,14] Such a prone sleeping position can only be used if the baby has had sufficient tummy time and physical therapy to gain adequate head control in a prone position. Prone sleepers with an uncorrected, consistent head turn will develop deformational plagiocephaly with frontal flattening on the same side as the torticollis; thus prone positioning without physical therapy is

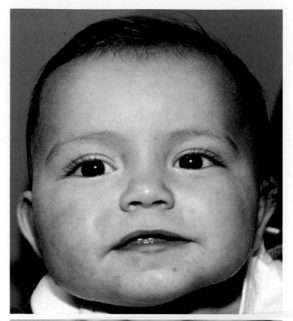

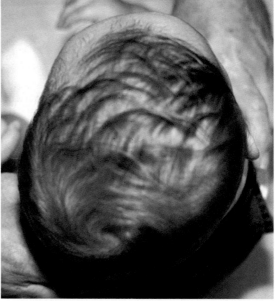

FIGURE 24-2. This infant has untreated left muscular torticollis at age 9 months, with associated deformational posterior plagiocephaly due to a persistent head turn to the right and associated left mandibular hypoplasia due to a persistent head tilt to the left. He responded well to physical therapy and cranial orthotic therapy.

unsafe and ineffective (Fig. 24-3). In the newborn infant with CMT, the position of comfort is usually with the head tilted toward the tight side and the chin turned away. A careful examination for hip dysplasia and truncal curvature is merited so that physical therapy can be directed toward correcting this asymmetric resting position.

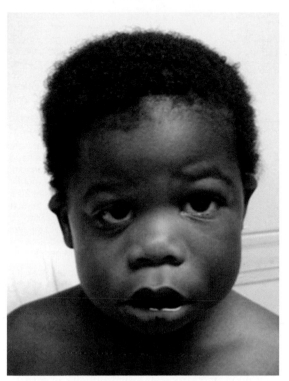

FIGURE 24-3. This 12-month-old boy has untreated right muscular torticollis with right facial flattening because he slept prone with his face turned to the left. He was considered too old to benefit from cranial orthotic therapy, but he responded well to physical therapy, with improved neck range of motion. His parents were instructed to position him for sleep in prone position with his head turned to the right.

Dunn has shown that torticollis is commonly associated with plagiocephaly, facial deformities, ipsilateral mandibular asymmetry, and positional foot deformities, and among infants with CMT, 56% were first-born (versus an expected 35% frequency) and 20% were in breech presentation (versus an expected 5% frequency); additionally, there was an association with oligohydramnios.[1] CMT occurs in 22% to 40% of infants born after difficult labors and deliveries, with the lower figure reflecting improved recent obstetric management.[14,15] Developmental dysplasia of the hip that requires orthopedic management occurs in 8% to 10% of children with CMT.[*] These findings implicate late gestational fetal constraint as a primary cause of torticollis, which also occurs frequently with multiple gestation (usually affecting the fetus who is bottom-most in the uterus) and with uterine structural abnormalities.[18]

*See references 2, 4, 8, 13, 14, 16, and 17.

## MANAGEMENT AND PROGNOSIS

Most cases of CMT are treated conservatively using active and passive neck-stretching exercises with repositioning so as to encourage head turning toward the less-preferred side (Fig. 24-4).[2,12-18] Because the SCM muscle has a vertical component as well as a horizontal (or rotational) component, the muscle must be actively stretched in both directions. In most instances it is best to stretch the muscle in both directions on both sides so as to achieve full and symmetric range of motion. For vertical stretching of a tight right CMT, position the infant in a supine position on a firm surface and push down on the right shoulder with one hand while slowly and evenly bringing the left ear toward the left shoulder; reverse the procedure for a tight left CMT. In right torticollis, the head is turned to the left, so neck rotation needs to be encouraged by placing a forearm across the upper chest and rotating the chin toward the right shoulder; the procedure is reversed for left torticollis. Each stretch for each of the four directions should be held for 30 to 60 seconds, and it is best to make it a habit to do these exercises with each diaper change so that the exercises are performed six to eight times per day.[18] Sudden giving-way or snapping of the sternomastoid muscle was observed with manual stretching in 8% of 452 patients with a sternomastoid tumor, particularly in infants younger than 1 month, with left-sided involvement and associated hip dysplasia. This snapping was associated with clinical signs of bruising and an increased range of motion, suggesting possible rupture of the muscle, but it was not associated with any increased need for operative treatment; also, 95% of patients with snapping had good or excellent results, which was not significantly different from those patients without snapping.[2]

Passive neck stretching can be facilitated by placing the infant on his or her stomach and directing the infant's gaze and head up and out on each side so that his or her chin and eyes follow an attractive object in a playful manner. Other forms of neck-stretching exercises consist of cradling the infant in one arm while gently rocking the infant and stretching the neck in each of the four directions. Some infants enjoy being held up by the ankles while gently bending the infant's head away from the shoulder while the head is against a firm surface or mattress. This exercise is especially helpful for vertical stretching, which is sometimes the most difficult direction to stretch.

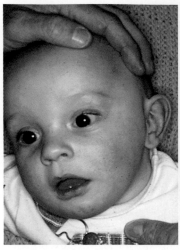 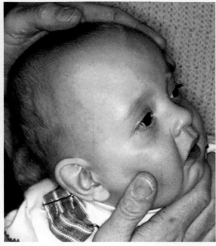

FIGURE 24-4. To restore SCM muscle symmetry and prevent progressive plagiocephaly, neck-stretching exercises should be done at least six times daily, preferably with each diaper change. For left torticollis, gently turn the infant's head toward the left side and try to get the chin slightly past the left shoulder. For the neck stretch, place your right hand on the infant's left shoulder, with your other hand on the left side of the infant's head. Gently stretch the neck, bringing the right ear to the right shoulder. Hold each stretch for at least 20 to 30 seconds. (Diagrams demonstrating stretching exercises for CMT can be found on the Orthoseek Web site at http://www.orthoseek. com/articles/congenmt.html.)

Encouraging the infant to feed toward his or her non-preferred side is another technique of passive neck stretching. Early encouragement of tummy time facilitates head turning and neck stretching, thereby helping prevent excessive brachycephaly or plagiocephaly as well as facilitating prone motor skills.[18]

If initiated before age 3 months, conservative treatment is very effective in restoring full range of motion, with minimal infant facial asymmetry in fully compliant families.[2,13,18] Severity of restricted lateral neck rotation and presence of a large palpable tumor are associated with a prolonged need for physical therapy and sometimes with the need for surgical correction.[13] Among 100 infants with CMT, the mean age of initial assessment for 25 infants with a palpable mass was 1.9 months versus 4.7 months for those without a mass. The mean duration of treatment to obtain full range of motion was 4.7 months, with a longer mean duration of treatment for those presenting with a mass (6.9 months for those with a mass versus 3.9 months for those without a mass). For those infants with a significant head tilt at 4.5 months, a tubular orthosis can be used to help correct vertical head position. Among 30 infants with a significant head tilt at 4.5 months, the mean duration of treatment was 7.2 months (versus 3.6 months for those without such head tilts). Thus, the more severe the neck restriction, the longer the required duration of conservative treatment to achieve full range of motion.[13] In other series, conservative treatment was successful in 95% of cases, with surgical correction undertaken only in resistant cases.[2,13-18]

When the severity of CMT was measured by the degree of limitation in passive neck rotation, the need for surgery was associated with patients who completed at least 6 months of manual stretching and still manifested deficits in passive rotation or lateral bending greater than 15 degrees.[2] Infants with a sternomastoid tumor were found to present earlier (within the first 3 months) and the group was associated with the highest incidences of breech presentation (19.5%), difficult labor (56%), and congenital hip dysplasia (6.8%).[21] Severity of limitation in neck rotation was significantly correlated with the presence of a sternomastoid tumor, larger tumor size, hip dysplasia, degree of head tilt, and craniofacial asymmetry. Infants with less than 10 degrees of limitation in passive neck rotation were treated at home with an active stimulation and positioning program. Infants with more than 10 degrees of limitation in passive neck rotation were treated with manual stretching three times per week by experienced physiotherapists. Those infants who failed to respond or improve after 6 months of physiotherapy with manual stretching were treated surgically with a unipolar open release and partial excision of the clavicular and sternal heads of the sternomastoid muscle. Malpresentation was noted in 14.6% of 1086 cases (13% breech, 1.6% other than breech or vertex presentation), hip dysplasia was found in 4.1%, foot deformations were noted in 6.5%, and craniofacial asymmetry was noted in 90.1%. There was a slight increase in left-sided torticollis (53%) and a 3:2 incidence of males to females. For the sternomastoid tumor group, the tumor occurred in the lower third in 35%, in the middle third in 40.4%, in the upper third in 11.9%, and over the entire muscle in 12.6%. The tumors ranged in size from 1 to 4 cm, and more than 70% of tumors were larger than 2 cm. Tumors were usually detected at 2 weeks, increased in size for the next 2 weeks, and then disappeared by 5 to 8 months. Cases requiring surgery were associated with late age at presentation, sternomastoid tumor, and more severe limitation in rotation. None of the patients with positional torticollis required surgery, and successful early treatment of CMT prevented secondary plagiocephaly.[19-22]

Indications for surgery include incorrect head posture persisting after 12 months (Figs. 24-5 to 24-7) and/or muscle fibrosis persisting after age 6 months (with reduced activity of the involved muscle demonstrated by electromyography).[21] Ultrasound has been useful in following sterno-mastoid pseudotumors, and ultrasound, MRI, and computed tomography (CT) have all been used to confirm fibrous replacement and predict the need for surgical correction (see Fig. 24-7).[7,23-25] In most cases, ultrasonography is the most cost-effective method for imaging and following ster-nomastoid changes.[24,25] Surgical management consists of tenotomy, unipolar or bipolar releases, or complete resection of the fibrotic muscle through incisions near the muscular insertions on the sternum and clavicle or near the origin on the mastoid bone, where the incision can be hidden in the hairline behind the ear.[26-28] Recent techniques emphasize smaller incisions and minimally invasive techniques via endoscopy, with early institution of postoperative physical therapy and splinting of the neck with a soft cervical collar.[27,28] Because early physical therapy is effective in the vast majority of CMT cases, there is scl-

dom any indication for surgery before the end of the first year since deformational posterior plagiocephaly can be prevented by persistent repositioning prior to 5 months and cranial ortho-sis is effective for most refractory cases after age 6 months.[18]

Failure to treat muscular torticollis can result in persistent mandibular asymmetry, facial scolio-sis, deformational plagiocephaly, and rotatory cervical spine subluxation on the side contralateral to the muscular torticollis (see Figs. 24-6 and 24-7).[29-32] The strict definition for CMT requires the presence of muscle fibrosis or a palpable knot, which may not be seen after the first month or so, but muscle imbalance is extremely common and is found in at least 64% of infants with deforma-tional plagiocephaly.[12] Among 232 patients with CMT, 82% had the diagnosis first established before age 3 months, but 87 children required sur-gery for CMT after the age of 12 months (mean age of surgery, 6 to 7 years). Breech presentation was reported in 28% of these 232 patients. Of those patients requiring surgery, classic features of CMT included head tilt (81%); limited range of motion (58%); an easily palpable, tight band in the area of the SCM muscle (33%); facial asymmetry (62%); and plagiocephaly (20%). Sur-gery was only recommended after physical ther-apy had failed in patients younger than 12 months or in patients who presented after that age with the previously described features.[31] Use of frontal cephalometric analysis or three-dimen-sional (3D) CT to assess craniofacial deformity in patients with late surgical correction of torticol-lis suggests that surgical treatment before age 5 to 6 years is most effective in preventing severe facial asymmetry, but neck range of motion could

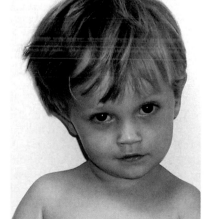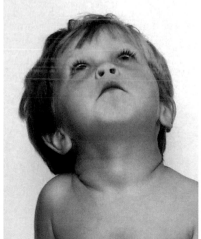

FIGURE 24-5. This boy has par-tially treated right muscular torti-collis at age 18 months. Because the deficits in lateral bending and neck rotation were less than 15 degrees, continued physical ther-apy was recommended with use of a tubular orthotic.

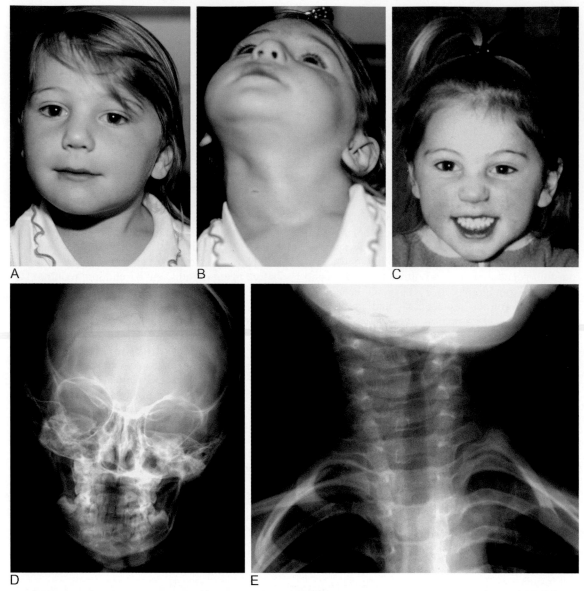

FIGURE 24-6. **A** and **B,** This 3-year-old girl *(top left and center)* has untreated severe torticollis-plagiocephaly deformation sequence with a fibrotic left SCM muscle and secondary deformation of her left lower face and clavicle. Her cranial diagonal difference was 2 cm with obvious right frontal prominence and a right epicanthal fold. She underwent surgical resection of her fibrotic SCM muscle through a hairline incision near her left mastoid bone. **C,** After surgery she received physical therapy and wore a cervical collar, resulting in much improved neck range of motion. **D** and **E,** Radiographs prior to surgery *(bottom left and right)* demonstrate obvious facial asymmetry with distortion of the left clavicular insertion point for the SCM muscle.

be improved by surgical correction at any age.[33,34] With untreated torticollis after age 3 years, there can be torsional rotation of the lower face toward the affected side, which starts with the mandible, progresses to involve the maxilla, and, ultimately, involves the orbits (see Figs. 24-6 and 24-7).[34]

Among 7609 Dutch infants screened in 1995 for positional plagiocephaly before age 6 months, the incidence of positional preference was 8.2% (n = 623), with flattening of the occiput noted in 10%, versus a 0.3% incidence of deformational plagiocephaly in Dunn's 1974 study of British infants.[1,35] These findings support the opinion that the prevalence of both positional preference and deformational plagiocephaly has risen dramatically in the past decade, with males more frequently

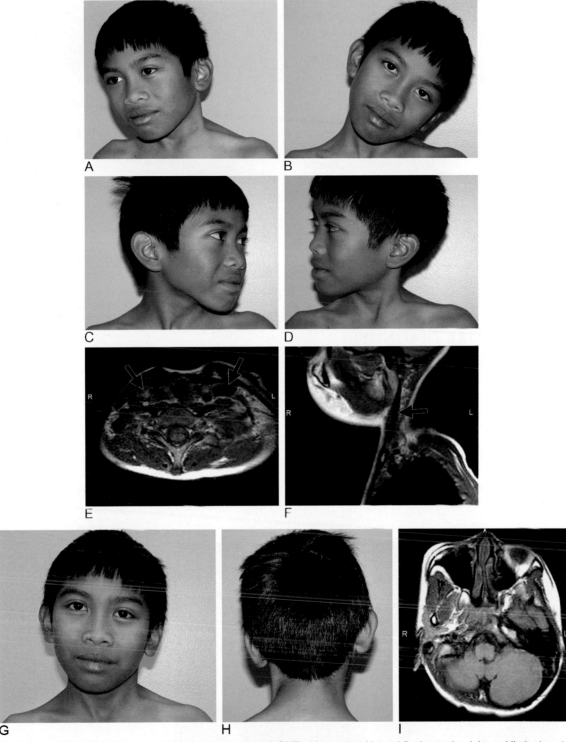

FIGURE 24-7. **A-D,** This 11-year-old boy has untreated left CMT with restricted lateral flexion to the right and limited neck rotation to the right. His left clavicle is higher and more prominent than the right clavicle, and the left SCM muscle is cord-like with a palpable mass (*arrows* in **E** and **F**) that is less intense than the contralateral muscle on T1-weighted MRI, suggesting fibrosis. **G** and **H,** A bipolar release of his left SCM muscle was required to correct his abnormal head posture. **I,** There is obvious persistent deformational plagiocephaly on cranial imaging.

(Courtesy of Robert M. Bernstein, Cedar Sinai Medical Center, Los Angeles, Calif.)

affected than females and a head turn to the right more common than to the left.[18] This is a direct result of the effort to position children in the supine position to prevent SIDS because prone and side sleeping positions have a protective effect for positional preference, which was noted in only 2.4% of prone-sleeping Swedish infants versus 19% of supine-sleeping infants.[36,37] Among the 623 infants with positional preference and deformational plagiocephaly, these features persisted in nearly one third when reexamined at age 2 to 3 years, resulting in a large number of referrals for additional diagnostic evaluations and/or treatment at much increased medical expense. These findings call for a primary pediatric preventive approach that includes early physical therapy for CMT and encouragement of tummy time when the infant is awake and under direct observation.[18] These findings and suggestions should in no way negate the recommendations of the "Back to Sleep" campaign.

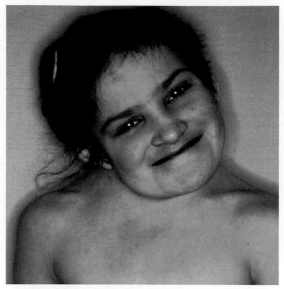

FIGURE 24-8. This girl has Klippel-Feil sequence with an osseous torticollis due to unbalanced cervical vertebral anomalies. Note her obviously short, wide neck.

## DIFFERENTIAL DIAGNOSIS

CMT is the most common type of congenital torticollis, but another cause of torticollis has been attributed to congenital fusion of cervical vertebrae (e.g., as in oculoauriculovertebral sequence or Klippel-Feil sequence), which is estimated to occur in 0.7% of newborns. Klippel-Feil sequence (Fig. 24-8) is found in 5% to 6% of patients with torticollis and may be associated with scoliosis, elevated scapula (Sprengel's deformity), renal anomalies, heart defects, and deafness, whereas CMT usually occurs in otherwise normal children. Acquired torticollis occurs infrequently in children when head and neck infection results in inflammation of cervical joints, with subsequent edema that causes C1-C2 subluxation with atlantoaxial rotatory displacement (Griscelli syndrome), resulting in contralateral stretching and spasm of the sternomastoid muscle (Fig. 24-9).[37] This is usually treated with muscle relaxants and cervical traction in a soft collar for patients who have been

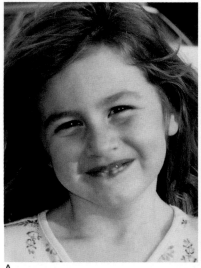
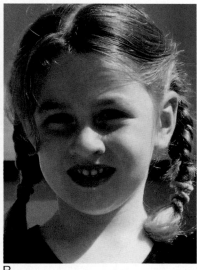

A                                B

FIGURE 24-9. **A,** This 6-year-old girl developed right torticollis in association with a cervical abscess (Griscelli syndrome). **B,** The torticollis resolved after treatment of the abscess.

symptomatic for less than 1 month, but, occasionally, posterior spinal fusion is necessary for refractory cases.[37] Benign paroxysmal torticollis is a self-limited disorder characterized by sudden, stereotypic head-tilting episodes that are often associated with pallor, agitation, nystagmus, and emesis; these episodes are sometimes mistaken for seizures. Episodes can be provoked by changes in position from upright to supine, which suggests a vestibular pathogenesis. Some patients have abnormal audiograms and go on to develop benign paroxysmal vertigo, cerebellar dysfunction, or migraine.[38] Familial spasmodic torticollis may not be distinct from dystonia musculorum because the latter sometimes presents first as torticollis, especially in the dominantly inherited variety. Ocular torticollis develops in some children with vertical ocular dystopia due to unilateral coronal synostosis, causing the child to tilt his or her head in a compensatory fashion; however, this does not occur in young infants. Posterior fossa tumors are a rare cause of acquired torticollis and are usually associated with neurologic signs and symptoms in older patients.[24] Among 6 children with torticollis and central nervous system lesions, all had abnormal neurologic examinations on initial presentation, and the youngest patient was 17 months old.[39] Torticollis associated with hiatal hernia (Sandifer's syndrome) may present as an intermittent and alternating head tilt.[40] Given the diversity of causes of torticollis, careful etiologic consideration is necessary before initiating treatment.

Engin et al[41] described a Turkish family that included five patients with torticollis among three generations. A 13-year-old boy and his 12-year-old sister had both suffered from right torticollis since birth, with the right SCM muscle resembling a fibrotic band. The cervical spine was radiographically normal, and facial asymmetry was not severe in the boy but was moderately severe in the girl. The parents were distantly related and unaffected, but on the father's side, the grandmother, an uncle, and a son of another uncle had suffered from left CMT. If the inheritance were autosomal dominant, then two males would represent skipped generations, but the possibility of autosomal recessive inheritance could not be ruled out.[41] Thompson et al[42] reported five affected girls from three sibships of an inbred kindred. Whether these case reports represent a familial susceptibility toward muscular fibrosis or the chance association of a common constraint-related deformation is unclear, but for most infants, CMT should not be considered to be inherited but may recur if constraint-related circumstances remain a factor. A family history of CMT is found in less than 5% of cases.[21]

For more extensive discussions of the diagnosis and treatment of torticollis, the reader is referred to Karmel-Ross's book on this topic.[43]

### References

1. Dunn PM: Congenital sternomastoid torticollis: an intrauterine postural deformity, *Arch Dis Child* 49:824–825, 1974.
2. Cheng JCY, Wong MWN, Tang SP, et al: Clinical determinants of outcome of manual stretching in the treatment of congenital muscular torticollis: a prospective study of 821 cases, *J Bone Joint Surg Am* 83:679–687, 2001.
3. Davids JR, Wenger DR, Mubarak SJ: Congenital muscular torticollis: sequellae of intrauterine or perinatal compartment syndrome, *J Pediatr Orthop* 13:141–147, 1993.
4. Hamanishi C, Tanaka S: Turned head–adducted hip–truncal curvature syndrome, *Arch Dis Child* 70:515–519, 1994.
5. Bredenkamp JK, Hoover LA, Berke GS, et al: Congenital muscular torticollis: a spectrum of disease, *Arch Otolaryngol Head Neck Surg* 116:212–216, 1990.
6. Tang S, Liu Z, Quan X, et al: Sternocleidomastoid pseudotumor of infants and congenital muscular torticollis: fine-structure research, *J Pediatr Orthop* 18:214–218, 1998.
7. Cheng JCY, Metrewell C, Chen TMK, et al: Correlation of ultrasonographic imaging of congenital muscular torticollis with clinical assessment in infants, *Ultrasound Med Biol* 26:1237–1241, 2000.
8. Tien YC, Su JY, Lin GT, et al: Ultrasonographic study of the coexistence of muscular torticollis and dysplasia of the hip, *J Pediatr Orthop* 21:343–347, 2001.
9. Carlson BM: The regeneration of skeletal muscle: a review, *Am J Anat* 173:119–150, 1973.
10. Vandenburgh HH, Hatfaludy S, Karlisch P, et al: Skeletal muscle growth is stimulated by intermittent stretch-relaxation in tissue culture, *Am J Physiol* 256:C674–C682, 1989.
11. Levine S, Salzman A: Neogenesis of skeletal muscle in the postinflammatory rat peritoneum, *Exp Mol Pathol* 60:60–69, 1994.
12. Golden KA, Beals SP, Littlefield TR, et al: Sternocleidomastoid imbalance versus congenital muscular torticollis: their relationship to positional plagiocephaly, *Cleft Palate Craniofac J* 36:256–261, 1999.
13. Emery C: The determinants of treatment duration for congenital muscular torticollis, *Phys Ther* 74:921–929, 1994.
14. Binder H, Eng G, Gaiser JF, et al: Congenital muscular torticollis: results of conservative management with long-term follow-up in 85 cases, *Arch Phys Med Rehab* 68:222–225, 1987.
15. Coventry MB, Harris LE: Congenital muscular torticollis in infancy: some observations regarding treatment, *J Bone Joint Surg Am* 41:85–822, 1959.
16. Walsh JJ, Morrissy RT: Torticollis and hip dislocation, *J Pediatr Orthop* 18:219–221, 1998.
17. Wei J, Schwartz K, Weaver A, et al: Pseudotumor of infancy and congenital muscular torticollis: 170 cases, *Laryngoscope* 11:688–695, 2001.
18. Graham JM Jr, Gomez M, Halberg A, et al: Management of deformational plagiocephaly: repositioning versus orthotic therapy, *J Pediatr* 146:258–262, 2005.
19. Cheng JC, Au AWY: Infantile torticollis: a review of 624 cases, *J Pediatr Orthop* 14:802–808, 1994.
20. Cheng JCY, Tang SP, Chen TMN, et al: The clinical presentation and outcome of congenital muscular torticollis in

infants—a study of 1086 cases, *J Pediatr Surg* 35: 1091–1096, 2000.

21. Cheng JCY, Tang SP, Chen TMK: Sternocleidomastoid pseudotumor and congenital muscular torticollis in infants: a prospective study of 510 cases, *J Pediatr* 134:712–716, 1999.

22. Celayir AC: Congenital muscular torticollis: early and intensive treatment is critical. A prospective study, *Pediatr Int* 42:504–507, 2000.

23. Singer C, Green BA, Bruce JH, et al: Late presentation of congenital muscular torticollis: use of MR imaging and CT scan in diagnosis, *Mov Disord* 9:100–103, 1994.

24. Parikh SN, Crawford AL, Choudhury S: Magnetic resonance imaging in the evaluation of infantile torticollis, *Orthopedics* 27:509–515, 2004.

25. Tang S, Hsu KH, Wong A, et al: Longitudinal follow-up study of ultrasonography in congenital muscular torticollis, *Clin Orthop* 1:179–185, 2002.

26. Wirth CJ, Hagena FW, Wuelker N, et al: Biterminal tenotomy for treatment of congenital muscular torticollis, *J Bone Joint Surg Am* 74:427–434, 1992.

27. Stassen LFA, Kerawala CJ: New surgical technique for the correction of congenital muscular torticollis (wry neck), *Br J Oral Maxillofac Surg* 38:142–147, 2000.

28. Burstein F: Long-term experience with endoscopic surgical treatment for congenital muscular torticollis in infants and children: a review of 85 cases, *Plast Reconstr Surg* 114:491–493, 2004.

29. Putnam GG, Postlethwaite KR, Chate RA, et al: Facial scoliosis: a diagnostic dilemma, *Int J Oral Maxillofac Surg* 22:324–327, 1993.

30. Slate RK, Posnick JC, Armstrong DC, et al: Cervical spine subluxation associated with congenital muscular scoliosis and craniofacial asymmetry, *Plast Reconstr Surg* 91:1187–1195, 1993.

31. Morrison DL, MacEwen GD: Congenital muscular torticollis: observations regarding clinical findings, associated conditions, and results of treatment, *J Pediatr Orthop* 2:500–505, 1982.

32. Canale ST, Griffin DW, Hubbard CN: Congenital muscular torticollis: a long-term follow-up, *J Bone Joint Surg Am* 64:810–816, 1982.

33. Arslan H, Gunduz S, Subasy M, et al: Frontal cephalometric analysis in the evaluation of facial asymmetry in torticollis, and outcomes of bipolar release in patients over 6 years of age, *Arch Orthop Trauma Surg* 122:489–493, 2002.

34. Yu CC, Wong FH, Lo LY, et al: Craniofacial deformity in patients with uncorrected congenital muscular torticollis: an assessment from three-dimensional computed tomography imaging, *Plast Reconstr Surg* 113:24–33, 2004.

35. Boere-Boonekamp MMM, van der Linden-Kuiper LT: Positional preference: prevalence in infants and follow-up after two years, *Pediatrics* 107:339–343, 2001.

36. Palmen K: Prevention of congenital dislocation of the hip: the Swedish experience of neonatal treatment of hip joint instability, *Acta Orthop Scand* 55 (suppl 208): 58–67, 1984.

37. Kautz SM, Skaggs DL: Getting an angle on spinal deformities, *Contemp Peds* 15:111–128, 1998.

38. Cataltepe SU, Barron TF: Benign paroxysmal torticollis presenting as "seizures" in infancy, *Clin Pediatr* 32:564–565, 1993.

39. Ballock RT, Song KM: The prevalence of non-muscular causes of torticollis in children, *J Pediatr Orthop* 16: 500–504, 1996.

40. Gorlin RJ, Cohen MM, Levin LS: *Syndromes of the head and neck*, ed 3, New York, 1990, Oxford University Press, p. 737.

41. Engin C, Yavuz SS, Sahin FI: Congenital muscular torticollis: is heredity a possible factor in a family with five torticollis patients in three generations? *Plast Reconstr Surg* 99:1147–1150, 1997.

42. Thompson F, McManus S, Colville J: Familial congenital muscular torticollis: case report and review of the literature, *Clin Orthop Relat Res* 202:193–196, 1986.

43. Karmel-Ross K, *Torticollis: differential diagnosis, assessment, surgical management and bracing*, New York, 1997, Haworth.

# 25 Torticollis-Plagiocephaly Deformation Sequence

## NONSYNOSTOTIC OR POSITIONAL PLAGIOCEPHALY

### GENESIS

Plagiocephaly, which literally translates from the Greek term *plagio kephale* as "oblique head," is a term used to describe asymmetry of the head shape when viewed from the top (Fig. 25-1). It is a nonspecific term that has been used to describe head asymmetry caused by either premature sutural fusion or postnatal head deformation resulting from a positional preference; hence, modifying terms such as *nonsynostotic, deformational,* and *positional* have been used to distinguish plagiocephaly without synostosis. The term *deformational plagiocephaly* should suffice to distinguish this type of defect and its proper management. The side of the plagiocephaly is usually indicated by the bone that has been most flattened by the deforming forces (see Figs. 24-2 and 24-3). During late fetal life, the head may become compressed unevenly in utero, but most deformational plagiocephaly occurs after delivery due to an asymmetric resting position. Such inequality of positional gravitational forces may result in asymmetric molding of the head and face.

Torticollis (see Chapter 24) is a condition in which the sternomastoid muscle is shorter and/or tighter on one side of the neck, causing the head to tilt toward the affected muscle and the head to turn away. This is the most frequent cause of deformational plagiocephaly, which results from progressive occipital flattening when an infant with torticollis is placed in supine position and preferentially turns his or her head to one side (see Fig. 25-1). Because the torticollis is usually on the side opposite the head turn, the forehead on the side of the torticollis may appear normal or recessed (see Fig. 24-3), whereas the forehead and ear ipsilateral to the flattened occiput appear to have been displaced anteriorly. If the infant sleeps on the stomach with a preferential head turn, then the frontal region on the side of the torticollis becomes flattened as the infant turns the head away

from the short or tight sternomastoid muscle (see Fig. 24-3). According to Dunn,[1] torticollis occurred with plagiocephaly once in every 300 live births prior to 1974, when many infants were positioned for sleep on their stomachs. Since the "Back to Sleep" campaign was initiated in 1992 for the prevention of sudden infant death syndrome (SIDS) by positioning infants on their backs for sleeping, the frequency of deformational posterior plagiocephaly has increased dramatically. This increase in deformational posterior plagiocephaly was first noted in 1996.[2-5]

Deformational plagiocephaly is not associated with premature closure of cranial sutures, but because craniosynostosis can be caused by fetal head constraint, diagnosis can be challenging when both deformational plagiocephaly and craniosynostosis occur together. Torticollis-plagiocephaly deformation sequence results from deformation of the infant's skull as normal brain growth combines with an asymmetric postnatal resting position to result in progressive cranial asymmetry (Fig. 25-2).[5] It is interesting to note that artificial deformation of infant heads has been practiced for thousands of years in many primitive cultures throughout the world (Fig. 25-3), and it is critical to remain cognizant of the impact of postnatal mechanical forces on the shape of an infant's head.[6] This previous practice of reshaping infant skulls with head-molding devices provides the basis for current therapy for infants with abnormal head shapes.

Deformational plagiocephaly is most likely to occur in first-born babies, in large babies, and among multiple-gestation infants.[7,8] In the torticollis-plagiocephaly deformation sequence, the infant usually has a head tilt toward the side of the shortened sternomastoid muscle.[5] The growth and development of the brain is usually normal; however, infants with macrocephaly and/or hypotonia are more likely to experience deformational

141

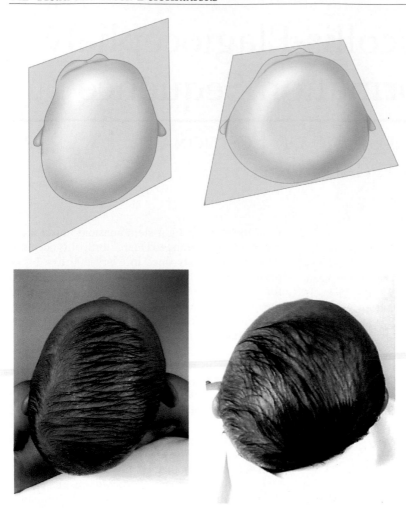

FIGURE 25-1. These infants demonstrate typical head shapes for deformational posterior plagiocephaly when viewed from the top (parallelogram on the left and trapezoidal on the right). The more brachycephalic head shape on the right suggests very little tummy time.
(Adapted from Pomatto JK, Calcaterra J, Kelly KM, et al: A study of family head shape: environment alters cranial shape, *Clin Pediatr* 45:55–64, 2006.)

plagiocephaly. Predisposing factors resulting in asymmetric head deformation include constraining intrauterine environment, poor muscle tone, torticollis, clavicular fracture, cervical/vertebral abnormalities, sleeping position, and incomplete bone mineralization. The importance of intrauterine positioning in determining both the occurrence and the severity of deformational plagiocephaly was demonstrated in a study of 140 twins treated with orthotic devices for positional plagiocephaly.[7,8] Among both discordant and concordant twin pairs, the bottom-most twin was more likely to be affected, and the more severely affected twin was more likely to manifest neck involvement and to be in a vertex position; there were no observed differences in sleep position (nearly all were supine sleepers) or gender (Fig. 25-4).[8] There was also a high incidence of fraternal twins born to older mothers who were pregnant for the first time using assisted reproductive technologies. Because twins are often born prematurely, when the cranium is less mineralized, they may be more susceptible to

deformational plagiocephaly due to incomplete calvarial mineralization. Thus intrauterine constraint is a predominant factor in the causation of deformational plagiocephaly, emphasizing the need for early diagnosis and intervention.

To reduce the incidence of SIDS, it is necessary to place infants on their backs for sleep except in cases of prematurity, gastroesophageal reflux, or obstructive sleep apnea; however, infants should be on their stomachs whenever they are awake and under direct adult supervision to facilitate the development of prone motor skills and to encourage the infant to turn his or her head from side to side. The development of positional brachycephaly, with or without plagiocephaly, can be an indication that parents are not providing their infants with adequate "tummy time." It is important to distinguish between deformational plagiocephaly and plagiocephaly due to premature sutural closure (or craniosynostosis) because therapy and management are very different for these conditions.

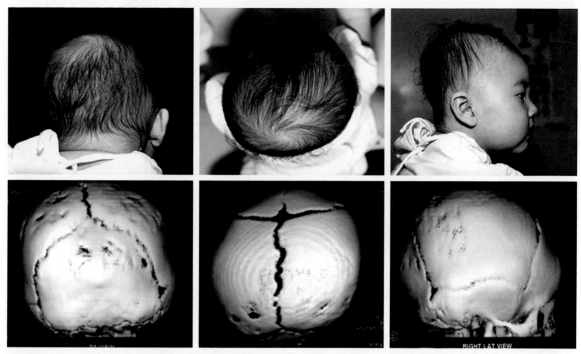

FIGURE 25-2. This 6-month-old infant was referred for an altered head shape due to deformational plagiocephaly with left torticollis and associated brachycephaly with right occipital flattening. A cranial 3D-CT scan had been done previously and clearly showed patent sutures. She responded well to neck physical therapy and cranial orthotic therapy.

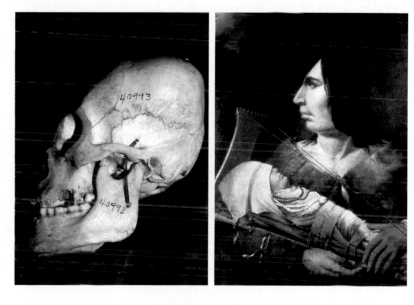

FIGURE 25-3. Northwest Pacific Coast Indians from the Kwakiutl tribe applied boards to the occiput and frontal regions from birth until 8 to 10 months. Once the boards were removed, the altered calvarial shape would persist for life.

## FEATURES

Deformational plagiocephaly is due to oblique molding of the head, and it is often accentuated by the tendency to remain exclusively supine and rest persistently on one side of the occiput. The classical parallelogram-shaped head is a combination of asymmetric flattening of the occiput with ipsilateral prominence of the forehead plus contralateral prominence of the other occiput with recession of the ipsilateral forehead (see Figs. 24-2, 25-1, and 25-2). This distorts the cranium in such a way that when the cranium is observed from above, it appears to be shaped like a parallelogram instead of having the normal, symmetrical oval shape. In cases in which the infant has received

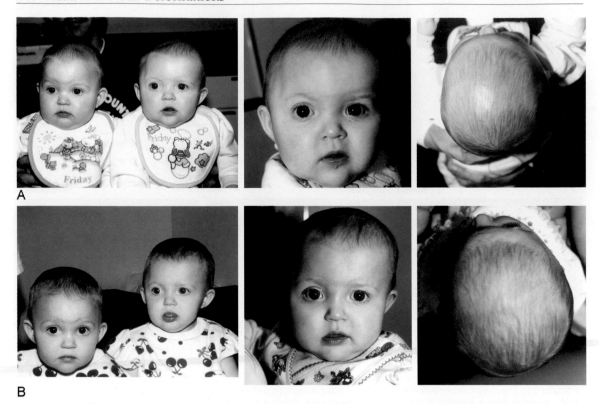

FIGURE 25-4. These monozygotic twins show how residual torticollis-plagiocephaly deformation sequence caused the twin on the right to manifest persistent craniofacial asymmetry between ages 6 **(A)** and 10 months **(B)**. The affected twin was beneath her co-twin in vertex presentation with her back to the mother's left side and her head turned to the right.

little or no tummy time, the head can become excessively flattened and somewhat trapezoidal in shape (see Fig. 25-1). The eye on the same side as the torticollis may appear less open because the soft tissues of the face are displaced superiorly on that side due to compression of the chin against the chest and persistent head tilting (see Fig. 25-4). The external ear may protrude and appear displaced anteriorly on the same side as the prominent forehead and flattened occiput, whereas the other ear appears pushed back with an uplifted lobule due to resting against the shoulder on the side with the recessed forehead, prominent occiput, and tight sternocleidomastoid muscle (Fig. 25-5).[5] This asymmetry of the ears is frequently noted by parents, and the ear on the side with the flattened occiput may also be significantly larger (as a manifestation of prolonged intrauterine compression) when compared with the ear on the side of the torticollis.[9] The position of the ears in deformational plagiocephaly differs from that seen in synostotic plagiocephaly due to unilateral lambdoid craniosynostosis, in which the ear may be vertically displaced downward on the synostotic side as a result of restricted sutural expansion (Fig. 25-6). Asymmetry of the cranium is most obvious when the

head is viewed from above; such asymmetry may be missed when the infant is examined face to face. The jaw is often pushed up on the side of the torticollis and may appear asymmetric and/or tilted.[5]

Other, more subtle characteristics may not be particularly noticeable on first glance but have been used to distinguish deformational plagiocephaly from synostotic plagiocephaly. These include asymmetry of the orbits with upward displacement on the side of the synostotic coronal suture, where the forehead and brow appear flattened. The presence of a unilateral epicanthal fold, usually ipsilateral to the side of occipital flattening, should prompt further investigation for the torticollis-plagiocephaly deformation sequence.[10] The degree of craniofacial distortion may be sufficient to cause abnormal placement of the eyes,[11] but usually one eye only appears to be less open due to vertical displacement of the soft tissues of the face on the side of the torticollis. Infants with torticollis often manifest other deformations such as dislocation of the hips, infantile scoliosis, and positional foot deformations due to late gestational constraint, especially if the baby was in breech presentation. The position of comfort is with the head tilted toward one side and the chin turned toward the

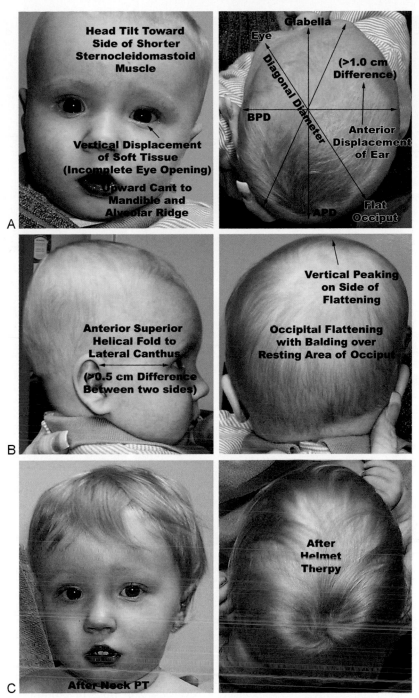

FIGURE 25-5. This infant shows all the key features of torticollis-plagiocephaly deformation sequence, with cranial measurements depicted on the top of his skull, before initiation of helmet therapy at age 5 months (**A** and **B**) and after completion of therapy at 14 months (**C**). *APD,* Anteroposterior diameter; *BPD,* biparietal diameter; *DD,* diagonal difference.

opposite side. Persistence of neck rotation due to lack of physical therapy and/or fibrosis of the muscle on that side will perpetuate the secondary effects of congenital muscular torticollis, but this can usually be prevented with early and persistent physical therapy.[5] A flattened cranium will foster a tendency for the infant to lie on this flattened area in his or her position of comfort, thus maintaining the deformity. Among 181 normal infants whose head shapes were observed at regular intervals

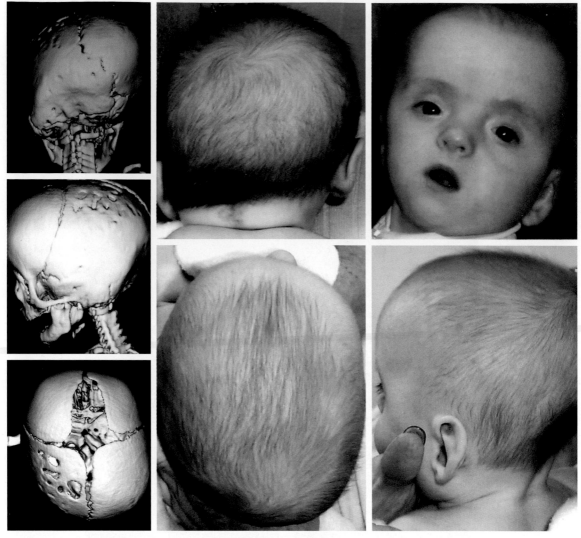

FIGURE 25-6. This infant was born with left lambdoid craniosynostosis and severe right congenital muscular torticollis, resulting in a very distorted cranium that required surgical correction with postoperative cranial orthotic therapy as well as prolonged physical therapy.

from birth through age 2 years in 2002, the prevalence of plagiocephaly or brachycephaly peaked at 4 months at 20% (associated with male gender, first-born, limited neck rotation, and inability to vary the infant's head position when putting the infant down to sleep) and then fell to 9% by age 8 months and to 3.3% by age 2 years.[12]

## MANAGEMENT, PROGNOSIS, AND COUNSEL

In most instances of deformational plagiocephaly with torticollis, observation of the infant's resting position and head shape during the first few weeks after birth will determine whether there is a preferential resting position. During this period of observation, a few procedures are worth considering. The surface upon which the infant's head rests should be relatively soft, and some cultures even use soft rings or pillows for all neonates to prevent infant head deformation (Fig. 25-7). The infant's crib should be placed so that visually attractive objects are on the side opposite to the preferential head turn. The head and neck should be moderately overstretched away from the side of the torticollis (see Chapter 24). With mild-to-moderate torticollis, early neck-stretching exercises usually correct the problem and prevent the postnatal plagiocephaly that would otherwise

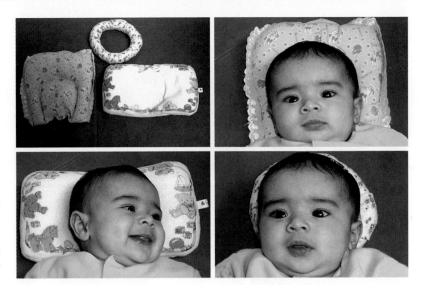

FIGURE 25-7. This infant required only neck physical therapy and head repositioning to maintain her normal head shape. She is shown here with a variety of infant positioning pillows from various parts of Asia.

result from always resting on the same area of the cranium (see Fig. 23-2).[5] Inability to nurse equally from both breasts may be the first clue to the presence of torticollis, and early referral to a physical therapist for treatment of torticollis is often the most effective treatment strategy. With torticollis, the head usually tilts to one side and the chin rotates toward the opposite side. For example, with a left torticollis, the head tilts to the left and the face turns to the right. To correct this posture, the neck should be stretched to the right so that the right ear is gradually brought toward the right shoulder and held there for 30 to 60 seconds. Then the chin should be rotated toward the left so that the chin is brought past the left shoulder and held there for 30 to 60 seconds (see Fig. 24-4). For the neck stretch to be effective, as the parent faces the baby, the parent's left hand should be on the left side of the baby's face and the right hand should be on the baby's shoulder, where it bears down firmly on the shoulder during the neck stretching. To correct torticollis appropriately, both exercises must be done together and regularly (at least 6 to 8 times each day). After a meal or diaper change is usually a good time to perform these exercises as a regular part of the daily routine. In cases of severe torticollis, it is particularly important to initiate early referral to a physical therapist for neck-stretching exercises to prevent muscle fibrosis and deformational plagiocephaly. Initial management always involves attempts to actively reposition the infant so as to correct any cranial asymmetry in addition to neck physical therapy to correct any associated torticollis (Fig. 25-8).[5] This can be accompanied by active

massaging of the tightened neck muscle, as well as alteration of the infant's sleep position.

Parents should be encouraged to correct deformational posterior plagiocephaly by placing the baby in the crib in such a position that the infant must lie opposite to his or her preferred position; however, this variation in resting position must be accompanied by neck physical therapy in order to be effective.[5] The development of excessive brachycephaly, with or without plagiocephaly, is an indication that parents are not providing their infants with adequate tummy time, which should be encouraged during waking periods while the infant is under adult supervision. Positioning of the infant's head can be accomplished with the use of an infant positioning device (see Fig. 25-8). The corrected head position can be maintained and facilitated by placing toys and other stimulating objects in the infant's field of view. By training the child not to lie on the already flattened parts of his or her head, those areas will be allowed to fill out and progression of occipital flattening will be prevented. Once significant occipital flattening occurs, it becomes difficult to reposition the infant, and failure to treat the underlying torticollis with physical therapy will also result in treatment failure.[5] Some parents find it useful to use an infant positioning device to control the infant's head position. One useful device consists of a long triangular wedge that runs along the infant's back and is connected to a shorter triangular wedge, which goes under the infant's axilla. The infant is then positioned on his or her back in a three-quarters turn so that he or she rests on the prominent aspect of the occiput. If repositioning is effective,

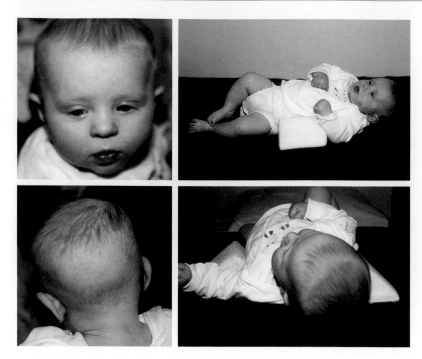

FIGURE 25-8. This girl with torti-collis-plagiocephaly deformation sequence was treated entirely with neck physical therapy and repositioning using an infant positioning device between ages 3 and 9 months. She is shown here partway through her therapy in a three-quarters turn, resting on her left occiput, with her bald spot shifted from the right, previously flattened occiput to the left occiput.

migration of the bald spot from the center of the previously flattened occiput toward the previously prominent occiput can be observed (see Fig. 25-8). It is important to warn the parents to not simply position the infant on the side of his or her head to prevent further occipital flattening, as this is not an effective way to use positioning and gravity to help correct cranial asymmetry. If the infant has had regular tummy time experience and is able to sleep safely in a prone position, parents must be cautioned to be sure the infant sleeps with his or her head turned toward the side of the torticollis so that the recessed forehead on that side does not become more recessed. Whenever possible, it is important to use the weight of the infant's head to correct cranial asymmetry by applying gravitational pressure to the prominent areas. The parents should be encouraged to follow through with physical therapy at home, particularly if the infant's condition is not being observed by a physical therapist.[5]

Management of infants who do not make progress with exercises and repositioning of the head, as well as of infants with moderately severe plagiocephaly that is still present at age 6 months, involves the use of a corrective helmet or cranial orthotic.[5,13-20] If the difference between cranial diagonal measurements is greater than 1 cm at age 6 months and/or the cephalic index is greater than 90% at age 5 months, then cranial orthotic

therapy is the most effective way to correct the abnormal head shape.[5,20] Cranial orthotic therapy is intended to re-mold the infant's head into a more normal, symmetric oval shape as the head grows, and it has been successfully used to correct infant head shapes for more than 30 years. The prominent parts are restrained while normal brain growth provides a corrective mechanical force from within the calvarium to round out the shallow or flattened regions. This method begins by making a plaster cast of the infant's deformed head with rapidly drying plaster splint material (Fig. 25-9). Using a stockinette cap, the plaster cast can be readily removed while maintaining its shape. This cast is then inverted and filled with plaster of Paris, into which a 1-inch pipe is inserted so that the completed bust can be mounted on a base for further work. After removing the cast from the bust, plaster of Paris is then added to the model where the head is shallow, but none is added where the head is unduly prominent (see Figs. 25-9 and 25-10). Thus, a more ideally shaped bust is modeled, and a plastic helmet resembling an American football helmet is made from the new model. The helmet is tight where the infant's head is prominent and allows for growth in the less prominent regions. Once brain growth has filled out the helmet, no further management is usually needed, and a corrected head shape will persist without further

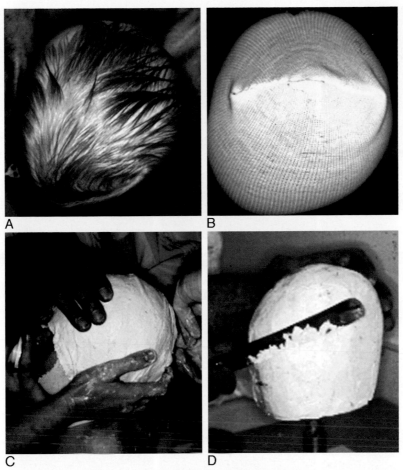

FIGURE 25-9. Following the procedures outlined by Clarren, when conservative measures proved unsuccessful in correcting this child's plagiocephaly by age 6 months **(A)**, a stockinette cap was placed over the infant's head **(B)** to prevent hair from becoming embedded in the rapidly drying plaster splint material used to make a mold of the infant's head **(C)**. Plaster of Paris is poured into the mold, and an iron pipe is placed in the bust, which is then allowed to dry overnight. The mold is removed, and the bust is mounted on a base so that it can be augmented into a symmetric shape **(D)**. Where the bust is flattened, plaster is added to the bust. In areas that are too prominent, the bust is left unchanged. Foam is stretched around the augmented bust to pad the inside of the helmet, to which ear spaces have been added. The foam is applied in two layers separated by talcum powder, and then ⅜ inch polypropylene plastic is molded around the bust in a vacuum oven. The helmet is cut off the bust, and the infant wears the helmet constantly (except for baths) until cranial symmetry has been restored.

(Procedures adapted from Clarren SK: Helmet therapy for plagiocephaly and congenital muscular torticollis, *J Pediatr* 94:43–46, 1979; and Clarren SK: Plagiocephaly and torticollis: etiology, natural history, and helmet therapy, *J Pediatr* 98:92–95, 1981.)

therapy (see Fig. 25-10), but sometimes additional physical therapy for torticollis is required (Fig. 25-11).[5,13-20]

Because deformational plagiocephaly is usually accompanied by muscular torticollis, it is important to institute active and passive neck-stretching and head-turning exercises to restore neck muscle symmetry.[5] If helmet therapy is used by 5 to 6 months of age, usually only 3 to 4 months are needed to reform the head to a more normal shape. However, if the helmet management is not used until 7 to 8 months of age, it may take 5 to 6 months to achieve the desired result. The pace of reformation relates to the rate of brain growth, which is much more rapid during the first 6 months than later in infancy, explaining why a

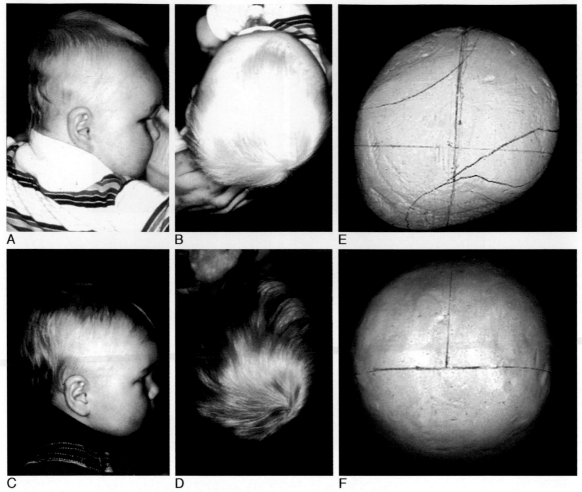

FIGURE 25-10. Before helmet therapy was begun at 6 months, this child had asymmetric occipital flattening, which resolved after 4 months of helmet therapy. His head is shown before (**A** and **B**) and after (**C** and **D**) helmet therapy, along with top views of his uncorrected (**E**) and corrected (**F**) busts.

preferential head turn combined with purposeful supine positioning can deform the head so quickly. This type of therapy is typically started at around 5 to 6 months of age, and the helmet is worn almost constantly for an average of 4 months (it is only removed for bathing). Follow-up must be maintained throughout this period to make adjustments to the inner padding of the helmet, allow for regular growth, and monitor progress.[5] An alternative type of helmet therapy termed *dynamic orthotic cranioplasty* (or simply the DOC helmet) is used in some centers.[21-25] This involves a concept similar to helmet therapy; however, it leaves the top of the appliance open to allow for aeration, and it actively remolds the cranium into a more symmetric shape. This technique also requires follow-up to adjust the device as the shape

changes, and approximately 10% of cases require a second helmet to achieve optimal results. Although no clinical trials have compared these two types of molding devices, results with both types of helmets have been excellent. Both techniques use the same principle of using mechanical forces to remold the cranium into a more symmetric shape as the head grows into the symmetric shape of the molding device, and both techniques have been approved by the Food and Drug Administration.[26]

For those children with moderately severe cranial deformation, if intervention is not attempted or is attempted too late, permanent distortion of the head may occur (see Figs. 24-6 and 24-7).[5] Of 98 infants with deformational plagiocephaly, only 3 had such severe and progressive deformation that

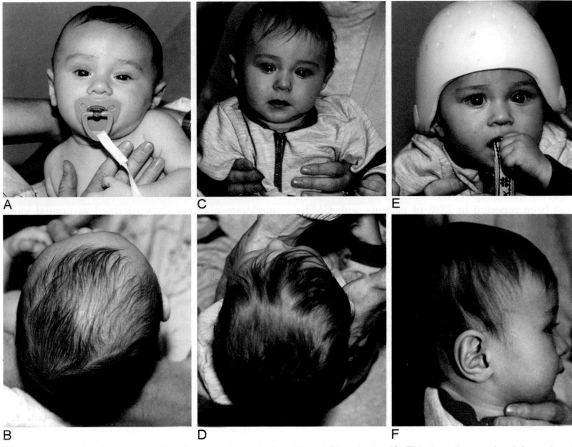

FIGURE 25-11. This infant with left torticollis is shown before (**A** and **B**) and after (**C–E**) helmet therapy for deformational plagiocephaly. Even though his head shape is fully corrected at age 10 months, he still needs continued neck physical therapy to correct his torticollis.

they required reconstructive cranial surgery (see the discussion on craniosynostosis for a description of this surgery). The remaining 95 infants were successfully managed with changes in sleeping position or helmet therapy.[17] In a prospective study of 114 infants treated with either head positioning in the crib (63 infants) or with helmet therapy (51 infants), posterior cranial symmetry was significantly better in infants managed with helmets than in those managed with positioning.[19] There is concern that residual facial asymmetry may, ultimately, lead to ocular disturbances. These ocular problems differ from those seen in craniosynostotic plagiocephaly, in which vertical displacement of the orbit occurs.[27] Unlike synostotic plagiocephaly, which is sometimes associated with genetic syndromes, deformational plagiocephaly is not a heritable disorder, and recurrence rates are usually low unless an underlying uterine factor, such as a bicornuate uterus, has caused the fetal head constraint.

The average length of treatment with helmet orthosis was 4.5 months for infants who averaged 6.5 months of age at the start of treatment, but younger infants were successfully treated with repositioning and physical therapy alone.[5] Orthotic treatment does not restrict cranial growth but rather redirects growth into a symmetric shape.[5,24] Efficacy of treatment is related to both the initial degree of asymmetry and the age at which orthosis is initiated, with earlier treatment more successful and late treatment of little or no benefit.[5,19-25] The practice of artificial postnatal head deformation is an ancient one that has been practiced by many older cultures (see Fig. 25-3).[6,28,29] These experiments of nature, as well as various clinical reports,[30,31] confirm that head deformation will persist throughout life if not managed appropriately.[5]

Failure to treat muscular torticollis can result in persistent facial asymmetry, cervical scoliosis, and

deformational posterior plagiocephaly has previously been confused with lambdoid synostosis, leading to unnecessary surgery and falsely elevated statistics concerning the frequency of lambdoid synostosis; however, the distinction between these conditions can now be made with certainty.[17-19] One study helped clarify the differential diagnosis and treatment for positional posterior plagiocephaly versus lambdoid synostosis.[17] During a 4-year period between 1991 and 1994, 102 patients with posterior plagiocephaly were assessed by a multidisciplinary team consisting of a dysmorphologist, pediatric neurosurgeon, and craniofacial surgeon. During this

same period, this team also assessed 130 patients with craniosynostosis that required surgery. Only 4 patients (3.1%) manifested clinical, imaging, and operative features of true unilambdoidal craniosynostosis. These features included a thick bony ridge over the fused lambdoid suture, with contralateral parietal and frontal bulging, and an ipsilateral occipitomastoid bulge leading to tilting of the ipsilateral skull base and a downward displacement of the ear on the synostotic side. These changes resulted in a trapezoidal head shape when viewed from above. In contrast, children with deformational, nonsynostotic posterior plagiocephaly had a parallelogram-shaped head, with

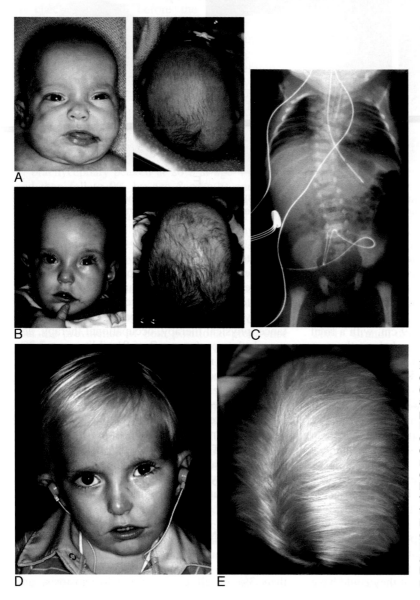

FIGURE 25-13. This infant with oculoauriculovertebral dysplasia **(A)** had severe cervical vertebral anomalies **(C)** that resulted in a persistent head turn to the right. **B,** By age 3 months, he had developed marked plagiocephaly as a consequence of his asymmetric resting position. Because his cervical vertebral anomalies could not be corrected, he was fitted with two consecutive helmets to maintain normal cranial symmetry during the period of most rapid head growth (through 2 years of age). **D** and **E,** At age 3 years, he had a persistent head turn and head tilt but relatively normal cranial symmetry.

forward displacement of the ear and frontal bossing on the side ipsilateral to the occipitoparietal flattening, accompanied by contralateral occipital bossing.[5] As shown in Fig. 25-6, some patients present with both unilateral lambdoid synostosis and torticollis-plagiocephaly deformation sequence, which suggests that both types of problems can result from fetal head constraint in utero and mandates a treatment program that includes surgery, physical therapy, and cranial orthotic therapy.

A malformation of the cervical vertebrae may be the primary cause of the head being turned to one side, in which case the deformational plagiocephaly and torticollis would be secondary to an intrinsic malformation problem (Fig. 25-13). In such infants, it is usually necessary to use more than one helmet to achieve the desired cranial symmetry because the torticollis does not respond to physical therapy. In severe bone dysplasias resulting in osteopenia, such as osteogenesis imperfecta type III or severe hypophosphatasia, the calvarium may be extremely soft and undermineralized to maintain its normal protective shape, with the result that the brain is actually compressed in an anteroposterior dimension, sometimes leading to communicating hydrocephalus. In such instances, prolonged helmet therapy may also be required.

A primary neuromuscular disorder may also be the primary cause of the torticollis, as in spastic torticollis, but these disorders are quite rare. After birth, neuromuscular disorders predisposing toward hypotonia and (occasionally) severe neglect may cause an infant to lie in one position long enough to give rise to asymmetric molding of the head. This can usually be distinguished from congenital muscular torticollis by physical examination and history after birth. Prematurely born infants may have poor muscle tone with a relatively malleable cranium. If such an infant lies persistently on a firm surface with the head turned to one side, he or she may develop deformational plagiocephaly. Such cases can usually be distinguished from postnatal constraint deformation by the history. If these principles of diagnosis and management are used, occipital plagiocephaly should no longer prove to be as controversial as it was in the 1990s, and much unnecessary surgery can be avoided.[39-41]

## References

1. Dunn PM: Congenital sternomastoid torticollis: an intrauterine postural deformity, *Arch Dis Child* 49:824–825, 1974.
2. Argenta LC, David LR, Wilson JA, et al: An increase in infant cranial deformity with supine sleeping position, *J Craniofac Surg* 7:5–11, 1996.
3. Turk AE, McCarthy JG, Thorne CHM, et al: The "Back to Sleep Campaign" and deformational plagiocephaly: is there cause for concern? *J Craniofac Surg* 7:12–18, 1996.
4. Kane AA, Mitchell LE, Craven KP, et al: Observations on a recent increase in plagiocephaly without synostosis, *Pediatrics* 97:877–885, 1996.
5. Graham JM Jr, Gomez M, Halberg A, et al: Management of deformational plagiocephaly: repositioning versus orthotic therapy, *J Pediatr* 146:258–262, 2005.
6. Dingwall EJ: *Artificial cranial deformations: a contribution to the study of ethnic mutilation*, London, 1931, John Bale, Sons, & Danielsson.
7. Littlefield TR, Kelly KM, Pomatto JK, et al: Multiple-birth infants at higher risk for development of deformational plagiocephaly, *Pediatrics* 103:565–569, 1999.
8. Littlefield TR, Kelly KM, Pomatto JK, et al: Multiple-birth infants at higher risk for development of deformational plagiocephaly. II. Is one twin at greater risk? *Pediatrics* 109:19–25, 2002.
9. Aase JM: Structural defects as a consequence of late intrauterine constraint: craniotabes, loose skin, and asymmetric ear size, *Semin Perinatol* 7:270–273, 1983.
10. Jones MC: Unilateral epicanthic fold: diagnostic significance, *J Pediatr* 108:702–704, 1986.
11. Frederick DR, Mulliken JB, Robb RM: Ocular manifestations of deformational frontal plagiocephaly, *J Pediatr Ophthalmol Strab* 30:92–95, 1993.
12. Hutchinson BL, Hutchinson LAD, Thompson JMD, et al: Plagiocephaly and brachycephaly in the first two years of life: a prospective cohort study, *Pediatrics* 114:970–980, 2004.
13. Clarren SK: Helmet therapy for plagiocephaly and congenital muscular torticollis, *J Pediatr* 94:43–46, 1979.
14. Clarren SK: Plagiocephaly and torticollis: etiology, natural history, and helmet therapy, *J Pediatr* 98:92–95, 1981.
15. Bruneteau RJ, Mulliken JB: Frontal plagiocephaly: synostotic, compensational, or deformational, *Plast Reconstr Surg* 89:21–31, 1992.
16. Cohen MM Jr: Frontal plagiocephaly: synostotic, compensational, or deformational—discussion, *Plast Reconstr Surg* 89:32–33, 1992.
17. Huang MHS, Gruss JS, Clarren SK, et al: The differential diagnosis of posterior plagiocephaly: true lambdoid synostosis versus positional molding, *Plast Reconstr Surg* 98:765–776, 1996.
18. Graham JM Jr: Craniofacial deformation, *Ballier Clin Pediatr* 6:293–315, 1998.
19. Mulliken JB, Vander Woude DL, Hansen M, et al: Analysis of posterior plagiocephaly: deformational versus synostotic, *Plast Reconstr Surg* 103:371–380, 1999.
20. Graham JM Jr, Kreutzman J, Earl D, et al: Deformational brachycephaly in supine-sleeping infants, *J Pediatr* 146:253–257, 2005.
21. Littlefield TR, Beals SP, Manwarring KH, et al: Treatment of craniofacial asymmetry with dynamic orthotic cranioplasty, *J Craniofac Surg* 9:11–17, 1998.
22. Kelly KM, Littlefield TR, Pornatto JK, et al: Importance of early recognition and treatment of deformational plagiocephaly with orthotic cranioplasty, *Cleft Palate Craniofac J* 36:127–130, 1999.
23. Golden KA, Beals SP, Littlefield TR, et al: Sternocleidomastoid imbalance versus congenital muscular torticollis: their relationship to positional plagiocephaly, *Cleft Palate Craniofac J* 36:256–261, 1999.

24. Kelly KM, Littlefield TF, Pomatto JK, et al: Cranial growth unrestricted during treatment for deformational plagiocephaly, *Pediatr Neurosurg* 30:193–199, 1999.
25. Ripley CE, Pomatto J, Beals SP, et al: Treatment of positional plagiocephaly with dynamic orthotic cranioplasty, *J Craniofac Surg* 5:150–159, 1994 [discussion, 160].
26. Littlefield TR: Food and Drug Administration regulation of orthotic cranioplasty, *Cleft Palate Craniofac J* 38:337–340, 2001.
27. Greenberg MF, Pollard ZF: Ocular plagiocephaly: ocular torticollis with skull and facial asymmetry, *Ophthalmology* 107:173–179, 2000.
28. Graham JM Jr, Charman CE, Chaisson R, et al: Postnatal head deformation: anthropological observations and applications to the treatment of postnatal plagiocephaly, *Proc Greenwood Genetic Center* 7:156–159, 1988.
29. Fitzsimmons E, Prost JH, Peniston S: Infant head molding: a cultural practice, *Arch Fam Med* 7:88–90, 1998.
30. Putnam GD, Postlethwaite KR, Chate RA, et al: Facial scoliosis—a diagnostic dilemma, *Int J Oral Maxillofac Surg* 22:324–327, 1993.
31. Slate RK, Posnick JC, Armstrong DC, et al: Cervical spine subluxation associated with congenital muscular scoliosis and craniofacial asymmetry, *Plast Reconstr Surg* 91:1187–1195, 1993.
32. Morrison DL, MacEwen GD: Congenital muscular torticollis: observations regarding clinical findings, associated conditions, and results of treatment, *J Pediatr Orthop* 2:500–505, 1982.
33. Boere-Boonekamp MMM, van der Linden-Kuiper LT: Positional preference: prevalence in infants and follow-up after two years, *Pediatrics* 107:339–343, 2001.
34. Palmen K: Prevention of congenital dislocation of the hip: the Swedish experience of neonatal treatment of hip joint instability, *Acta Orthop Scand* 55 (Suppl 208):58–67, 1984.
35. Moss S: Nonsurgical, nonorthotic treatment of occipital plagiocephaly: what is the natural history of the misshapen neonatal head? *J Neurosurg* 87:667–670, 1997.
36. Pollack I, Losken H, Fasick P: Diagnosis and management of posterior plagiocephaly, *Pediatrics* 99:180–185, 1997.
37. Bridges SJ, Chambers TL, Pople IK: Plagiocephaly and head binding, *Arch Dis Child* 86:144–145, 2002 [commentary, 145–146].
38. Miller RI, Clarren SK: Long-term developmental outcomes in patients with deformational plagiocephaly, *Pediatrics* 105:e26, 2000.
39. Jones BM, Hayward R, Evans R, et al: Occipital plagiocephaly: an epidemic of craniosynostosis? *Pediatr Neurosurg* 24:69–70, 1996.
40. Pope IA, Sanford RA, Muhlbauer MS: Clinical presentation and management of 100 infants with occipital plagiocephaly, *Pediatr Neurosurg* 25:1–6, 1996.
41. Fernbach S: Craniosynostosis 1998: concepts and controversies, *Pediatr Radiol* 28:722–728, 1998.

# 26 Infant Sleeping Position and Sudden Infant Death Syndrome

## GENESIS

The postmortem diagnosis of sudden infant death syndrome (SIDS) was introduced midway through the 20th century, but its association with infant sleeping position was not evident until the 1990s. SIDS is considered to have a multifactorial basis whereby some infants are born with risk factors that make them more vulnerable to dying during infancy. African-American and Native American infants are more than twice as likely to die of SIDS than are Caucasian babies, and infant sleeping position has recently emerged as a major risk factor for SIDS. It has been hypothesized that abnormalities in the arcuate nucleus, which controls breathing and waking, might be involved in some cases of SIDS. Normal infants sense inadequate air intake, which triggers them to awaken, cry, and change cardiorespiratory function to compensate for insufficient oxygen and excess carbon dioxide. This situation might result from infants sleeping on their stomachs and re-breathing exhaled air that is trapped in underlying bedding, and a baby with defective functioning of the arcuate nucleus might lack this protective mechanism and succumb to SIDS. There are also other predisposing factors for SIDS, such as chronic hypoxia induced by maternal cigarette smoking during pregnancy or concurrent respiratory infection in the infant. Also, more SIDS cases occur in the colder months, when such infections are more common. Increases in cellular and protein immune responses have also been suggested to play a role. Arousal thresholds are significantly higher in both active and quiet sleep when infants sleep prone at 2 to 3 weeks or 2 to 3 months (the age of peak susceptibility to SIDS) but not at 5 to 6 months (the age when susceptibility to SIDS has decreased). Thus the prone position significantly impairs arousal from sleep during the time when infants are most likely to die from SIDS, which is the major cause of death for infants between ages 1 and 12 months.[1]

## FEATURES

Between 1989 and 1991, epidemiologic studies showed a strong association between infants sleeping on their stomachs and death from SIDS.[2-6] In 1992 the American Academy of Pediatrics (AAP) formed a Task Force on Infant Positioning and SIDS, which determined that infants who slept prone on their stomachs had as much as an 11.7 times higher risk for SIDS than infants who slept supine on their backs. Hence in 1992 the recommendation was made to position infants on their backs or sides for sleep, except in cases of prematurity, gastroesophageal reflux, or obstructive sleep apnea.[7] By 1993, similar risk reduction efforts in Australia, England, and New Zealand had resulted in a 50% reduction in SIDS deaths over a 1- to 2-year period.[8-10] In addition, there was no apparent increase in doctor visits or adverse respiratory events for infants placed on their sides or backs.[11,12] When side positioning was compared with placing infants on their backs, it became evident that the risk for SIDS was greater when infants were placed on their sides, possibly because of a higher likelihood of spontaneously turning onto their stomachs. Thus in 1996 the recommendation was revised to avoid side positioning.[13] Further recommendations were made to position babies on a firm surface free of soft bedding, pillows, or comforters because sleeping with these items also increases the risk of SIDS[14] (and possibly explains the increased frequency of SIDS during the colder months).

As a consequence of the "Back to Sleep" campaign, the predominant sleeping pattern in the United States changed from 70% prone in 1992 to 24% prone in 1996, with a concomitant 38% decrease in SIDS during the same time interval.[15] Between 1994 and 1998, prone placement declined from 44% to 17% among Caucasian infants and from 53% to 32% among African-American infants, with supine positioning increasing from 27% to 58% among Caucasian infants and 17% to 31%

157

among African-American infants.[16] From 1992 to 1994, the prevalence of prone sleep positioning decreased from 70% to 13%.[17] In 2001 the prevalence of prone positioning among Caucasian infants was 11% compared with 21% among African-American infants, and the rate of SIDS among African-American infants was 2.5 times that of Caucasian infants.[17] This decrease in supine positioning among African-American versus Caucasian infants may account for the increased frequency of SIDS among African-American infants. Despite recommendations for supine sleep positioning, some caregivers persist with prone positioning because they believe the infant is more comfortable and sleeps better. Finally, side and prone sleeping positions increase the risk of SIDS, particularly in infants who are unused to prone sleeping, with an adjusted odds ratio (OR) of 6.9 and 8.2, respectively.[18] The end result of this public education effort was a decline in the prevalence of prone sleeping position from 70% in 1992 to 13% in 2004, with a concomitant reduction in the rate of SIDS from 1.2 per 1000 in 1992 to 0.56 per 1000 in 2001 (a decrease of 53% over this 10-year period).[17] During this same time period, for specific subgroups, the risk of SIDS for low-birth-weight infants rose from an OR of 2.1 to 3.6; for infants born to smoking mothers, from 2.7 to 3.7; for infants born to unmarried mothers, from 1.4 to 2.5; for infants born to African-American mothers, from 1.4 to 2.5; and for infants born to mothers with limited prenatal care, from 1.5 to 2.5. Thus the recent reduction in SIDS deaths associated with changes in sleeping practices has strengthened the association of SIDS with these other risk factors. These findings emphasize the interplay between SIDS, lung disease, socioeconomic factors, and exposure to tobacco smoke and suggest that some population subgroups remain unaware of recent medical advice regarding optimal sleep positioning for infants.[19]

## MANAGEMENT

Given the strong association between prone sleeping positioning and SIDS, it is advisable to position infants on their backs for sleep, except in cases of prematurity, gastroesophageal reflux, or obstructive sleep apnea. The key to effective management is to position infants in supine position, with regular variation in the position of the infant's head so as to avoid undue flattening.[17,20-22] Aberrant head shapes can be avoided by early initiation of neck physical therapy at the first sign of plagiocephaly development, with effective positioning to both

sides of the occiput. Supine sleepers attain several motor milestones later than prone sleepers (e.g., rolling prone to supine, tripod sitting, creeping, crawling, and pulling to stand); however, all milestones are eventually attained within the expected normal range.[23]

Encouraging "tummy time" when infants are awake and under observation may help to minimize these differences in normal motor development by strengthening the infant's neck muscles and facilitating prone motor activities. Because most supine-sleeping infants are unused to viewing their world from the stomach, they need this visual experience to facilitate their motor development. It is also important to note that recent studies have shown that 53% of SIDS victims who had always slept in a non-prone position died shortly after they were placed prone by a parent or other caretaker. In 56% of these cases, a secondary caretaker other than the parents was responsible for the change; this emphasizes the importance of stressing proper infant sleep positioning to everyone involved in the care of infants. These findings also stress the importance of giving infants adequate "tummy time" experience while they are awake in order to facilitate development of head turning while prone as a key protective mechanism in case the infant turns from supine to prone during sleep.[20-24] Taking all these data together, it is clear that the "Back to Sleep" campaign has been one of the modern triumphs of preventive medicine in reducing the incidence of SIDS by more than 50%, but primary care providers should deliver a broader message: It is essential to place infants on their backs for sleep, except in cases of prematurity, gastroesophageal reflux, or obstructive sleep apnea, but infants should be on their stomachs whenever they are awake and under direct adult supervision to develop their prone motor skills and full range of neck motion.

## DIFFERENTIAL DIAGNOSIS

Rarely an underlying genetic disease causes SIDS, such as certain metabolic or genetic diseases. Medium-chain acyl-CoA dehydrogenase deficiency may be mistaken as SIDS. This deficiency prevents proper processing of fatty acids, leading to build-up of fatty acid metabolites that disrupt cardiorespiratory function. Another report suggests that 50% of infants who died of SIDS had prolonged QT on electrocardiograms performed during the first week of life.[25] Furthermore, one infant with near-miss SIDS was found to have a fresh dominant mutation in the *SCN5A* cardiac sodium channel gene responsible for the LQT3 subtype of long-QT syndrome.[26] In light of such etiologic heterogeneity, there should be a comprehensive death scene evaluation for any child dying of SIDS.[27] Primary care physicians should discuss safe sleep environments with their patients, including the avoidance of cigarette smoke exposure, overheating, and soft bedding, the use of a safe crib, and the use of a supine sleep position and avoidance of unsafe side or prone sleeping positions.[17,28-30]

## References

1. Horne RC, Ferens D, Watts AM, et al: The prone sleeping position impairs arousability in term infants, *J Pediatr* 138:811–816, 2001.
2. Lee NN, Chan YF, Davies DP, et al: Sudden infant death in Hong Kong: confirmation of low incidence, *Br Med J* 298:721, 1989.
3. Fleming PJ, Gilbert R, Azaz Y, et al: Interaction between bedding and sleeping position in the sudden infant death syndrome: a population-based case-control study, *Br Med J* 301:85–89, 1990.
4. Mitchell EA, Scragg R, Stewart AW, et al: Results from the first year of the New Zealand cot death study, *NZ Med J* 104:71–76, 1991.
5. Dwyer T, Ponsonby A-L, Newman NM, et al: Prospective cohort study of prone sleeping position and sudden infant death syndrome, *Lancet* 337:1244–1247, 1991.
6. Dwyer T, Ponsonby A-L, Newman NM, et al: Prone sleeping position and SIDS: evidence from recent case-control and cohort studies in Tasmania, *J Paediatr Child Health* 27:340–343, 1993.
7. AAP Task Force on Infant Positioning and SIDS. Positioning and SIDS, *Pediatrics* 89:1120–1126, 1992.
8. Dwyer T, Ponsonby A-L, Blizzard L, et al: The contribution of changes in prevalence of prone sleeping position to the decline in sudden infant death syndrome in Tasmania, *JAMA* 273:783–789, 1995.
9. Gilbert R: The changing epidemiology of SIDS, *Arch Dis Child* 70:445–449, 1994.
10. Mitchell EA, Brunt JM, Everard CM: Reduction in mortality from sudden infant death syndrome in New Zealand: 1986–1992, *Arch Dis Child* 70:291–294, 1994.
11. Ponsonby A-L, Dwyer T, Cooper D: Sleeping position, infant apnea, and cyanosis: a population-based study, *Pediatrics* 99:e3, 1997.
12. Willinger M, Hoffman HJ, Hartford RB: Infant sleep position and risk for sudden infant death syndrome: report of meeting held January 13–14 1994, National Institutes of Health, Bethesda, MD, *Pediatrics* 93:814–820, 1994.
13. AAP Task Force on Infant Positioning and SIDS: Positioning and sudden infant death syndrome (SIDS), *Pediatrics* 92:1216–1218, 1996.

14. Scheers NJ, Daytron M, Kemp JS: Sudden infant death with external airways covered: case-comparison study of 206 deaths in the United States, *Arch Pediatr Adolesc Med* 152:540–547, 1998.
15. Willinger M, Hoffman HJ, Wu K-T, et al: Factors associated with the transition to nonprone sleep positions of infants in the United States, *JAMA* 280:329–335, 1999.
16. Willinger M, Ko C-W, Hoffman HJ, et al: Factors associated with caregiver's choice of infant sleep position: 1994–1998, *JAMA* 283:2135–2142, 2000.
17. AAP Task Force on Sudden Infant Death Syndrome: The changing concept of sudden infant death syndrome: diagnostic coding shifts, controversies regarding the sleep environment, and new variables to consider in reducing risk, *Pediatrics* 116:1245–1255, 2005.
18. Li DK, Petitti DB, Willinger M, et al: Infant sleeping position and the risk of sudden infant death syndrome in California, 1997–2000, *Am J Epidemiol* 157:446–455, 2003.
19. Paris C, Remler R, Daling JR: Risk factors for sudden infant death syndrome: changes associated with sleep position recommendations, *J Pediatr* 139:771–777, 2001.
20. Persing J, James H, Swanson J, et al: Prevention and management of positional skull deformities in infants, *Pediatrics* 112:199–202, 2003 [Letters to the editor, *Pediatrics* 113:422–424, 2003].
21. Graham M, Gomez JM Jr, Halberg A, et al: Management of deformational plagiocephaly: repositioning versus orthotic therapy, *J Pediatr* 146:258–262, 2005.
22. Graham J, Kreutzman JM Jr, Earl D, et al: Deformational brachycephaly in supine-sleeping infants, *J Pediatr* 146:253–257, 2005.
23. Cote A, Gerez T, Brouillette RT, et al: Circumstances leading to a change to prone sleeping in sudden infant death syndrome victims, *Pediatrics* 106:e86, 2000.
24. Davis BE, Moon RY, Sachs HC, et al: Effects of sleep position on infant motor development, *Pediatrics* 102:135–140, 1998.
25. Schwartz PJ, Stramba-Badiale M, Sergantini A, et al: Prolongation of QT interval and the sudden infant death syndrome, *N Engl J Med* 338:1709–1714, 1998.
26. Schwartz PJ, Priori SG, Dumaine R, et al: A molecular link between the sudden infant death syndrome and the long-QT syndrome, *N Engl J Med* 343:262–267, 2000.
27. Iyasu S, Rowley DL, Hanzlick RL, et al: Guidelines for death scene investigation of sudden unexplained infant deaths: recommendations of the interagency panel on sudden infant death syndrome, *MMWR* 45:1–22, 1966.
28. Moon RY, Grinras JL, Erwin R: Physician beliefs and practices regarding SIDS and SIDS risk reduction, *Clin Pediatr* 41:391–395, 2002.
29. Matthews T, McDonnell M, McGarvey C, et al: A multivariate "time-based" analysis of SIDS risk factors, *Arch Dis Child* 89:267–271, 2004.
30. Malloy M, Freeman D: Age at death, season, and day of death as indicators of the effect of the Back to Sleep Program on Sudden Infant Death Syndrome in the United States, 1992–1999, *Arch Pediatr Adolesc Med* 158:359–365, 2004.

# 27 Positional Brachycephaly

## GENESIS

*Brachycephaly* translates literally to "short head" and refers to a head that is shortened in the anteroposterior dimension and wide between the biparietal eminences when viewed from above. The most frequent cause of brachycephaly is constant supine positioning during infancy (Fig. 27-1). The increasing prevalence of brachycephaly in recent years is a consequence of the success of efforts to prevent sudden infant death syndrome (SIDS). The "Back to Sleep" campaign was initiated by the American Academy of Pediatrics in June 1992, with the initial recommendation to place infants to sleep on their sides or backs to prevent SIDS. After 1996, the more stringent recommendation for only supine sleep positioning was made because it was recognized that some side-sleeping infants were still dying from SIDS after assuming a prone sleeping position during the night.[1] The end result of this public education effort has been a decline in the prevalence of prone sleeping position from 70% in 1992 to 10.5% in 1997, with a concordant reduction in SIDS from 2.6 per 1000 in 1986 to 1.0 per 1000 in 1998.[2] When infants remain in a persistently supine position without any preferential head turn due to torticollis and without the developmental benefits of turning their heads from side to side during regular periods of "tummy time" while awake and under direct adult observation, their heads become progressively flattened through the impact of gravity and persistent occipital mechanical pressure.

A 1995 study of 7609 Dutch infants, who were screened for positional preference before age 6 months, revealed that 8.6% manifested positional preference with resultant deformational plagiocephaly; an additional 10% manifested occipital flattening, 45% of whom showed persistent asymmetric occipital flattening at age 2 to 3 years.[3] Among 181 otherwise normal New Zealand infants whose head shapes were followed at regular intervals from birth through age 2 years in 2002, the prevalence of plagiocephaly or brachycephaly peaked at 4 months at 20% (associated with male gender, first-born, limited neck rotation, and inability of caregivers to vary the infant's head position when putting the infant down to sleep) and then fell to 9% by age 8 months and 3.3% by age 2 years. Despite continued advice by family doctors and community child health nurses to encourage neck rotation, tummy time, and repositioning, 13% of the 4-month cases, were still cases at age 2 years, and 33% of the 8-month cases were still cases at age 2 years.[4] The supine-sleeping infants in this 2002 cohort were significantly more brachycephalic at each assessment interval (cephalic index 4% to 5% greater) than a 1977 cohort of prone sleeping infants, and these investigators used a cephalic index cutoff of 93% as the point at which the abnormal head shape was obvious. This high prevalence of persistent plagiocephaly in predominantly supine-sleeping

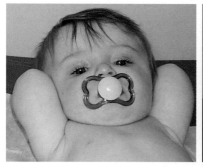
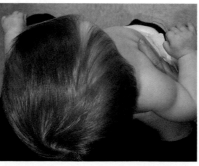

FIGURE 27-1. This 9-month-old boy was one of a set of quadruplets who were delivered close to term, and his position of comfort after birth was with both arms positioned behind his head. Persistent prone positioning resulted in brachycephaly with a cranial index of 98%.

infants compares with the previous 0.3% incidence of deformational plagiocephaly in Dunn's 1974 study of predominantly prone-sleeping British infants.[5] Thus, the prone sleeping position manifests a protective effect for both positional preference and deformational brachycephaly. This was confirmed in a 1984 Swedish study in which 2.4% of children with a prone sleeping position and 19% of children with a supine sleeping position showed a positional preference.[6]

Taking all of these data together, it is clear that the "Back to Sleep" campaign has been a major success in reducing the incidence of SIDS by more than 50%, but primary care providers also need to emphasize the importance of tummy time to parents. It is essential to place infants on their backs for sleep, except in cases of prematurity, gastroesophageal reflux, or obstructive sleep apnea. However, infants should be placed on their stomachs whenever they are awake and under direct adult supervision in order to develop their prone motor skills and to encourage the full range of neck rotation. The development of positional brachycephaly, with or without plagiocephaly, is an indication that parents may not be providing their infants with adequate tummy time.

## FEATURES

*Brachycephaly* refers to a head that is shortened in the anteroposterior dimension and wide between the biparietal eminences, with a cranial index (CI = width ÷ length × 100%) greater than 81% (see Fig. 25-5).[7] The normal CI ranges from 76% to 81%, and dolichocephaly is present when the CI is less than 76%. Positional brachycephaly results from gravitational deformation of the infant's skull during exclusive or persistent supine positioning during both sleeping and waking hours (see Fig. 27-1). Normal brain growth combined with a constant supine postnatal resting position can result in progressive cranial widening with occipital flattening. The malleable neonatal cranium, which arises from within the dura mater surrounding the growing brain, reflects the mechanical interaction between internal brain growth and external deforming forces. Although excessive brachycephaly is considered abnormal today, it may not have been so in the past. The purposeful use of external mechanical forces to deform the shape of an infant's head was practiced by various cultures for thousands of years, and a variety of head shapes were intentionally created using various external-shaping devices (Fig. 27-2).[8,9] Six main techniques were used for intentional cranial

deformation: manual cranial massage, wooden boards, banding, pads, stones, and cradle boards. Positioning infants in hard wooden cradles may also have unintentionally created brachycephalic heads in some Middle Eastern cultures,[9] and binding an infant's head to a stiff surface has similarly altered head shapes in many primitive cultures throughout the world.[8]

Certain wooden cribs and cradle boards with flat bottoms were particularly likely to deform an infant's head. Other cultures used pads and bindings to create deforming devices made from various materials. In some regions of the world, manual massaging of the infant's head was done to achieve a perfectly round effect. In addition, brachycephaly has a worldwide distribution because of supine positioning on a hard surface. Immobility or cradling also resulted in brachycephaly because many cultures bound their infants in a supine position. The inability of a swaddled infant to reposition itself, combined with constant supine positioning on a firm surface, often resulted in brachycephaly.[9] Because both unintentional and deliberate cranial deformations persist throughout life, it is essential for pediatricians to recognize the impact of postnatal mechanical forces in shaping infant heads. Primitive practices of head molding from older cultures also provide the basis of current therapy for infants who have developed misshapen heads. The typical brachycephalic head shape is flat in the back and quite wide, with peaking of the vertex. Sometimes the head is so flattened that it is wider than it is long, with a CI greater than 100% in the most severe cases.

Cultures in which infants are placed for sleeping in supine position have a higher incidence of brachycephaly than do cultures in which infants are placed in prone position.[10] The CI is 80% for term neonates delivered by cesarean section, which is similar to that of prone-sleeping cultures. The CI during infancy in India (where infants sleep supine) is higher than during later childhood. Of note, child-rearing practices in India promote frequent tummy time when the infant is awake and under observation. Prone-sleeping cultures have a normocephalic CI (mean CI = 80% with a range from 76% to 81%), while school children in Japan and Korea (supine-sleeping cultures) are brachycephalic (85%–91%).[10] With the continued success of the "Back to Sleep" campaign, infants will have a more rounded head shape than was seen among cultures that put their infants to sleep on their stomachs. The current normative CI is 86% to 88%, and it is relatively rare to encounter a case of dolichocephaly among infants who sleep supine unless the infant

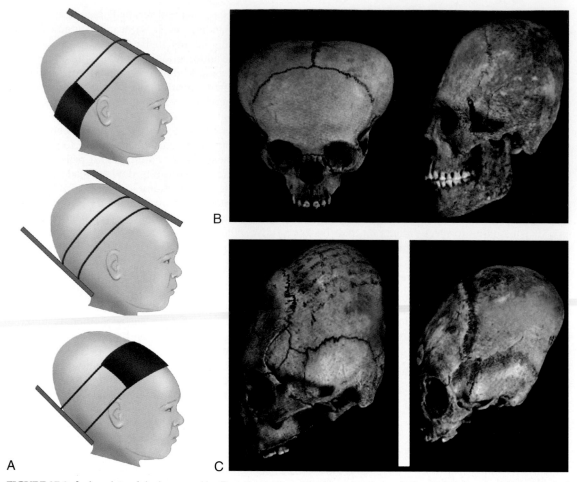

FIGURE 27-2. **A,** A variety of devices used by Peruvian Indians to achieve brachycephalic skull shapes, as demonstrated by adult skulls from these cultures. Highland Peruvians apparently applied circumferential bandages to the calvarium to achieve a conical head shape **(B),** while Coastal Peruvians applied boards to the occiput and pads to the frontal region, along with circumferential banding **(C).**

(Adapted from Dingwall EJ: *Artificial cranial deformation. A contribution to the study of ethnic mutilation,* London, 1931, John Bale, Sons, & Danielson.)

has sagittal craniosynostosis or congenital hypotonia. In a study of 39 infants with plagiocephaly, 30% of the infants had head widths more than two standard deviations above the mean for age, and 4.6% exceeded three standard deviations.[11] The mean CI for these infants was 88.5% (whereas the mean CI for their fathers was 75% and the mean CI for their mothers was 74%), and 14% of the infants had a CI great than 100%.[11] Thus, infants who sleep supine have significantly more brachycephaly than their prone-sleeping parents.

Some parents who become concerned about their infant's brachycephaly from prolonged supine positioning consider positioning their infant in a side-sleeping position, which is a dangerous sleep position for SIDS in an infant who has had little or no tummy time. Infants who experience no periods of consistent tummy time become very distressed when placed in prone position, and their parents readily agree that their infant has never tolerated being on his or her stomach. The best management is to institute regular periods of tummy time beginning in early infancy while the infant is awake and under direct observation.[12]

## MANAGEMENT, PROGNOSIS, AND COUNSEL

Because the primary cause of brachycephaly is constant supine positioning, the most important method of treatment is to vary the infant's head position during sleep. Repositioning may be accomplished with the use of an infant positioning device, and toys and other stimulating objects can be placed in the infant's field of view to encourage him or her to turn from side to side during sleep. Another essential form of treatment is providing the infant with adequate tummy time each day throughout infancy. Although it is recommended that infants sleep on their backs, placing an infant on its stomach (under adult supervision) is an excellent method to not only prevent cranial flattening but also to facilitate good neck muscle rotation and tone while stimulating the development of prone motor skills. Many brachycephalic infants in our clinic were deprived of tummy time by well-meaning parents who followed advice to keep infants on their backs to prevent SIDS. Such infants experienced no periods of regular tummy time and became very distressed when placed in prone position. The cure is to institute regular periods of tummy time throughout each day, beginning shortly after birth, while the infant is awake and under direct observation.

One prospective study from 1998 through 1999 randomized the treatment of 74 infants with positional plagiocephaly with either repositioning (45 infants) or cranial orthotic therapy (29 infants).[13] Some infants were initially repositioned and then later put into helmets when they failed to respond; their subsequent responses to helmets were included among the helmeted group. Outcomes were similar in both groups, but repositioning took three times as long as helmet therapy, and the groups were too small for statistical analysis.[13] Cranial orthotic therapy has proven to be effective in correcting deformational posterior plagiocephaly,[14] and it has also been used to correct brachycephaly.[10] With extreme occipital flattening, a helmet can often be difficult to fit or require prolonged treatment; thus, prevention is of paramount importance.[15] At the first sign of occipital flattening, repositioning and tummy time should be promptly initiated to correct brachycephaly,

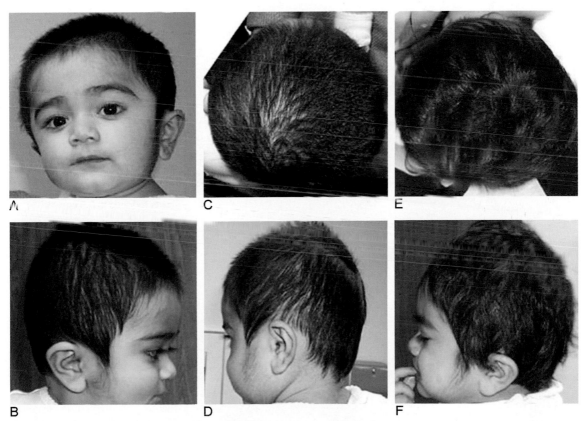

FIGURE 27-3. At 10.5 months, this male infant presented with a CI of 103% **(A-D)**. After 5 months of orthotic helmet therapy, his CI was brought into the normal range **(E, F)**.

and routine use of these practices during the first 6 weeks and thereafter should prevent this deformity.[12,14]

For those infants who do not make progress with repositioning and tummy time and have severe persistent brachycephaly (CI >90%) at age 5 months, use of an orthotic helmet will correct the brachycephaly (Fig. 27-3) and any associated plagiocephaly (Fig. 27-4).[10,14] The CI cut-off for clinical abnormality in one recent study was 93%,[4] but attempts to reposition brachycephalic heads after age 5 months demonstrate only slight improvement in CI[10]; hence, significant brachycephaly at age 5 to 6 months is likely to persist with cranial orthotic therapy. Reassurance is appropriate for parents of those infants with a CI <90% at age 5 months because brachycephaly is unlikely to develop or worsen after this age.[10]

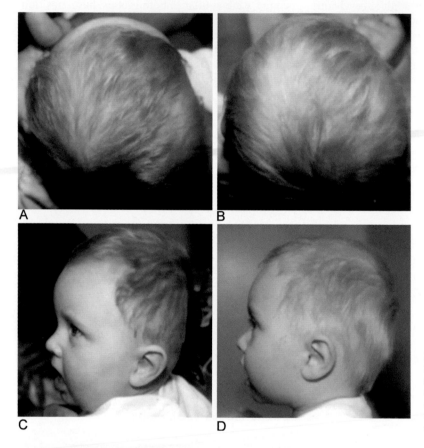

FIGURE 27-4. **A** and **B,** This 7-month male infant with right torticollis had a CI of 93% with a DD of 1.5 cm. **C** and **D,** After 5 months of helmet orthotic therapy, his CI was improved to 91% and his DD was reduced to 0.5 cm.

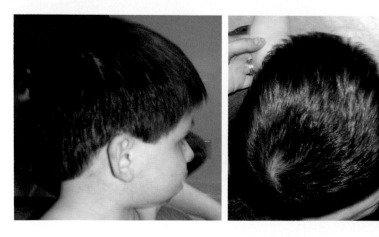

FIGURE 27-5. This child was adopted from a Russian orphanage where brachycephalic plagiocephaly was not managed, resulting in a 95% CI and 1-cm DD at age 18 months.

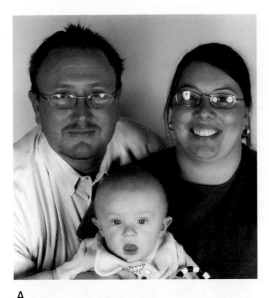

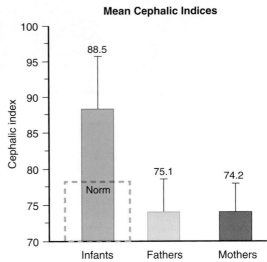

**Mean Cephalic Indices**

A

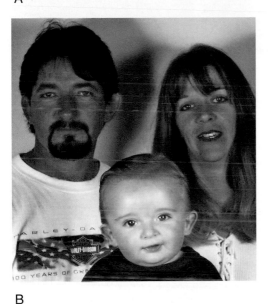

B

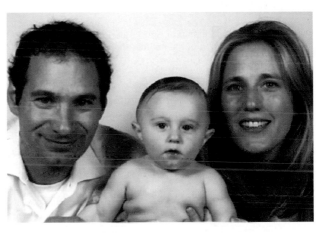

C

FIGURE 27-6. These infants with brachycephalic plagiocephaly had a CI that was dramatically different from that of their parents.
    (Adapted from Pomatto JK, Littlefield TR, Calcaterra J, et al: A study of family head shape: environment alters cranial shape, *Clin Pediatr* 45:55–63, 2006.)

Helmet therapy can remold the infant's head into a more normal, symmetric oval shape, and it has been successfully used to correct infant head shapes for more than 30 years.[10-18] The prominent lateral parts of the infant's head are restrained from becoming any wider while normal brain growth provides the corrective mechanic anteroposterior forces from within the calvarium to round out the shallow or flattened regions. Brachycephalic plagiocephaly persists without treatment (see Figs. 25-12 and 27-5), and it can lead to a head shape that is dramatically different from either parent (Fig. 27-6).

## DIFFERENTIAL DIAGNOSIS

Brachycephaly can be associated with bilateral coronal craniosynostosis, and cranial orthotic therapy after corrective surgery can be helpful in

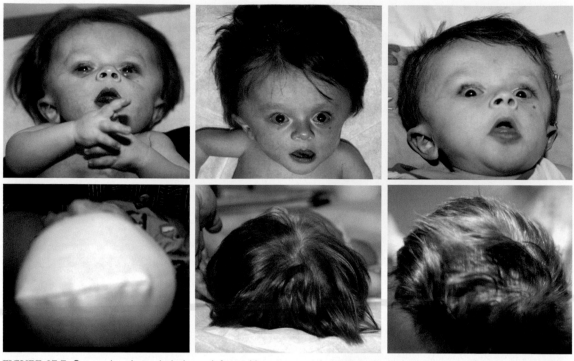

FIGURE 27-7. Severe brachycephaly in an infant with osteogenesis imperfecta type III and associated communicating hydrocephalus. The infant was first treated at age 11 months, and over the course of the next year, his neurologic state improved after initiation of helmet therapy.

directing head growth into a more optimal shape. Some surgical techniques for bicoronal synostosis actually duplicate the mechanic effects of helmet molding by surgically producing transverse tension across the skull and letting it expand anteriorly by means of a superiorly hinged fronto-orbital flap and expand posteriorly via an inferiorly based occipital flap. This may be particularly useful for genetic types of bicoronal synostosis with defective fibroblast growth factor receptor responses.[19,20] It is important to distinguish deformational brachycephaly from bilateral coronal craniosynostosis because therapy and management are very different for each condition. It is also important to note that brachycephaly may be associated with various syndromes that increase pliability of the infant skull through calvarial demineralization or increase an infant's tendency to remain recumbent for prolonged periods of time. Thus, conditions associated with skull demineralization, such as osteogenesis imperfecta or hypophosphatasia, lead to deformational brachycephaly because the cranium is much more malleable (Fig. 27-7). Conditions resulting in congenital hypotonia, such as Down syndrome, lead to brachycephaly, as do conditions associated with limited neck mobility, such as Klippel-Feil sequence (see Fig. 24-8).

## References

1. AAP Task Force on Infant Positioning and SIDS: Positioning and sudden infant death syndrome (SIDS), *Pediatrics* 92:1216–1218, 1996.
2. Paris C, Remler R, Daling JR: Risk factors for sudden infant death syndrome: changes associated with sleep position recommendations, *J Pediatr* 139:771–777, 2001.
3. Boere-Boonekamp MM, van der Linden-Kuiper LT: Positional preference: prevalence in infants and follow-up after two years, *Pediatrics* 107:339–343, 2001.
4. Hutchinson BL, Hutchinson LA, Thompson JM, et al: Plagiocephaly and brachycephaly in the first two years of life: a prospective cohort study, *Pediatrics* 114:970–980, 2004.
5. Dunn PM: Congenital sternomastoid torticollis: an intrauterine postural deformity, *Arch Dis Child* 49:824–825, 1974.
6. Palmen K: Prevention of congenital dislocation of the hip: the Swedish experience of neonatal treatment of hip joint instability, *Acta Orthop Scand* 55(Suppl 208):58–67, 1984.
7. Hall JG, Froster-Iskenius UG, Allanson JE: *Handbook of normal physical measurements*, New York, 1995, Oxford University Press, p 108.
8. Dingwall EJ: *Artificial cranial deformation*, London, 1931, John Bale, Sons, & Danielson.
9. Ewing JF: Hyperbrachycephaly as influenced by cultural conditioning, *Papers of the Peabody Museum of American*

*Archaeology & Ethnology*, vol XXIII, no 2, Cambridge, MA, 1950, Harvard University.

10. Graham JM Jr, Kreutzman J, Earl D, et al: Deformational brachycephaly in supine-sleeping infants, *J Pediatr* 146:253–257, 2005.

11. Pomatto JK, Littlefield TR, Calcaterra J, et al: A study of family head shape: environment alters cranial shape, *Clin Pediatr* 45:55–63, 2006.

12. Graham JM Jr: Tummy time is important, *Clin Pediatr* 45:119–122, 2006.

13. Loveday BP, de Chalain T: Active counterpositioning or orthotic device to treat positional plagiocephaly? *J Craniofac Surg* 12:308–313, 2001.

14. Graham JM Jr, Gomez M, Halberg A, et al: Management of deformational plagiocephaly: repositioning versus orthotic therapy, *J Pediatr* 146:258–262, 2005.

15. Ripley CE, Pomatto J, Beals SP, et al: Treatment of positional plagiocephaly with dynamic orthotic cranioplasty, *J Craniofac Surg* 5:150–159, 1994 [discussion, 160].

16. Persing J, James H, Swanson J, et al: Prevention and management of positional skull deformities in infants, *Pediatrics* 112:199–202, 2003.

17. Clarren SK: Helmet therapy for plagiocephaly and congenital muscular torticollis, *J Pediatr* 94:43–46, 1979.

18. Clarren SK: Plagiocephaly and torticollis: etiology, natural history, and helmet therapy, *J Pediatr* 98:92–95, 1981.

19. Lauritzen C, Friede H, Elander A, et al: Dynamic cranioplasty for brachycephaly, *Plast Reconstr Surg* 98:7–14, 1996.

20. Guimaraes-Ferreira J, Gewall F, Sahlin P, et al: Dynamic cranioplasty for brachycephaly in Apert syndrome: long-term follow-up study, *J Neurosurg* 94:757–764, 2001.

# 28 Other Postnatal Head Deformations

## PREMATURE INFANT

The liability toward deformation depends on the magnitude and duration of the forces applied and the pliability of the fetus. The prematurely born infant is more malleable than the term baby, and prior to the "Back to Sleep" campaign, postnatal cranial deformation was primarily a problem of premature infants, with severe deformation inhibiting parental attachment and bonding in some cases.[1,2] In addition, the premature infant is less active and more likely to lie in one position persistently. If the surface on which he or she lies is relatively firm, often the premature infant will develop flattening on both sides of the head, with a dolichocephalic, narrow head shape (Figs. 28-1 and 28-2). This head shape can persist into adulthood and inhibit parental attachment and bonding in some cases[1-4]; it can be avoided by placing premature infants on pressure-relief mattresses or waterbeds to prevent adverse molding.[2,5,6] Early studies documented that preterm infants in prone position with resultant lateral flattening had more dolichocephaly than term infants placed in supine position.[7] As infants have been persistently positioned on their backs to prevent SIDS since 1994, the incidence of dolichocephaly related to

prematurity has markedly decreased, but other head shapes have taken its place, such as plagiocephaly in infants with torticollis, oxycephaly in infants with persistent vertex molding, and brachycephaly in infants with constant supine positioning. The risk for such deformations in prematurely born infants can be minimized to some extent by careful positioning of premature infants on water-filled cushions or other pressure-relief mattresses rather than the relatively firm surfaces in standard incubators.[2,5,6]

Developmental care of prematurely born infants has become standard in today's modern neonatal intensive care units, in which skilled nurses rotate the infant's head position on a regular basis, especially for those neonates who cannot do so themselves. Without such changes in resting position, the premature baby may persistently lie on one side of the head and develop plagiocephaly as a result. This is particularly likely to occur in premature infants who undergo surgical procedures that limit their opportunities for repositioning or in neurologically damaged infants. Obviously, gentle physical therapy and repositioning can help prevent postnatal deformations in premature infants.

## FULL-TERM INFANT

A term infant with a neurologic deficiency or who is seriously neglected may tend to lie in one position and may develop asymmetric flattening on one side of the head (Fig. 28-3). Thumb sucking seldom causes deformation in early infancy; however, once the teeth have developed, thumb sucking can deform the upper jaw. This is especially true when the child "pulls out" on the teeth. Growth of the mandible tends to catch up to that of the maxilla during the first few years, and the mandibular teeth normally conform to the maxillary teeth. Supernumerary teeth or the absence of teeth can lead to mild deformation, including malocclusions between the maxilla and mandible. Nowhere have the principles of mechanic treatment been more effectively used than in the

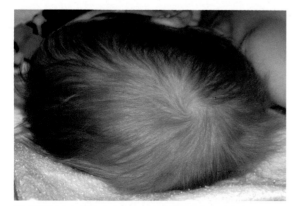

FIGURE 28-1. This is a fairly typical premature infant head shape from 30 years ago, long and narrow, with a cranial index less than 76%.

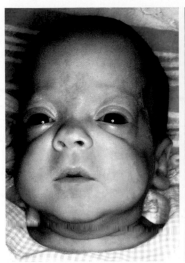
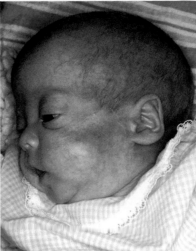
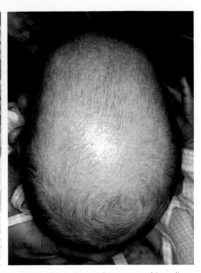

FIGURE 28-2. This infant was born prematurely at 28 weeks and positioned on the sides of her head for most of her first few months due to the need for respiratory therapy and venous access. As she rested on one side or the other, her head became progressively more dolichocephalic, with frontal bossing. As her head became longer and narrower, she lacked sufficient neck strength to rest on her occiput without a positioning ring. This is about as close as infants come today to a true premature infant head shape.

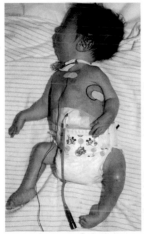
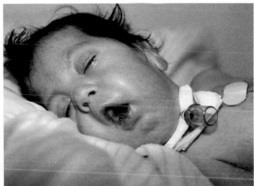

FIGURE 28-3. This infant was born with profound congenital hypotonia of undetermined etiology. The head is turned on one side or the other and has become progressively flattened due to the infant's inability to move. This infant is at risk for idiopathic infantile scoliosis with inability to suck or swallow; prominent lateral palatine ridges due to lack of tongue movement; inability to control secretions, necessitating tracheostomy; and a poor long-term prognosis.

mouth. Once the teeth have fully erupted, they may be used as anchors for a variety of devices to alter the growth and/or alignment of the maxilla, mandible, or both. Intraoral devices that provide rather small pressures on developing teeth can have a considerable affect on form. In India, mothers often massage infants' alveolae in an effort to help align the unerupted teeth buds into an even row. Current anthropologic data also indicate that infant head molding, through the application of pressure or bindings to the cranial bones to alter their shapes, is still prevalent among certain Caribbean, Latino, European, African-American, Asian, and Native American groups.[8] The use of cranial orthotics to correct aberrant head shapes is discussed in Chapters 25 and 27.

## References

1. Budreau G: Postnatal cranial molding and infant attractiveness: implications for nursing, *Neonatal Network* 4:13–19, 1987.
2. Chan J, Kelley M, Khan J: The effects of pressure relief mattress on postnatal head molding in very low birth weight infants, *Neonatal Network* 12:19–22, 1993.
3. Chan J, Kelley M, Khan J: Predictors of postnatal head molding in very low birth weight infants, *Neonatal Network* 14:47–52, 1995.
4. Baum J, Searls D: Head shape and size of preterm low-birth-weight infants, *Develop Med Child Neurol* 13:576–581, 1971.
5. Hemingway MM, Oliver SK: Waterbed therapy and cranial molding of the sick preterm infant, *Neonatal Network* 10:53–56, 1991.
6. Schwirian PM, Eesley T, Cuellar L: Use of water pillows in reducing head shape distortion in preterm infants, *Res Nursing Health* 9:203–207, 1986.
7. Largo RN, Duc G: Head growth changes in head configuration in healthy preterm and term infants during the first six months of life, *Helvetica Paediatrica Acta* 32:431–442, 1977.
8. Fitzsimmons E, Prost J, Peniston S: Infant head molding: a cultural practice, *Arch Fam Med* 7:88–90, 1998.

# Craniosynostosis

# 29 Craniosynostosis: General

## GENESIS

The term *craniostenosis* (literally translating as "cranial narrowing") is used to describe the abnormal head shape that results from premature fusion of one or more sutures, whereas *craniosynostosis* is the process of premature sutural fusion that results in craniostenosis. The term *craniosynostosis* is used more widely, perhaps in an effort to distinguish deformational nonsynostotic head shapes from those caused by underlying sutural synostosis, but the two terms can be used interchangeably. Plagiocephaly is a nonspecific term used to describe an asymmetric head shape, which can result from either craniosynostosis or cranial deformation, and differentiation between these two processes is critical to determining the proper mode of treatment (i.e., surgery versus physical techniques). Synostotic plagiocephaly is usually corrected by a neurosurgical procedure, whereas deformational plagiocephaly responds to early physical therapy, repositioning, and cranial orthotic therapy if these early measures are unsuccessful.

In an otherwise normal fetus, prenatal limitation of normal growth stretch across a suture during late fetal life can result in craniosynostosis (Fig. 29-1). Synostosis can also occur when the lack of growth stretch is caused by a deficit in brain growth, as in severe primary microcephaly. Experimental prolongation of gestation, which resulted in fetal crowding after installation of a cervical clip in pregnant mice, has been shown to lead to craniosynostosis.[1] The frequency of craniosynostosis was greatest among mouse fetuses located proximally in the uterine horns, where the crowding was most severe. The most common cause of craniosynostosis in an otherwise normal infant is constraint of the fetal head in utero.[2-7] When external fetal head constraint limits growth stretch across a cranial sutural area between the constraining points, it may lead to craniosynostosis of an intervening suture (see Fig. 29-1). With sagittal craniosynostosis (the most common type), this event usually occurs in an otherwise normal child. The constrained suture tends to develop a bony ridge, especially at the point of maximum constraint between the biparietal eminences. Such ridging can easily be palpated or visualized on skull radiographs, and three-dimensional cranial computed tomography (3D-CT) allows the ridge to be seen even more clearly.

In general, craniosynostosis begins at one point and then spreads along a suture.[6,8] At the center of the fused suture, there is complete sutural obliteration with nonlamellar bone extending completely across the sutural space, while further away from the initial site of fusion, the sutural margins are closely approximated with ossifying connective tissue. The longer the time before the craniosynostosis is surgically corrected, the greater the tendency for more of the suture to become synostotic, with synostosis beginning at only one location in most cases.[6] Pronounced sutural ridging tends to occur primarily over midline end-to-end sutures (i.e., in sagittal and metopic synostosis). Ridging also occurs with coronal and lambdoidal synostosis, but it may be less prominent than that seen with synostotic midline end-to-end sutures. Synostosis

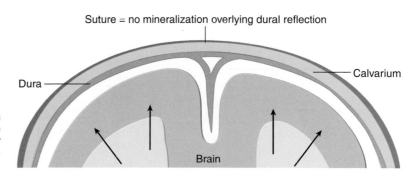

FIGURE 29-1. As long as there is continued growth stretch from the expanding brain, the sites over the dural reflections remain unossified, thereby forming the sutures.

173

prevents future expansion at that site, and the rapidly growing brain then distorts the calvarium into an aberrant shape, depending on which sutures have become synostotic. The various sutures and fontanelles are shown in Fig. 29-2, and the specific head shapes that result from each type of sutural fusion are shown in Figs. 29-3 and 29-4. The earlier the synostosis takes place, the greater the effect on skull shape, but the precise mechanisms that lead to sutural synostosis are heterogeneous and incompletely understood. For example, craniosynostosis may result from mutant gene function, storage disorders, hyperthyroidism, or failure of normal brain growth. The topic of craniosynostosis has been comprehensively reviewed by Cohen.[8]

The frequency of craniosynostosis is 3.4 per 10,000 births, and it is usually an isolated, sporadic anomaly in an otherwise normal child. About 8% of all craniosynostosis cases are familial. Familial types of craniosynostosis occur most frequently in coronal synostosis and account for 14.4% of coronal synostosis, 6% of sagittal synostosis, and 5.6% of metopic synostosis.[9-11] Whereas lambdoidal synostosis is almost never familial. The frequency of associated twinning is increased, and most twin pairs are discordant, especially in sagittal and metopic synostosis; this would tend to support fetal crowding as a cause of these types of synostosis, whereas concordance for coronal synostosis is much higher for monozygotic twins than for dizygotic twins.[8] Familial craniosynostosis is usually transmitted as an autosomal dominant trait with incomplete penetrance and variable expressivity. A wide variety of chromosomal anomalies have also been associated with craniosynostosis, a fact that emphasizes the importance of chromosomal analysis for those patients with syndromic craniosynostosis in whom a recognizable monogenic syndrome is not apparent, particularly when there is associated developmental delay and growth deficiency. In addition, craniosynostosis can also occur as a component of numerous syndromes, many of which manifest phenotypic overlap and genetic heterogeneity.

Named syndromes with a demonstrated mutational basis include Apert's syndrome, Crouzon syndrome, Pfeiffer's syndrome, Saethre-Chotzen syndrome, Jackson-Weiss syndrome, Boston craniosynostosis, Beare-Stevenson cutis gyrata syndrome, and FGFR3-associated coronal synostosis; however, the efficiency of actually detecting a mutation for a given syndrome varies from about 60% for Crouzon syndrome to 98% for Apert's syndrome. Secondary craniosynostosis can occur with certain primary metabolic disorders (e.g., hyperthyroidism, rickets), storage disorders (e.g., mucopolysaccharidosis), hematologic disorders (e.g., thalassemia, sickle cell anemia, polycythemia vera, congenital hemolytic icterus), brain malformations (e.g., holoprosencephaly, microcephaly, encephalocele, overshunted hydrocephalus), and selected teratogenic exposures (e.g., diphenylhydantoin, retinoic acid, valproic acid, aminopterin, fluconazole, cyclophosphamide).[8]

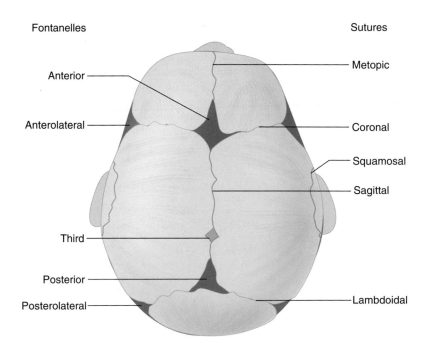

FIGURE 29-2. Diagram showing the named cranial sutures and fontanelles.

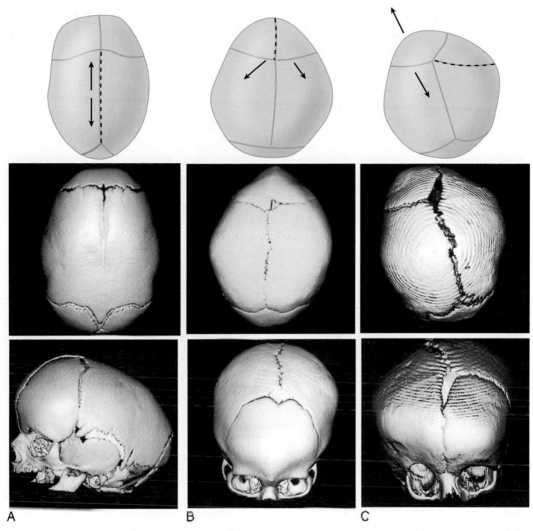

FIGURE 29-3. Diagrams and 3D-CT scans depicting sagittal **(A)**, metopic **(B)**, and right coronal **(C)** synostosis.

## FEATURES

The impact of craniosynostosis on skull shape is dependent on which sutures are synostotic, the extent of craniosynostosis, and the timing of the problem. The earlier the craniostenosis occurs, the more profound its impact on subsequent craniofacial development. Craniosynostosis of multiple sutures may limit overall brain growth and result in increased intracranial pressure.[7] Elevated intracranial pressure occurs more commonly with syndromic craniosynostosis and multiple sutural synostosis. On skull radiographs, increased intracranial pressure due to craniosynostosis may be associated with a "beaten copper" appearance. The precise reason for this phenomenon is not known, but it may be the result of the altered

magnitude and direction of forces on the bony trabecular organization within the calvarium. In children older than 8 years, the finding of papilledema indicates the presence of increased intracranial pressure, but the absence of papilledema in younger children is not predictive of normal pressure. Pronounced sutural ridging occurs primarily in sagittal and metopic synostosis, and these midline, end-to-end sutures may be predisposed toward ridging when they become synostotic.[8] It is important to distinguish craniosynostosis in normal-appearing infants from that which occurs in association with genetic syndromes.[8-11] Ridging of one lambdoid suture occurs commonly with lambdoid synostosis, and such ridging helps distinguish lambdoidal synostosis from deformational posterior plagiocephaly.[12,13] Ridging occurs infrequently in

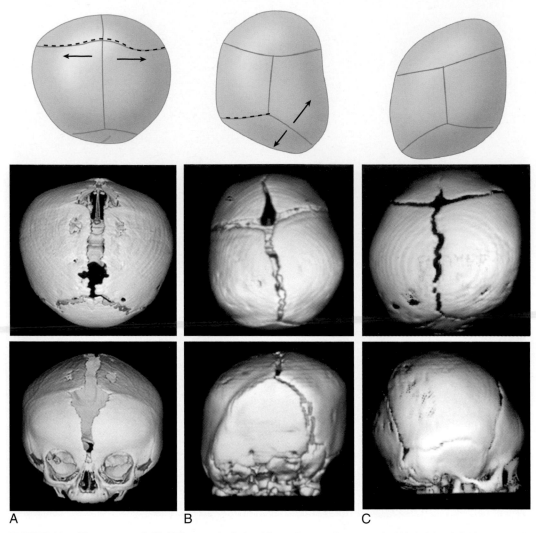

FIGURE 29-4. Diagrams and 3D-CT scans depicting bilateral coronal synostosis **(A)**, left lambdoid synostosis **(B)**, and right occipital deformational plagiocephaly **(C)**.

unilateral coronal craniosynostosis, suggesting that some of these cases may have a constraint-related phenotype, but unless a mutation is detected, it is virtually impossible to distinguish between coronal synostosis due to fetal head constraint and genetic craniosynostosis.

Inability to demonstrate a mutation does not rule out a genetic basis for the craniosynostosis, and not every person with a mutation manifests craniosynostosis. Bilateral coronal synostosis often lacks sutural ridging and usually has a genetic pathogenesis, which suggests that all such patients should be screened for mutations. Among 57 patients with bilateral coronal synostosis, mutations were found in fibroblast growth factor receptor (FRGR) genes for all 38 patients with a syndromic form of craniosynostosis. Even more

interesting were the observations that among 19 patients with unclassified brachycephaly, mutations in or near exon 9 of FGFR2 were found in 4 patients, a common Pro250Arg mutation in exon 7 of FGFR3 was detected in 10 patients, and only 5 patients (9%) manifested brachycephaly without a detectable mutation in FGFR 1, 2, or 3.[14] These findings suggest that mutation analysis should be performed in all patients with coronal synostosis.

## MANAGEMENT AND PROGNOSIS

Mild degrees of craniostenosis may not always require surgery; however, early surgical therapy is usually warranted in most cases. With the exception of instances in which both the coronal and sagittal sutures are synostotic (thereby impairing brain growth early in infancy), the predominant indication for surgery is the restoration of normal craniofacial shape and growth, thus reducing neurologic and ophthalmologic complications associated with increased intracranial pressure and inadequate orbital volume as well as improving childhood psychosocial development. A variety of neurosurgical techniques have been developed for the treatment of craniosynostosis.[8] Most of these techniques involve removing the aberrant portion of the bony calvarium from its underlying dura, including the area that surrounds the synostotic suture(s). If this is done within the first few months after birth, a new bony calvarium usually develops within the remaining dura mater, following the same principles that normally guide prenatal calvarial morphogenesis.[8] As long as there is continued growth stretch from the expanding brain, the sites over the dural reflections remain unossified, thereby forming the sutures (see Fig. 29-1). Thus, the calvarium and its sutures usually develop normally after a partial calvarectomy for constraint-induced craniosynostosis. The new bony calvarium begins to develop within 2 to 3 weeks after surgery and is usually firm by 5 to 8 weeks. If the procedure is performed after 3 to 4 months of age, the approach is similar, with the exception that pieces of the calvarium are usually replaced in a mosaic over the dura mater to act as niduses for the mineralization of new calvarium. New endoscopic repair techniques have been developed, as well as postoperative orthotic molding techniques; such procedures are most effective if done relatively early in infancy. These techniques are most useful in otherwise normal infants who do not manifest a syndromic type of craniosynostosis with impaired responses to normal growth factors. With or without endoscopic surgical techniques, the use of postsurgical cranial remodeling devices has improved cosmetic results and in some circumstances has avoided the need for a second surgical procedure.[15]

After early surgery for isolated craniosynostosis (primary frontoorbital advancement and/or calvarial vault remodeling at a mean age of 8 months), only 13% of 104 patients (10 bilateral coronal, 57 unilateral coronal, 29 metopic, and 8 sagittal) required a second cranial vault operation for residual defects at a mean age of 23 months. Perioperative complications were minimal (5%), with 87.5% of patients considered to have at least satisfactory craniofacial form and with low rates of hydrocephalus (3.8%), shunt placement (1%), and seizures (2.9%). Among cases of isolated craniosynostosis, unilateral coronal synostosis was the most problematic type due to vertical orbital dystopia, nasal tip deviation, and altered craniofacial growth problems with residual craniofacial asymmetry.[16] In a second study of 167 children with both nonsyndromal (isolated) and syndromal craniosynostosis (12 bilateral coronal, 18 unilateral coronal, 39 metopic, and 46 sagittal), reoperation was necessary in only 7%, with reoperation occurring more often in syndromic cases (27.3%) than in cases of nonsyndromic craniosynostosis (5.6%).[17] One series of 256 patients underwent endoscopic-assisted craniectomies for craniosynostosis (134 sagittal, 57 coronal, 50 metopic, and 9 lambdoid) followed by postoperative helmet therapy.[17] Of the patients with sagittal synostosis, 87% had excellent results with a cephalic index (CI) >75, and only 4.3% had poor results with a CI <70 (mostly attributed to poor parental compliance with helmet therapy). Helmet therapy consisted of three phases: the first helmet was worn for 1 to 2 months after surgery to achieve a normal CI; the second helmet was worn for 3 to 6 months to overcorrect the CI; and the third helmet was worn for 7 to 12 months to maintain a normal CI.[18]

Although intracranial pressure can be elevated in patients with nonsyndromic craniosynostosis, they usually do not have decreased cranial volumes either before or after surgical repair, and as a group they show slightly larger intracranial volumes when compared with normal controls.[19] This could reflect the impact of fetal constraint on fetuses with larger heads, or it might relate to the known association of macrocephaly with nonsyndromic coronal craniosynostosis due to the common Pro250Arg mutation in FGFR3 (which was not analyzed in these studies). Hydrocephalus occurs in 4% to 10% of patients with craniosynostosis and is more common with syndromic and multiple sutural craniosynostosis. In nonsyndromic patients, the rate of cerebral ventricular dilatation is the same as that observed in the general population and appears to be related to venous hypertension induced by jugular foramen stenosis, which usually stabilizes spontaneously and rarely requires shunting. Some cases of progressive hydrocephalus among syndromic craniosynostosis cases were related to multiple sutural involvement that constricted cranial volume as well as to alterations in the skull base, crowding in the posterior fossa, and jugular foraminal stenosis.[20] These findings were most frequent among patients with Crouzon, Pfeiffer, or Apert syndromes, especially in association with cloverleaf skull abnormalities. A diffuse, beaten-copper pattern on skull radiographs, in addition to obliteration of anterior sulci or narrowing of basal cisterns in children younger than age 18 months, is predictive of increased intracranial pressure in more than 95% of cases.[21]

It is possible to visualize cranial sutures and fontanelles at 15 to 16 weeks of gestation, but the sagittal suture is difficult to visualize using two-dimensional ultrasonography, and 3D ultrasonography appears to be the best method for its demonstration.[22] It is unlikely that most cases of isolated craniosynostosis arise this early in gestation. Very few cases of craniosynostosis have been diagnosed prenatally, and in most of these cases, the diagnosis was made through association with other malformations.[23]

## DIFFERENTIAL DIAGNOSIS

The numerous causes of craniostenosis can be divided into several general categories, such as problems of the brain or mesenchymal tissues and metabolic disorders.[9,11] Recent apparent "epidemics" of craniosynostosis in Colorado, where the birth prevalence was more than twice that found in Atlanta, Georgia, highlight the impact of differing diagnostic techniques and illustrate how misdiagnosis can lead to inappropriate surgery.[8,12,13,24] In Colorado and York-Selby, United Kingdom, almost half of all craniosynostosis cases were diagnosed as having lambdoid synostosis, a type that usually constitutes less than 5% of all cases. Overdiagnosis of nonsynostotic deformational posterior plagiocephaly as unilateral lambdoid synostosis accounted for most instances of this misdiagnosis. Thus, it is critically important to validate the diagnosis of posterior craniosynostosis either through an independent second opinion or via 3D-CT scan. Categorization of the craniosynostosis (i.e., as isolated or syndromic, sporadic or familial, and primary or secondary) can also help clarify the diagnosis in most cases. There are several categorical causes for craniosynostosis.

## Brain Problems

Basic problems in early brain morphogenesis may cause a lack of dural reflection and hence the lack of a suture, thereby resulting in the inability of the calvarium to grow laterally in that region.[10] Observed examples[1] include holoprosencephaly (single ventricle) with no anterior interhemispheric fissure and consequently no metopic suture[2]; unilateral deficiency of the early cerebrum with no insular sulcus and hence no sphenoid wing; or unilateral deficiency of the dural reflection and hence no coronal suture. Deficit of brain growth, such as occurs in severe microcephaly, may result in a lack of expansile brain force, with craniostenosis as a secondary consequence. More localized brain growth deficiency may cause a particular suture to become prematurely craniostenotic; for example, frontal brain growth deficiency may result in metopic craniostenosis. Excessive shunting of hydrocephalus may also result in lack of growth stretch at the suture lines, enhancing the tendency toward craniostenosis.[9]

## Mesenchymal Tissue Problems

In a number of disorders, various types of craniosynostosis occur because of an aberration in mesenchymal tissues. In many of these syndromes, there are associated anomalies in limbs, such as syndactyly, brachydactyly, or broad deviated thumbs and halluces, suggesting a specific syndrome with a known pathogenesis and natural history (e.g., Apert, Crouzon, Pfeiffer, or Saethre-Chotzen syndromes). Most of these syndromic disorders are genetically determined, and mutational analysis for disorders resulting from mutations in FGFR1, FGFR2, FGFR3, and TWIST is now available through several clinical molecular genetic testing facilities. It is beyond the scope of this text to discuss these syndromes in detail, and the reader is referred to other sources.[8]

## Metabolic Problems

Early rickets, regardless of its cause, can result in craniosynostosis in about one third of cases. The prolonged use of aluminum-containing antacids along with the ingestion of soy-based formulas, both of which prevent phosphate absorption and lead to rickets, has been reported to cause secondary craniosynostosis.[25] In rare instances, early hyperthyroidism has also caused craniosynostosis, as has hypercalcemia.[9] Secondary craniosynostosis can also occur with storage disorders, such as mucopolysaccharidosis, and with various hematologic disorders, such as thalassemia, sickle cell anemia, polycythemia vera, and congenital hemolytic icterus.

### References

1. Koskinen-Moffett L, Moffet BC: Sutures and intrauterine deformation. In: Pershing JA, Edgerton MT, Jane JA, eds: *Scientific foundations and surgical treatment of craniosynostosis,* Baltimore, 1989, Williams & Wilkins, pp 96–106.

Craniosynostosis: General 179

2. Graham JM Jr, deSaxe M, Smith DW: Sagittal craniostenosis: fetal head constraint as one possible cause, *J Pediatr* 95:747–750, 1979.
3. Graham JM Jr, Badura R, Smith DW: Coronal craniostenosis: fetal head constraint as one possible cause, *Pediatrics* 65:995–999, 1980.
4. Graham JM Jr, Smith DW: Metopic craniostenosis and fetal head constraint: two interesting experiments of nature, *Pediatrics* 65:1000–1002, 1980.
5. Higgenbottom MC, Jones KL, James HE: Interuterine constraint and craniosynostosis, *Neurosurgery* 6:39–49, 1980.
6. Koskinen-Moffet LK, Moffet BC, Graham JM Jr: Cranial synostostosis and intra-uterine compression: a developmental study of human sutures. In: Dixon AD, Sarnat BG, eds: *Factors and mechanisms influencing bone growth*, New York, 1982, Alan R. Liss, pp 365–378.
7. Graham JM Jr: Craniofacial deformation, *Ballier Clin Pediatr* 6:293–315, 1998.
8. Cohen MM Jr, MacLean RE, eds: *Craniosynostosis: diagnosis, evaluation, and management*, ed 2, New York, 2000, Oxford University Press.
9. Lajeunie E, Le Merrer M, Bonati-Pellie C, et al: Genetic study of nonsyndromic coronal craniosynostosis, *Am J Med Genet* 55:500–504, 1995.
10. Lajeunie E, Le Merrer M, Bonati-Pellie C, et al: Genetic study of scaphocephaly, *Am J Med Genet* 62:282–285, 1996.
11. Lajeunie E, Arnaud E, Le Merrer M, et al: Syndromal and nonsyndromal primary trigonocephaly: analysis of a series of 237 patients, *Am J Med Genet* 55:500–504, 1998.
12. Huang MH, Gruss JS, Clarren SK, et al: The differential diagnosis of posterior plagiocephaly: true lambdoid synostosis versus positional molding, *Plast Reconstr Surg* 98:765–776, 1996.
13. Dias MS, Klein DM, Backstrom JW: Occipital plagiocephaly: deformation or lambdoid synostosis, *Pediatr Neurosurg* 24:61–68, 1996.
14. Mulliken JB, Steinberger D, Kunze S, et al: Molecular diagnosis of bilateral coronal synostosis, *Plast Reconstr Surg* 104:1603–1615, 1999.
15. Littlefield TR: Cranial remodeling devices: treatment of deformational plagiocephaly and postsurgical applications, *Semin Pediatr Neurol* 11:268–277, 2004.
16. McCarthy JG, Glasberg SB, Cutting CB, et al: Twenty-year experience with early surgery for craniosynostosis: isolated craniofacial synostosis—results and unsolved problems, *Plast Reconstr Surg* 96:273–283, 1995.
17. Williams JK, Cohen SR, Burstein FD, et al: A longitudinal, statistical study of reoperation rates in craniosynostosis, *Plast Reconstr Surg* 100:305–310, 1997.
18. Jimenez DF, Barone CM, McGee ME: Design and care of helmets in postoperative craniosynostosis patients: our personal approach, *Clin Plastic Surg* 31:481–487, 2004.
19. Polley JW, Charbel FT, Kim D, et al: Nonsyndromal craniosynostosis: longitudinal outcome following cranio-orbital reconstruction in infancy, *Plast Reconstr Surg* 102:619–628, 1998.
20. Cinalli G, Sainte-Rose C, Kollar EM, et al: Hydrocephalus and craniosynostosis, *J Neurosurg* 88:209–214, 1998.
21. Tuite GF, Evanston J, Chong WK, et al: The beaten copper cranium: a correlation between intracranial pressure, cranial radiographs, and computed tomographic scans in children with craniosynostosis, *Neurosurgery* 39:691–699, 1996.
22. Ginath S, Debby A, Malinger G: Demonstration of cranial sutures and fontanelles at 15 to 16 weeks of gestation: a comparison between two-dimensional and three-dimensional ultrasonography, *Prenat Diagn* 24:812–815, 2004.
23. Miller C, Losken HW, Towbin R, et al: Ultrasound diagnosis of craniosynostosis, *Cleft Palate Craniofac J* 39:73–80, 2002.
24. Alderman B, Fernbach SK, Greene C, et al: Diagnostic practice and the estimated prevalence of craniosynostosis in Colorado, *Arch Pediatr Adolesc Med* 151:159–164, 1997.
25. Shetty AK, Thomas T, Raoet J, et al: Ricketts and secondary craniosynostosis associated with long term antacid use in an infant, *Arch Pediatr Adolesc Med* 152:1243–1245, 1998.

# 30 Sagittal Craniosynostosis

## GENESIS

Early descent of the fetal head into the maternal pelvis (as early as 4 to 6 weeks before delivery) with fetal head entrapment that results in biparietal constraint is considered the most common cause of sagittal craniostenosis.[1,2] This mode of genesis is shown in Fig. 29-1. Synostosis limits lateral cranial expansion, resulting in dolichocephaly with progressive frontal and/or occipital prominence (Fig. 30-1), and ridging is usually palpable along the posterior portion of the sagittal suture (Fig. 30-2). The platypelloid pelvis, which is relatively small in the anteroposterior dimension compared with its lateral dimensions, would hypothetically constitute the greatest risk for this type of entrapment head constraint. Prolongation of gestation in pregnant mice via placement of a cervical clip resulted in fetal crowding and craniosynostosis.[3] Further support for the importance of

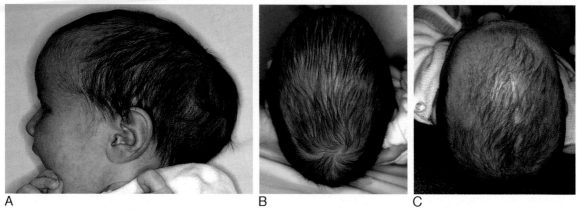

A           B           C

FIGURE 30-1. Side **(A)** and top **(B)** views of sagittal craniosynostosis, demonstrating a prominent occipital bulge with prominent forehead resulting in dolichocephaly. **C,** Postoperative top view of this same infant, demonstrating resolution of the initial dolichocephaly.

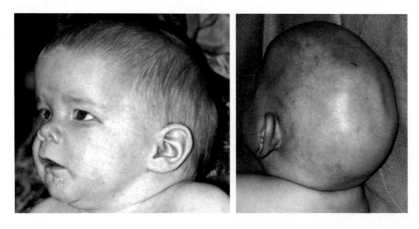

FIGURE 30-2. Prominent forehead with ridging of the sagittal suture along the posterior sagittal suture between the biparietal eminences in the plane of presumed lateral head constraint.

180

biomechanical forces in sagittal craniosynostosis derives from a study of sutural histology in completely synostotic and nonsynostotic sagittal sutures that were removed at the time of surgery. There is a definite qualitative difference in the trabecular pattern for both the vector and direction of suture

fusion initiation for the partially and completely synostotic suture compared with the open portion of the same suture (Fig. 30-3). Within the synostotic suture, the trabecular pattern is more disorganized and less polarized than it is within the open suture, where trabeculae are oriented parallel to

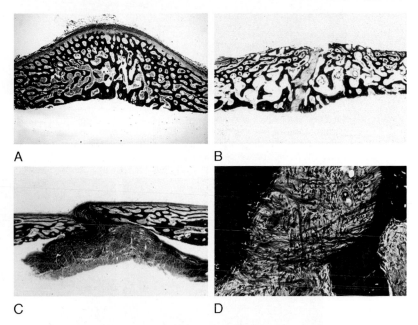

FIGURE 30-3. There is a definite qualitative difference in the trabecular pattern for both the vector and direction of suture fusion initiation for the partially and completely synostotic suture **(A)** versus the open portion of the same suture **(B)**. Within the closing suture **(C)**, the trabecular pattern was more disorganized and less polarized than it was within a completely open sagittal suture from an infant who died of an unrelated cause. In this normal open sagittal suture **(D)**, the trabeculae were oriented parallel to the direction of biomechanical growth-stretch forces.

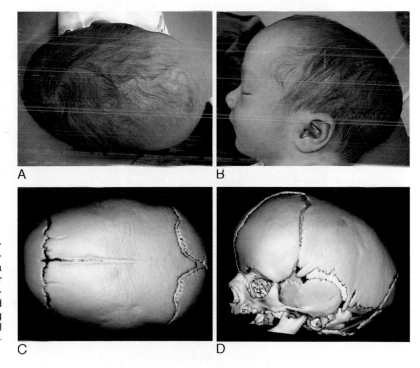

FIGURE 30-4. **A** and **B,** This 6-week-old infant has typical features of sagittal synostosis with a palpable ridge along the posterior sagittal suture. **C** and **D,** Three-dimensional cranial computed tomography scans demonstrating obliteration of the posterior sagittal suture with compensatory expansion of other cranial sutures.

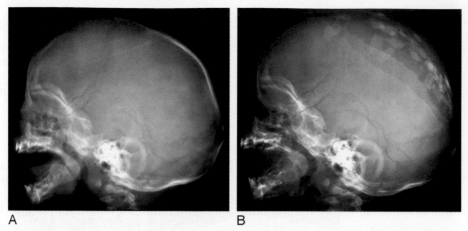

A        B

FIGURE 30-5. **A,** Skull radiographs before surgical correction, demonstrating scaphocephaly with hyperostosis of the sagittal suture. **B,** Skull radiographs after subtotal calvarectomy. Pieces of cranial bone are placed over the dura to serve as niduses for the reformation of new cranial bones with reformation of a new sagittal suture.

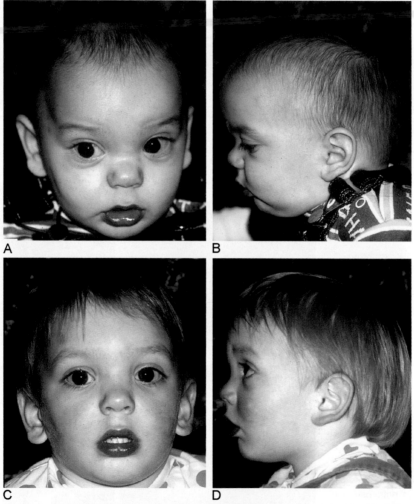

FIGURE 30-6. Infant with sagittal synostosis before **(A, B)** (age 6 months) and after surgery **(C, D)** (age 10 months). Note the dramatic change in the bifrontal versus biparietal dimensions in the top view of the head.

the direction of biomechanical growth–stretch forces.[4,5] Bony ridging is most prominent in the posterior half of the synostotic sagittal suture (in the plane of the widest cranial diameter), consistent with this being the initiation site of synostosis and the site of the most longstanding sutural fusion.[5]

Sagittal craniostenosis is the most common type of craniostenosis, accounting for 50% to 60% of cases and occurring in 1.9 per 10,000 births, with a 3.5:1 male:female gender ratio.[6] Only 6% of cases are familial, with 72% of cases sporadic and no paternal or maternal age effects noted. Twinning occurred in 4.8% of 366 cases, with only 1 monozygotic twin pair being concordant, and intrauterine constraint was considered a likely cause in many cases.[6] The predilection for occurrence in males has been attributed to the more rapid rate of head growth in the male fetus during the last trimester of gestation.[1,2] The larger head is more likely to become seriously constrained, and the associated twinning also contributes toward fetal head constraint.

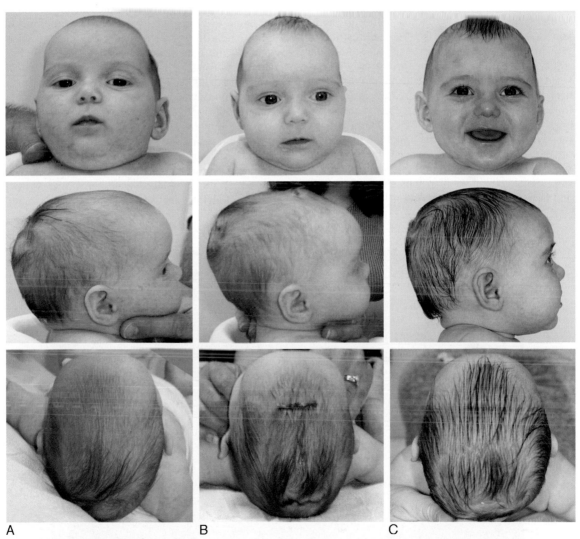

A      B      C

FIGURE 30-7. **A,** This infant with sagittal synostosis is shown just prior to endoscopic strip craniectomy at 2.5 months with a cephalic index of 73% and frontal bossing. **B,** Two weeks after surgery, she had persistent frontal bossing with a cephalic index of 75%, at which time she was fitted with a cranial orthotic. **C,** After 3 months of orthotic therapy, her frontal bossing had resolved and her cephalic index had improved to 76%, and the orthotic was discontinued. She maintained her correction with a cephalic index of 75% at age 9 months.

## FEATURES

The head is long and narrow (dolichocephalic) with a prominent forehead and occiput (see Fig. 30-1). There is usually a ridge along the mid- to posterior sagittal suture that is most prominent between the biparietal eminences (see Fig. 30-2). The term *scaphocephaly* comes from the Greek word *scaphos*, which refers to the keel of a boat. In older children, endocranial ridging is sometimes observed on skull radiographs, suggesting a change in the distribution of intracranial and extracranial biomechanical forces over time; this may be accompanied by calvarial thinning just lateral to the most ridged suture. Relatively excessive anteroposterior growth may partially spread the coronal, temporosquamosal, and/or lambdoidal sutures (Fig. 30-4), and restraint of growth along the posterior sagittal suture may result in flattening between the occiput and the vertex (see Fig. 30-1). The head circumference may appear to be falsely increased, providing a mistaken impression of macrocephaly or possibly even hydrocephalus. Histologic examination of the synostotic suture reveals complete obliteration of the sutural ligament with endocranial bone resorption and ectocranial bone deposition (see Fig. 30-3).[4,5] Skull radiographs show obliteration and hyperostosis of the sagittal suture (Fig. 30-5).

## MANAGEMENT, PROGNOSIS, AND COUNSEL

(See also Chapter 29.) Craniosynostosis of the sagittal suture alone imposes a moderate cranial structural problem, and it may sometimes be difficult for the parents and physicians to resolve the question of whether surgical intervention is indicated. Sagittal synostosis does not affect the neurologic function of the infant or toddler.[7] However, older children may demonstrate moderately severe speech and language difficulties in as many as 37% of cases, and the tendency toward such problems is associated with a positive family history for such difficulties and later age of surgical correction.[8–10] In a study of 30 older untreated children (average age, 9.25 years) with sagittal synostosis, almost all patients and parents were pleased with their decision, and the affected children demonstrated normal cognitive and school performance as well as normal behavior and psychological adjustment on standardized testing.[11]

Various surgical techniques have been used to correct sagittal craniosynostosis. With extended strip craniectomy, an H-shaped strip of calvarium is excised along the sagittal suture, just above the lambdoid sutures and just behind the coronal sutures. With subtotal calvarectomy and cranial vault remodeling, the excised frontal, parietal, and

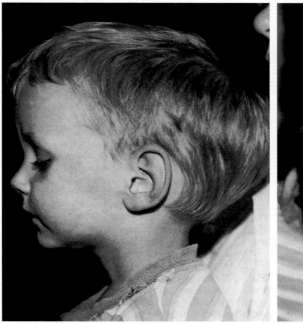
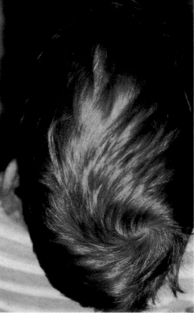

FIGURE 30-8. This 6-year-old boy has unoperated sagittal craniosynostosis (note scaphocephaly with prominent occipital bulge).

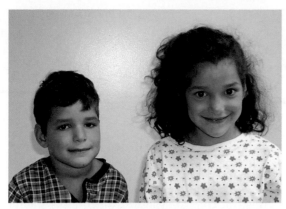

FIGURE 30-9. This brother and sister with sagittal synostosis and late surgical correction demonstrate residual dolichocephaly with frontal prominence.

occipital bones are trimmed, reshaped, and relocated using absorbable sutures (see Figs. 30-1, 30-5, and 30-6). Subtotal calvarectomy will normalize head shape for the majority of children when performed around ages 4 to 6 months.[9,12,13] Another technique uses endoscopic strip craniectomy with postoperative cranial remodeling helmets. Extended strip craniectomy can achieve a comparable head shape when performed before 4 months of age and accompanied by prompt postoperative orthotic molding (Fig. 30-7). It is still unclear whether strip craniectomy is as effective in correcting the cephalic index as is subtotal calvarectomy, and comparison studies are currently underway. Timely surgery corrects the craniofacial deformation, whereas late or untreated sagittal synostosis results in persistent dolichocephaly (Fig. 30-8). Most constraint-induced instances of sagittal craniostenosis are sporadic; however, there are some rare instances of familial sagittal craniostenosis (Fig. 30-9).[14] It is not clear whether such familial cases are a consequence of inherited pelvic type, large head size, or a gene that specifically affects the sagittal suture and results in early closure.

## References

1. Graham JM Jr, deSaxe M, Smith DW: Sagittal craniostenosis: fetal head constraint as one possible cause, *J Pediatr* 95:747–750, 1979.
2. Graham JM Jr: Craniofacial deformation, *Balliere Clin Paediatr* 6:293–315, 1998.
3. Koskinen-Moffett L, Moffet BC: Sutures and intrauterine deformation. In: Pershing JA, Edgerton MT, Jane JA, eds: *Scientific foundations and surgical treatment of craniosynostosis*. Baltimore, 1989, Williams & Wilkins, pp 96–106.
4. Ozaki W, Buchman SR, Muraszko KM, et al: Investigation of the influences of biomechanical force on the ultrastructure of human sagittal craniosynostosis, *Plast Reconstr Surg* 102:1385–1394, 1998.
5. Koskinen-Moffett LK, Moffett BC Jr, Graham JM Jr: Cranial synostosis and intrauterine compression: a developmental study of human sutures. In: Graham AD, Sarnat BG, eds: *Factors and mechanisms influencing bone growth*, New York, 1982, Alan R. Liss, pp 365–378.
6. Lajeunie E, Le Merrer M, Bonati-Pellie C, et al: Genetic study of scaphocephaly, *Am J Med Genet* 62:282–285, 1996.
7. Kapp-Simon KA, Figueroa A, Jocher CA, et al: Longitudinal assessment of mental development in infants with non-syndromic cranial synostosis with and without cranial release and reconstruction, *Plast Reconstr Surg* 92:831–839, 1993.
8. Virtanen R, Korhonen T, Fagerholm J, et al: Neurocognitive sequelae of scaphocephaly, *Pediatrics* 103:791–795, 1999.
9. Panchal J, Marsh JL, Park TS, et al: Sagittal craniosynostosis outcome assessment for two methods and timing of intervention, *Plast Reconstr Surg* 103:1574–1584, 1999.
10. Shipster C, Hearst D, Somerville A, et al: Specch, language and cognitive development in children with isolated sagittal synostosis, *Devel Med Child Neurol* 45:34–43, 2003.
11. Boltshauser E, Ludwig S, Dietrich F, et al: Sagittal craniosynostosis: cognitive development, behaviour, and quality of life in unoperated children, *Neuropediatrics* 34:293–300, 2003.
12. Panchal J, Marsh JL, Park TS, et al: Photographic assessment of head shape following sagittal synostosis surgery, *Plast Reconstr Surg* 103:1585–1591, 1999.
13. Jimenez DF, Barone CM, McGee ME: Design and care of helmets in postoperative craniosynostosis patients: our personal approach, *Clin Plast Surg* 31:481–487, 2004.
14. McGillivray G, Savarirayan R, Cox TC, et al: Familial scaphocephaly syndrome caused by a novel mutation in the FGFR2 tyrosine kinase domain, *J Med Genet* 42:656–662, 2005.

# 31 Coronal Craniosynostosis

## GENESIS

Coronal craniosynostosis is the second most common type of craniosynostosis, accounting for 20% to 30% of cases. Constraint-induced unilateral coronal craniosynostosis can be secondary to early descent of the fetal head into a constraining pelvis, aberrant fetal lie, or constraint within a bicornuate uterus.[1-3] It is known that 71% of unilateral coronal craniosynostosis is right-sided,[4] and this nonrandom predilection may relate to the fact that 67% of vertex presentations are in the left occiput transverse position, with the left coronal suture against the sacral prominence.[1] If the fetal head descends early and is maintained in the most common position (i.e., left occiput transverse), the result may be more constraint across the right coronal suture as it lies against the pubic bone as compared with the left coronal suture as it lies against the sacral prominence. This may explain the increased prevalence of right-sided, unilateral coronal craniosynostosis. Nonsyndromic coronal craniosynostosis occurs in 0.94 per 10,000 births, with 61% of cases sporadic and 14.4% of 180 pedigrees familial. Bilateral cases occur much more frequently than unilateral cases, and coronal synostosis is more common in females (male: female ratio, 1:2). The paternal age is significantly older than average (32.7 years), with average paternal age of 26 to 27 years and the advent of testicular aging at age 30 years. Most sperm banks discourage donors over age 40 years. These data have been interpreted as being consistent with autosomal dominant inheritance, with 60% penetrance when the synostosis has a genetic basis.[5]

When craniosynostosis occurs as part of a syndrome, it is most important to examine the patient carefully for associated anomalies. Evaluation of the limbs, ears, eyes, and cardiovascular system yields the most significant data for diagnosing syndromes associated with craniosynostosis. Limb defects such as syndactyly, brachydactyly, or broad, deviated thumbs and halluces suggest the presence of an associated syndrome. It is also important to examine both parents for digital anomalies, carpal coalition, and/or facial asymmetry because these findings may represent variable expression of an altered gene in a parent.

Bilateral coronal synostosis often lacks sutural ridging and usually has a genetic basis, which suggests that all such patients should be screened for mutations. Among 57 patients with bilateral coronal synostosis, mutations were found in fibroblast growth factor receptor (FRGR) genes for all 38 patients who had a syndromic form of craniosynostosis. Among 19 patients with unclassified brachycephaly, mutations in or near exon 9 of FGFR2 were found in 4 patients, and a common Pro250Arg mutation in exon 7 of FGFR3 was detected in 10 patients. Only five patients (9%) manifested brachycephaly without a detectable mutation in FGFR 1, 2, or 3.[6] These findings suggest that mutation analysis of FGFR and TWIST genes should be performed in all patients with coronal synostosis. It is also important to obtain hand and foot radiographs in older children and their parents because subtle digital changes and carpal/tarsal coalition can be seen in individuals with the Pro250Arg mutation in FGFR3, even if they lack findings of coronal craniosynostosis.[7] An estimated 10% of patients with unilateral coronal synostosis carry this mutation; some parents carry this mutation but demonstrate few clinical manifestations.[8] In a prospective study of 47 patients with synostotic frontal plagiocephaly (unilateral coronal synostosis), mutations were found in 8 patients (17%): 2 with FGFR 2, 3 with FGFR3 Pro250Arg, and 3 with TWIST mutations.[9] Two clinical features were strongly associated with mutation detection: (1) asymmetric brachycephaly with retrusion of both orbital rims and (2) orbital hypertelorism. In addition, four patients had such clinical findings and either unilateral or bilateral coronal synostosis in an immediate relative in whom no mutation could be found.[9] It is important to emphasize that inability to demonstrate a mutation does not rule out a genetic cause for the craniosynostosis, and not every person with a mutation manifests craniosynostosis.

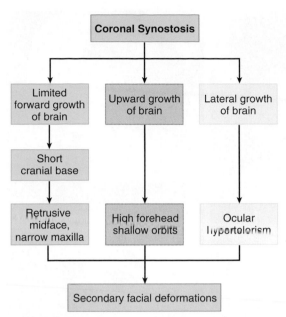

FIGURE 31-1. Diagram depicting the manner in which bilateral coronal craniostenosis results in secondary facial effects.

# FEATURES

In patients with bilateral coronal craniosynostosis, the forehead is high and broad. The impact of bilateral coronal synostosis on the craniofacial region is summarized in Figs. 31-1 and 31-2. When there is unilateral coronal craniosynostosis (also termed *synostotic frontal plagiocephaly*), the impact on the facial structures is asymmetric, resulting in significant facial distortion that may complicate surgical correction (Figs. 31-3 and 31-4). On the side of the synostotic suture, the forehead is tall and flattened, with vertical upward displacement of the orbit and ear on that side. The forehead on the side opposite the synostosis usually bulges forward, and the nasal root deviates toward the flattened side. The affected supraorbital rim is retruded, elevated, and slightly displaced laterally on the side of the flattened forehead. These features persist and worsen in patients who are not treated surgically, with orbital distortion affecting the visual system. There may be marked thickening and up-tilting of the sphenoid wings, with an oval obliquity to the orbital margins (called the

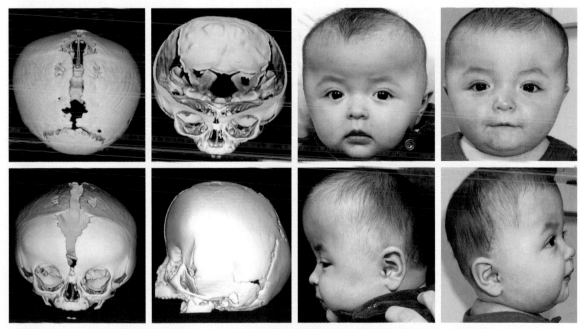

FIGURE 31-2. As shown on the this three-dimensional cranial computed tomography scan, there is complete obliteration of both coronal sutures, resulting in a high, broad forehead with brachycephaly and ocular hypertelorism.

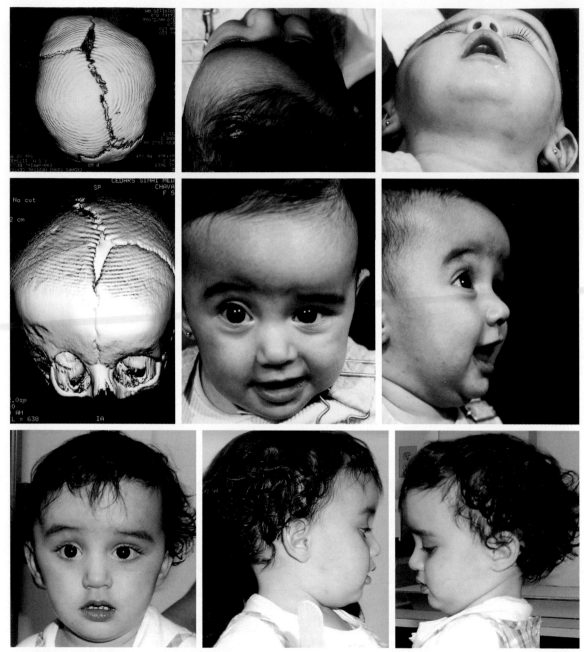

FIGURE 31-3. This girl has right coronal synostosis with a tall, flattened forehead on the side of the synostotic suture, resulting in vertical upward displacement of the orbit and ear on that side. The forehead on the side opposite the synostosis is prominent, and the nasal root deviates toward the flattened side. The supraorbital rim on the side of the flattened forehead is retruded, elevated, and laterally displaced.

*harlequin sign*). With syndromes such as Crouzon, Pfeiffer (Fig. 31-5), and Apert syndromes, the orbits are shallow and wide-set, often with pronounced proptosis. The synostosis is often initiated at the lower end of the coronal suture (near the sphenoid wing), and it progresses superiorly. There is a head tilt toward the nonsynostotic side (sometimes termed *ocular torticollis* or *pseudopalsy of the superior oblique muscle*) in about half the affected children because the foreshortened superomedial orbital wall on the affected side displaces the trochlea posteriorly, which weakens the action of the superior oblique tendon. This results in relative overactivity of the inferior oblique muscle compared with the superior oblique muscle. Thus, in an attempt to compensate for the diplopia, the head may begin to tilt toward the nonsynostotic side.

## MANAGEMENT, PROGNOSIS, AND COUNSEL

The impact of coronal synostosis on adjacent facial structures, such as the orbit, is of such magnitude that surgical intervention during the first half of infancy is generally warranted. Furthermore the child with untreated coronal craniosynostosis may have a restricted nasopharynx fostering middle ear infections, an abnormal oral cavity contributing to speech problems, dental malocclusion, and obstructive sleep apnea. Because intracranial volume almost triples within the first year and by age 2 years is four times greater than the cranial capacity at birth, asymmetric cranial expansion due to unilateral coronal synostosis can have a major impact on the symmetry of facial structures. Surgery for unilateral coronal craniosynostosis (or synostotic frontal plagiocephaly) seeks to correct the progressive distortions affecting the forehead and orbits and to align the nasal root. Three basic variations in surgical techniques have evolved (listed in order of their development):

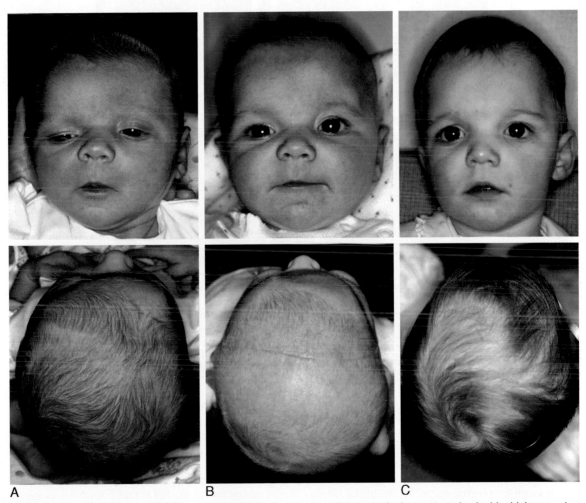

A                B                C

FIGURE 31-4. At age 9 days, this infant with unilateral left coronal craniosynostosis demonstrated palpable ridging over her synostotic left coronal suture **(A)**. Frontal calvarectomy at 6 weeks of age resulted in a complete restoration of normal features, as demonstrated by similar head views 6 weeks after surgery **(B)** and at age 17 months **(C)**.

*Continued*

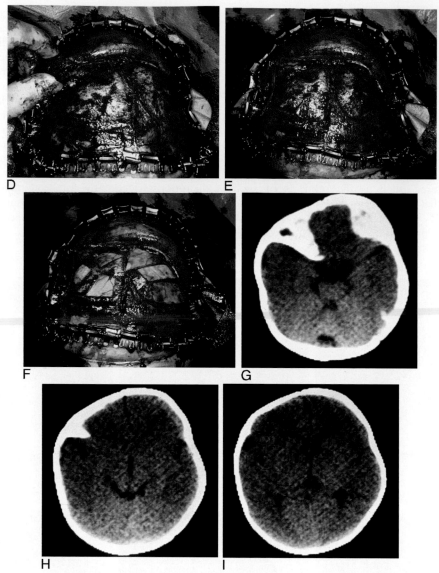

FIGURE 31-4. *Continued* Exposure of cranial bone at the time of surgery revealed that the left coronal suture was densely ridged with restriction of the left frontal region (**D** and computed tomography scans in **G-I**). The left orbital rim was advanced (**E**), and pieces of cranial bone were replaced over the dura to serve as niduses for the reformation of new cranial bone (**F**). The nose is at the top of each view of the exposed cranium.

1. Unilateral frontoorbital advancement
2. Bilateral frontoorbital advancement without nasal straightening
3. Bilateral frontoorbital advancement with closing wedge nasal osteotomy[10]

Measurable postoperative frontoorbital asymmetry remains most marked in the first group, which leads most surgeons to advance both sides even though only one side may be synostotic. Postoperative symmetry is most ideal with slight overcorrection of the vertical and anteroposterior supraorbital rim deformity on the affected side, along with nasal straightening.[10] In children with bilateral coronal craniosynostosis, particularly when it occurs as part of a syndrome (e.g., Pfeiffer, Apert, or Crouzon syndromes), primary frontoorbital advancement during infancy must be exaggerated to compensate for diminished frontal growth potential.[11]

Because binocular vision develops at 3 months when the retina reaches maturity and because the

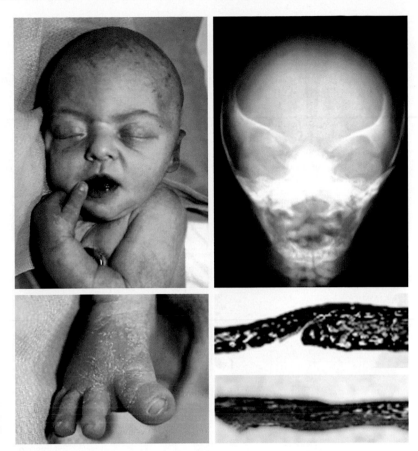

FIGURE 31-5. This infant with Pfeiffer syndrome shows laterally deviated thumbs and halluces with bilateral harlequin sign on skull radiographs. (Note the facial differences compared with the infants shown in Figs. 31-2 to 31-4, who have nonsyndromic bilateral coronal synostosis.)

eye reaches its adult size by age 3 years, with a doubling of ocular volume during the first 12 months, early surgical correction of plagiocephaly is necessary to prevent strabismus due to synostosis-related traction on the ocular globe. Even when surgery is undertaken between 3 and 6 months of age, the ocular problems are not always prevented or alleviated, and careful ophthalmologic follow-up is indicated.[12-14] In a study of 39 children with unicoronal synostosis, vertical strabismus was explained by initial traction on the lateral rectus muscles, with secondary stretching of the inferior oblique muscle and associated underaction of the superior oblique muscle on the side of the synostosis. When strabismus was followed over time and correlated with time of surgical repair, it was clear that strabismus was initially horizontal and then became vertical if the synostosis was not released early. Children who were surgically treated after 11 months of age showed vertical strabismus, and those surgically treated before this age had horizontal strabismus. The later that reconstructive surgery was performed, the more pronounced was the degree of measurable astigmatism because of continuing compen-

satory bone growth.[15] Thus primary frontoorbital advancement is usually performed between 3 and 9 months of age; some surgeons operate as early as 3 months due to the increased pliability of cranial bone and predictable reossification of cranial defects, and others wait until 6 to 9 months, when bone is stronger and fixation is more stable.[11,16] Early surgery allows the cranial base (the roof of the face) to grow forward, carrying the midface with it. The forward growth of the cranial base is normally 56% complete by birth and 70% complete by 2 years of age.

When mutations in FGFR genes limit the forward growth of the anterior cranial base, surgery may be less effective in restoring facial features to normal.[17,18] A study of 76 patients with nonsyndromic isolated coronal synostosis revealed that 29 of these patients (38%) had the Pro250Arg mutation in FGFR3. Reoperation for functional reasons (raised intracranial pressure) was nearly five times more common in the patients with this mutation than in those with no mutation. Within the entire group of 76 patients, the reoperation rate was 11.8% (10.5% for functional reasons). Presence of the Pro250Arg mutation in FGFR3 was the only factor that reached significance for predicting reoperation. This suggests that the risk of functional sequelae and thus the need for reoperation is higher in syndromic craniosynostosis as well as in nonsyndromic coronal synostosis with the Pro250Arg mutation in FGFR3.[18] For these reasons, preoperative mutation evaluation is strongly recommended. Syndromic craniosynostosis has been associated with mutations in FGFR1, FGFR2, FGFR3, TWIST, MSX2, and EFNB1, and nonsyndromic coronal craniosynostosis has been associated with the Pro250Arg mutation in FGFR3 and with mutations in EFNB4.

## DIFFERENTIAL DIAGNOSIS

Coronal synostosis may occur as an isolated finding or as part of a variety of genetic disorders that affect the growth of craniofacial structures and limbs.[6,9,18] It is beyond the scope of this text to review these syndromes in any detail; the reader

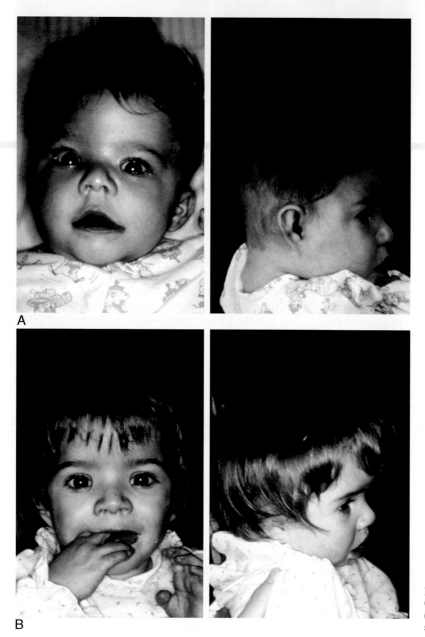

FIGURE 31-6. This girl with Saethre-Chotzen syndrome is shown before (A) and after (B) surgical reconstruction.

Continued

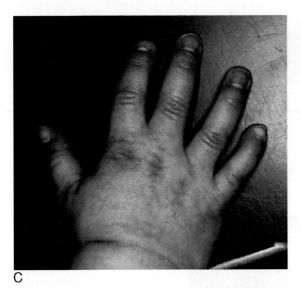

C

FIGURE 31-6. *Continued* Note partial syndactyly of second and third fingers with fifth finger clinodactyly **(C)**.

is referred to Cohen and MacLean's comprehensive book on craniosynostosis for an extensive discussion of this topic.[18] Mutations are found in virtually all patients with Apert, Crouzon, or Pfeiffer syndrome, and a mutation was also found in 75% of patients with unclassified brachycephaly.[6] Mutations in TWIST are found in 80% of patients with Saethre-Chotzen syndrome (Fig. 31-6).[9] Patients with macrocephaly; a high, broad forehead; down-slanting palpebral fissure; distal brachydactyly; and/or anomalous toes may demonstrate the FGFR3 Pro250Arg mutation (Figs. 31-7 and 31-8).[7] Patients with unilateral coronal synostosis have a 6% to 11% likelihood of demonstrating this mutation.[8,9] Approximately 54% of patients with craniofrontonasal syndrome (Fig. 31-9) demonstrate synostotic frontal plagiocephaly,[18] and mutations have been found in the X-linked gene EFNB1, which is located at Xq13.1.[19] Loss of function mutations in EFNB1 result in a paradoxically greater severity in heterozygous females than

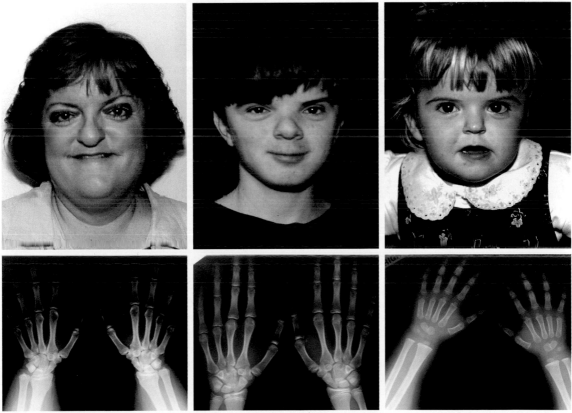

FIGURE 31-7. This mother and her two children have the FGFR3 Pro250Arg mutation that results in macrocephaly with variable coronal synostosis and capitate-hamate coalition.

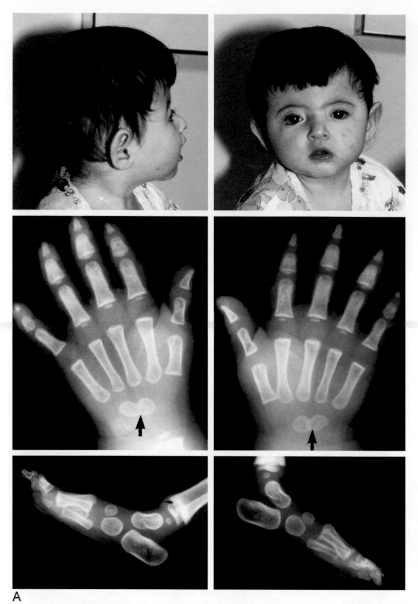

FIGURE 31-8. This infant with the FGFR3 Pro250Arg mutation has coronal synostosis and capitate-hamate coalitions with hypoplastic distal phalanges **(A)**. Her affected mother also required surgery for bilateral coronal synostosis and demonstrates capitate-hamate coalitions, calcaneo-cuboid coalitions, and hypoplastic distal phalanges **(B)**.

*Continued*

in hemizygous males. Constraint limitation of craniofacial growth in late gestation may occasionally yield an appearance at birth quite similar to that of coronal synostosis, especially in patients with face presentations or persistent transverse lie or who were constrained in one horn of a bicornuate uterus. If the coronal sutures are not fused, such patients demonstrate rapid spontaneous restitution toward normal form in the first few postnatal weeks, which would not be expected with coronal craniosynostosis. For this single reason, it is probably best to wait a few weeks before making a decision about calvarial surgery unless the pro-

blem is obvious and severe with evidence of increased intracranial pressure.

The discovery of a common point mutation in FGFR3 (Pro250Arg) in patients with "nonsyndromic" coronal craniosynostosis warrants consideration in any patient with this disorder (Figs. 31-7 and 31-8). In a study of 62 familial and sporadic cases of nonsyndromal coronal craniosynostosis, this mutation was found in 42% of cases.[20] Among 35 sporadic cases, 17% had the FGFR3 Pro250Arg mutation (with an average paternal age of 39.7 years at the time of birth, which suggests fresh dominant mutation) whereas 74% of

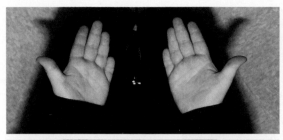

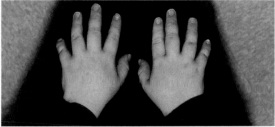

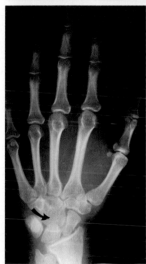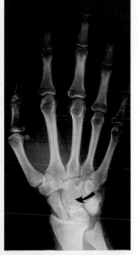

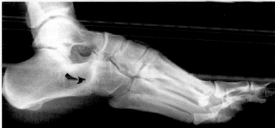

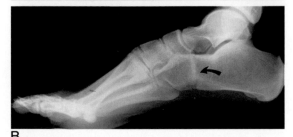

B

FIGURE 31-8. *Continued*

27 familial cases revealed this mutation. Of the 62 cases, 30% had plagiocephaly and 70% had brachycephaly, and females were significantly more severely affected than males (which possibly explains much of the observed female excess in coronal craniosynostosis).[20] When associated findings were examined, many patients manifested severe forehead retrusion with hypertelorism and bulging of the temporal fossae (possibly reflecting poorer postoperative results in older patients who underwent outdated surgical procedures). The mean intelligence quotient (IQ) among affected persons was 97, but 26 patients had an IQ less than 80, and 1 patient with associated hydrocephalus had an IQ of 63. No effort was made to correlate efficacy of surgical repair with cognitive outcomes.[20] Brachydactyly was observed in 22 of 32 cases, most commonly affecting the middle phalanges; carpal fusion was noted in only 3 of 22 radiographs, with tarsal fusion in 2 cases and calcaneo-cuboid fusion in 1 case. In one familial case, both parents had normal skull radiographs and craniofacial examinations, but both the proband and her father carried the mutation and demonstrated carpal and tarsal fusions on radiographs.[20] Among 4 of 37 patients with unicoronal synostosis due to this FGFR3 mutation, 3 fathers were identified as carrying the same mutation but had only subtle hand radiographic findings and no craniofacial findings.[8] Thus, not only should this mutation be searched for in patients with nonsyndromic coronal craniosynostosis, but both parents should also be analyzed if the mutation is found, even if they appear clinically normal. If mutation screening is negative for this common mutation in FGFR3, screening for FGFR1, FGFR2, and TWIST should be done because mutations in these genes can also cause coronal craniosynostosis with variable, subtle associated facial and distal limb anomalies.

Saethre-Chotzen syndrome is caused by mutations that result in haploinsufficiency for TWIST, and it can usually be distinguished on clinical grounds from Muenke syndrome, which results from a gain-of-function mutation in FGFR3 due to the point mutation Pro250Arg.[21,22] Patients with Saethre-Chotzen syndrome have a low frontal hairline, microcephaly (37%), ptosis, small ears, dilated parietal foramina, intradigital webbing, hallux valgus, and/or broad great toes with a wide distal phalanx. They must be observed for progressive multisuture fusion, which occurs in 53% of patients and can lead to intracranial hypertension (35% of patients at a median age of 30 months).[22] The presence of intracranial hypertension leads to reoperation in 18% of patients with Saethre-Chotzen syndrome, and papilledema

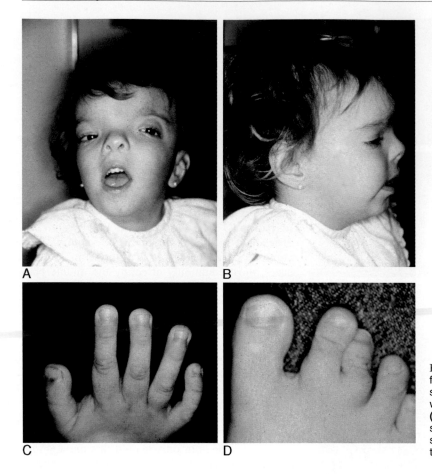

FIGURE 31-9. This girl with cranio-frontonasal syndrome demonstrates left coronal synostosis with severe ocular hypertelorism **(A, B)**, characteristic longitudinal splitting of the nails **(C)**, and partial syndactyly of the second and third toes **(D)**.

was the most frequent sign of this complication. In five patients who were not treated early enough, visual loss occurred due to irreversible optic nerve damage; therefore such patients should be observed with annual eye exams.[22] Patients with Muenke syndrome had mild to moderate mental retardation in 34% of cases, with sensorineural hearing loss in 32% of cases; thus, these patients should receive early intervention and annual hearing exams.[21]

## References

1. Graham JM Jr, Badura R, Smith DW: Coronal craniostenosis: fetal head constraint as one possible cause, *Pediatrics* 65:995–999, 1980.
2. Higginbottom MC, Jones KL, James HE: Intrauterine constraint and craniosynostosis, *Neurosurgery* 6:39–44, 1980.
3. Graham JM Jr: Craniofacial deformation, *Balliere Clin Paediatr* 6:293–315, 1998.
4. Hunter AG, Rudd NL: Craniosynostosis: II. Coronal synostosis: its familial characteristics and associated clinical findings in 109 patients lacking bilateral polysyndactyly or syndactyly, *Teratology* 15:301–310, 1977.
5. Lajeunie E, Le Merrer M, Bonati-Pellie C, et al: Genetic study of nonsyndromic coronal craniosynostosis, *Am J Med Genet* 55:500–504, 1995.
6. Mulliken JB, Steinberger D, Kunze S, et al: Molecular diagnosis of bilateral coronal synostosis, *Plast Reconstr Surg* 104:1603–1615, 1999.
7. Graham JM Jr, Braddock SR, Mortier GR, et al: Syndrome of coronal craniosynostosis with brachydactyly and carpal-tarsal coalition due to Pro250Arg mutation in FGFR3 gene, *Am J Med Genet* 77:322–329, 1998.
8. Gripp KW, McDonald-McGinn DM, Gaudenz K, et al: Identification of the first genetic cause for isolated unilateral-coronal synostosis: a unique mutation in the fibroblast growth factor receptor 3 (FGFR3), *J Pediatr* 132:714–716, 1998.
9. Mulliken JB, Gripp K, Stolle CA, et al: Molecular analysis of patients with synostotic frontal plagiocephaly (unilateral coronal synostosis), *Plast Reconstr Surg* 113:1899–1909, 2004.
10. Hansen M, Padwa BL, Scott BL, et al: Synostotic frontal plagiocephaly: anthropometric comparison of three techniques for surgical correction, *Plast Reconstr Surg* 100:1387–1395, 1997.
11. Pai L, Kohout MP, Mulliken JB: Prospective anthropometric analysis of sagittal orbital-globe relationship following fronto-orbital advancement in childhood, *Plast Reconstr Surg* 103:1341–1346, 1999.
12. Robb RM, Boger WP: Vertical strabismus associated with plagiocephaly, *J Pediatr Ophthalmol Strabis* 20:58–62, 1983.
13. Gosain AK, Steele MA, McCarthy JG, et al: A prospective study of the relationship between strabismus and head

posture in patients with frontal plagiocephaly, *Plast Reconstr Surg* 97:881–891, 1996.

14. Lo L-J, Marsh JL, Kane AA, et al: Orbital dysmorphology in unicoronal synostosis. *Cleft Palate Craniofac J* 33:190–197.

15. Denis D, Genitori L, Conrath J, et al: Ocular findings in children operated on for plagiocephaly and trigonocephaly, *Child Nerv Syst* 12:683–689, 1996.

16. Posnick JC: Unilateral coronal synostosis (anterior plagiocephaly): current clinical perspectives, *Ann Plast Surg* 36:430–447, 1996.

17. Reinhart E, Muhling J, Michel C, et al: Craniofacial growth characteristics after bilateral fronto-orbital advancement in children with premature craniosynostosis, *Child Nerv Syst* 12:690–694, 1996.

18. Thomas GP, Wilkie AO, Richards PG, et al: FGFR3 P250R mutation increases the risk of reoperation in appar-ent "nonsyndromic" coronal synostosis, *J Craniofacial Surg* 16:347–352, 2005.

19. Cohen MM Jr, MacLean RE, eds: *Craniosynostosis: diagnosis, evaluation, and management*, ed 2, New York, Oxford University Press, 2000.

20. Twigg SRF, Kan R, Babbs C, et al: Mutations of ephrin-B1 (*EFNB1*), a marker of tissue boundary formation, cause craniofrontonasal syndrome, *Proc Natl Acad Sci U S A* 101:8652–8657, 2004.

21. Lajeunie E, El Ghouzzi V, Le Marrer M, et al: Sex-related expressivity of the phenotype in coronal craniosynostosis caused by the recurrent P250R FGFR3 mutation, *J Med Genet* 36:9–13, 1999.

22. Kress W, Schropp C, Lieb G, et al: Saethre-Chotzen syndrome caused by TWIST 1 gene mutations: functional differentiation from Muenke coronal synostosis syndrome, *Eur J Hum Genet* 14:39–48, 2006.

# 32 Metopic Craniosynostosis

## GENESIS

Metopic synostosis occurs in about 0.67 per 10,000 births, making it the third most common type of craniosynostosis (accounting for 10%–20% of patients). Like sagittal synostosis, metopic synostosis occurs more frequently in males, with a 3.3:1 male:female ratio, and only 5.6% of cases were familial in a study by Laverne et al.[1] There was no maternal or paternal age effect, and the frequency of associated twinning was 7.8% of 179 pedigrees studied, with two twin monozygotic pairs concordant.[1] The similarity of epidemiologic features in sagittal and metopic craniosynostosis suggests that prenatal lateral constraint of the frontal part of the head is a frequent cause of metopic craniosynostosis (Figs. 32-1 to 32-4). Examples of constraint-induced metopic synostosis have included a monozygotic triplet whose forehead was wedged between the buttocks of her two co-triplets in utero (see Fig. 32-3) and an infant whose head was compressed within one horn of his mother's bicornuate uterus (see Fig. 32-4).[2] There is also some evidence to suggest that fetal head constraint can alter expression of transforming growth factor beta (TGF-B) and fibroblast growth factor (FGF) receptors, resulting in nonsyndromic craniosynostosis.[3]

Metopic synostosis represented only 7% of craniosynostosis cases that required surgery.[4,5] The metopic suture is the first cranial suture to close, and analysis of computed tomography scans in patients with and without metopic synostosis demonstrated that the metopic suture normally begins to close at 3 to 4 months and is usually completely closed by 8 to 9 months. Normal fusion commences at the nasion and proceeds superiorly, concluding at the anterior fontanelle.[4,5] In a study of 76 unrelated patients with syndromic (36 patients) and nonsyndromic trigonocephaly (40 patients) caused by metopic synostosis, molecular screening for microdeletions at 9p22-p24 and 11q23-q24 revealed deletions in 7 syndromic patients (19.4%), but no deletions were found in the nonsyndromic patients.[6] The ratio of affected males to females was 5:1 in the syndromic group and 1.8:1 in the nonsyndromic group, which suggests that genes in these deleted regions and on the X-chromosome play a major role in syndromic trigonocephaly.[6]

Trigonocephaly is usually an isolated anomaly in an otherwise normal child, but it can occur as part of a syndrome, such as Opitz C trigonocephaly syndrome (Fig. 32-5) or result from a wide range of chromosome abnormalities, such as deletions of 9p22-p24 or 11q23-q24, the latter deletion also

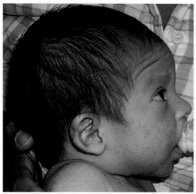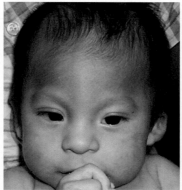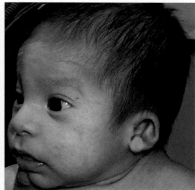

FIGURE 32-1. This child shows characteristic features of metopic craniosynostosis. Findings include bitemporal narrowing and a palpable midline ridge from the nasion to the anterior fontanelle over the site of the fused suture, resulting in a prow-shaped, triangular anterior cranial vault (termed *trigonocephaly*). There is also up-slanting of the palpebral fissures with ocular hypotelorism.

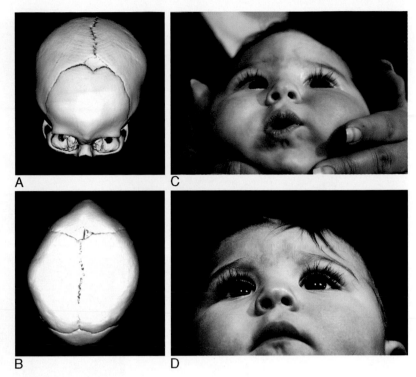
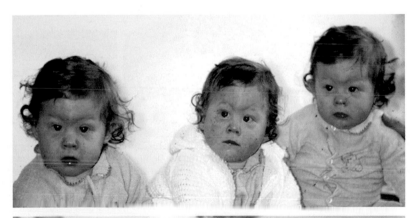

FIGURE 32-2. Three-dimensional computed tomography scans (**A** and **B**) demonstrating the ridged metopic suture, which is most evident in the worm's-eye view of this patient before (**C**) and after (**D**) surgery.

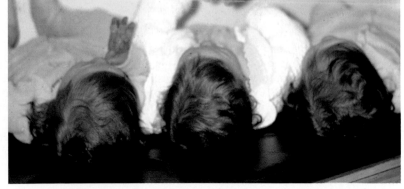

FIGURE 32-3. One of monozygotic triplets born to a 104-lb (prepregnancy weight) woman who gained 64 pounds during the pregnancy. Prenatal radiographs had shown this triplet to have the frontal portion of her head wedged between the buttocks of her co-triplets. This was considered the source of the constraint that yielded the metopic craniostenosis with secondary narrowed forehead and up-slanting palpebral fissures, features that were not shared by her monozygotic co-triplets.

(From Graham JM Jr, Smith DW: Metopic craniostenosis as a consequence of fetal head constraint. Two interesting experiments of nature, *Pediatrics* 65: 1000, 1980.)

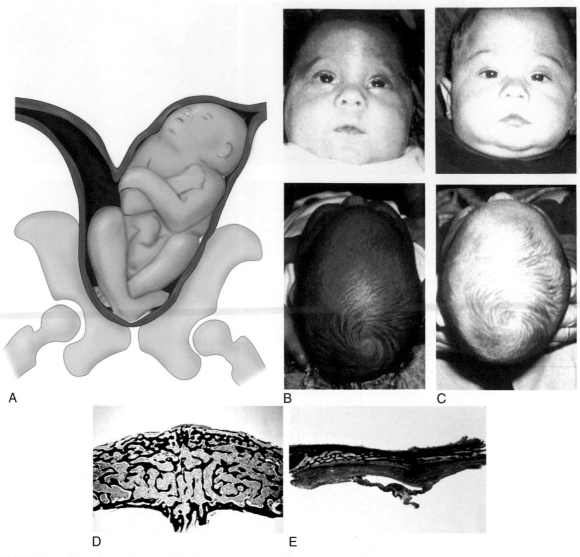

FIGURE 32-4. Metopic craniostenosis in an infant who was reared in a bicornuate uterus (B). During cesarean section, it took several minutes to dislodge the head from its tightly entrapped position in one upper uterine horn (illustrated in A). C, Postoperative status of the infant following calvarectomy of the frontal bone region down to the supraorbital ridges, which allowed the brain to remold the forehead while a more normally shaped bony calvarium was formed. Histologic section through the dense metopic ridge of the patient shows complete replacement of the normal sutural ligament with dense thickened bone (D) compared with control suture material from a deceased infant of the same age (E).

called *Jacobsen syndrome* (Fig. 32-6).[7–9] In a study of 25 infants with trigonocephaly and metopic synostosis, 6% were familial, 16 (64%) had isolated metopic synostosis, 2 (8%) had metopic synostosis combined with sagittal synostosis, and 7 (28%) had metopic synostosis as part of a syndrome (2 with Jacobsen syndrome due to chromosomal deletion of 11q23-q24, 1 with Opitz C trigonocephaly syndrome, 1 with Say-Meyer trigonocephaly syndrome, 1 with I-cell disease, and 2 others with

unknown syndromes).[7] In a previous study of 278 cases of metopic synostosis, 75% were non-syndromic, and 6% were familial.[1] Metopic synostosis has also been associated with fetal exposure to valproic acid but not with exposure to other anticonvulsants.[9,10] The mean intelligence quotient (IQ) of 17 patients with metopic synostosis was 75; significantly higher IQs were noted in infants who were surgically treated before age 6 months.[10]

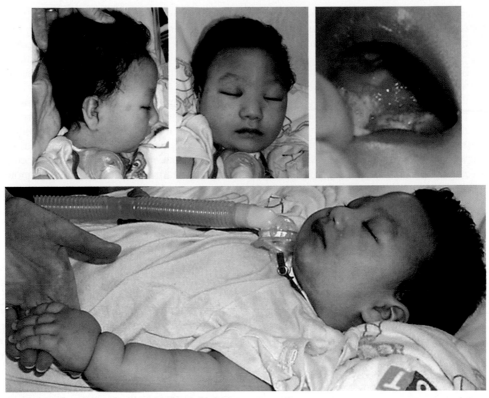

FIGURE 32-5. This patient with Opitz C trigonocephaly syndrome was one of three infants born into a family with this autosomal recessive syndrome and normal chromosomes via comparative genomic hybridization.

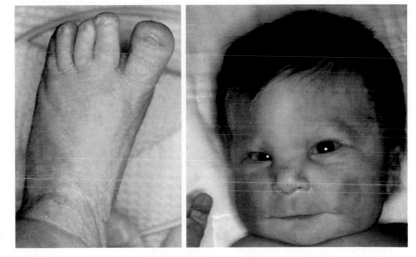

FIGURE 32-6. This patient with trigonocephaly, developmental delay, and broad thumbs and great toes has Jacobsen syndrome due to chromosomal deletion of 11q23-q24.

## FEATURES

The diagnosis of metopic synostosis is made clinically and confirmed by radiographic studies. Findings include bitemporal narrowing, a palpable midline ridge from the nasion to the anterior fontanelle over the site of the fused suture, and a prow-shaped, triangular anterior cranial vault (termed *trigonocephaly*). There may be progressive up-slanting of the palpebral fissures with ocular hypotelorism (see Figs. 32-1 to 32-4). Normal metopic sutural closure is usually associated with an endocranial bony spur, but premature metopic synostosis is associated with an endocranial metopic notch in 93% of cases.[5] The synostotic metopic suture is markedly thickened on histologic sections when compared with age-matched neonates who died from other causes (see Fig. 32-4). Milder degrees of metopic ridging occur fairly frequently at birth, but unless there is progressive distortion of the orbits, such mild ridging usually resolves spontaneously without treatment. This mild metopic ridging without synostosis is very common (occurring in 10%–25% of normal neonates), and it should not be misdiagnosed as metopic synostosis.[7]

## MANAGEMENT AND PROGNOSIS

Generally, no treatment is required in mild cases without associated orbital deformity. Moderate to severe metopic synostosis often warrants active forehead reshaping with recontouring of the frontoorbital bar down to and including the supraorbital ridges via a frontal calvarectomy. In the more severe cases with ocular hypotelorism, the brows and orbital roofs are removed and relocated. These procedures are usually undertaken between ages 3 and 9 months. When surgery is restricted to just the forehead and supraorbital rims, the hypotelorism remains uncorrected and narrowness of the forehead also persist, so most surgeons prefer more extended frontoorbital procedures that correct both the trigonocephaly and the hypotelorism by inserting an interpositional bone graft into the middle of the supraorbital bar, thus providing additional fullness in the temporal regions.[11,12] Of 1713 patients treated for craniosynostosis in Paris, 237 (14%) were trigonocephalic, and 76 patients over age 3 years were studied for long-term neurodevelopmental outcome (at a mean age of 6.5 years) and associated malformations (patients with known syndromes and chromosomal alterations were excluded). The mean age of surgery was 11.5 months, and 22.6% of those surgically treated before age 12 months showed impaired mental development versus 52.2% in those surgically treated after age 12 months. Children with brain malformations such as hydrocephalus or hypoplastic corpus callosum had poorer cognitive outcomes, and 18.4% had associated extracranial malformations. Children with associated malformations were more often delayed in development (57%) than children with isolated trigonocephaly (26%). Overall, 31% of trigonocephaly patients had delayed development; this appeared to be related to the severity of the problem and the presence of associated malformations. Isolated patients who were operated on at an early age had the best cognitive outcomes.[13] Among 14 children surgically treated for trigonocephaly, the incidence of ocular disorders increased with age at the time of corrective surgery due to prolonged stretching of the lateral rectus muscles, with strabismus noted in 2 of the 14 patients. Most patients presented with bilateral astigmatism, and the later the reconstructive surgery was performed, the more pronounced the astigmatism.[14]

## DIFFERENTIAL DIAGNOSIS

It is important to exclude primary defects of the brain such as the holoprosencephaly malformation sequence and syndromes such as Opitz C trigonocephaly syndrome (see Fig. 32-5). The latter condition includes unusual facial features, hypotonia, multiple frenula, limb defects, visceral anomalies, and mental deficiency, and it is inherited in an autosomal recessive fashion. Metopic craniosynostosis can also result from various chromosomal abnormalities, such as deletions of chromosome 9p22-p24 and 11q23-q24 (Jacobsen syndrome), as demonstrated in Fig. 32-6.[6,7,15] Because some of these chromosomal abnormalities can be quite subtle, high-resolution chromosomal studies or comparative genomic hybridization studies are indicated in children with associated malformations and neurodevelopmental problems.

### References

1. Laverne E, Arnaud E, Le Merrier M, et al: Syndromal and nonsyndromal primary trigonocephaly: analysis of a series of 237 patients, *Am J Med Genet* 55:500–504, 1998.
2. Graham JM Jr, Smith DW: Metopic craniostenosis as a consequence of fetal head constraint: two interesting experiments of nature, *Pediatrics* 65:1000, 1980.
3. Hunenko O, Karmacharya J, Ong G, et al: Toward an understanding of non-syndromic craniosynostosis: altered patterns of TGF-B receptor and FGF receptor expression induced by fetal head constraint, *Ann Plast Surg* 46:546–554, 2001.
4. Vu HL, Panchal J, Parker EE, et al: The timing of physiologic closure of the metopic suture: a review of 159 patients using reconstructed 3D CT scans of the craniofacial region, *J Craniofac Surg* 12:527–532, 2001.
5. Weinzweig J, Kirschner RE, Farley A, et al: Metopic synostosis: defining the temporal sequence of normal suture fusion and differentiating it from synostosis on the basis of computed tomography images, *Plast Reconstr Surg* 112:1211–1218, 2003.
6. Jehee JS, Johnson D, Alonso LG, et al: Molecular screening for microdeletions at 9p22-p24 and 11q23-q24 in a

large cohort of patients with trigonocephaly, *Clin Genet* 67:503–510, 2005.

7. Azimi C, Kennedy SJ, Chitayat D, et al: Clinical and genetic aspects of trigonocephaly: a study of 25 cases, *Am J Med Genet* 117:127–135, 2003.

8. Cohen MM Jr, MacLean RE, eds: *Craniosynostosis: diagnosis, evaluation, and management*, ed 2, New York, 2000, Oxford University Press.

9. Chabrolle JP, Bensouda B, Bruel H, et al: La craniostenose de la metopique, effet probable de l'exposition intrauterine a un traitement maternel par le Valproate, *Arch Pediatr* 8:1333–1336, 2001.

10. Lejeunie E, Barcik U, Thorne JA, et al: Craniosynostosis and fetal exposure to sodium Valproate, *J Neurosurg* 95:778–782, 2001.

11. Collmann H, Sorenson N, Kraub J: Consensus: trigonocephaly, *Child Nerv Syst* 12:664–668, 1996.

12. Havlik RJ, Azurin DJ, Bartlett SP, et al: Analysis and treatment of severe trigonocephaly, *Plast Reconstr Surg* 103:381–390, 1999.

13. Bottero L, Lajeunie E, Arnaud E, et al: Functional outcome after surgery for trigonocephaly, *Plast Reconstr Surg* 102:952–958, 1998.

14. Denis D, Genitori L, Conrath J, et al: Ocular findings in children operated on for plagiocephaly and trigonocephaly, *Child Nerv Syst* 12:683–689, 1996.

15. Penny LA, Dell'Aquila M, Jones MC, et al: Clinical and molecular characterization of patients with distal 11q deletions, *Am J Hum Genet* 56:676–683, 1995.

# 33 Lambdoidal Craniosynostosis

## GENESIS

Lambdoidal craniosynostosis accounts for 2% to 4% of all cases of craniosynostosis, and misdiagnosis of nonsynostotic deformational posterior plagiocephaly with occipital flattening as lambdoidal synostosis resulted in apparent epidemics of craniosynostosis, in which the proportion of lambdoid synostosis cases was more than 40% of total craniosynostosis cases in Colorado and more than 70% in York-Selby, England.[1-5] Both of these "epidemics" of craniosynostosis arose during the time when Western cultures were shifting their infant sleeping position from prone to supine in an effort to reduce the incidence of sudden infant death syndrome (SIDS). With this change, infants no longer move their heads from one side to the other as they do in the prone sleeping position; thus placing infants on their backs quickly magnified any inequity in resting position such that asymmetric occipital flattening developed in infants with positional torticollis. Because the lambdoid sutures are not readily visualized on skull radiographs, nonvisualization of these sutures in an asymmetrically flattened occiput was interpreted as lambdoid synostosis. Further complicating this diagnosis is the fact that most lambdoid synostosis occurs as an isolated anomaly in an otherwise normal child and is frequently associated with muscular torticollis, which suggests that many cases of lambdoid synostosis are a consequence of fetal compression. Synostosis can result from constraint of the posterior cranium associated with abnormal fetal lie or presentation. There are also reports of children with chromosome abnormalities who manifest lambdoid synostosis as one component of a broader pattern of altered morphogenesis.[2,6]

## FEATURES

Unilateral lambdoid synostosis results in plagiocephaly, which differs from that seen in deformational posterior plagiocephaly or synostotic anterior plagiocephaly due to unicoronal synostosis. Unlike coronal synostosis, facial structures and orbits are usually not initially affected by lambdoid synostosis, although unilateral involvement results in ipsilateral occipital flattening with ridging of the involved lambdoid suture and downward vertical displacement of the auricle (Fig. 33-1).[3,7] Radiographic and clinical signs include trapezoidal cranial asymmetry when viewed from the vertex position, small posterior fossa, and sutural sclerosis, but sole reliance on skull radiographs and clinical signs alone has led to misdiagnosis, so it is best to confirm the diagnosis of suspected lambdoid synostosis with three-dimensional computed tomography (3D-CT) scans, which clearly image the involved suture(s) and allow a secure diagnosis to be made (Fig. 33-2). Parents and physicians may note apparent protrusion of the mastoid bone on the involved side, as well as palpable sutural ridging.

During the 4-year period between 1991 and 1994, a multidisciplinary team consisting of a dysmorphologist, a pediatric neurosurgeon, and a craniofacial surgeon assessed 102 patients with posterior plagiocephaly. During this same period, the team also assessed 130 patients with craniosynostosis who required surgery.[3] Only four patients (3.1%) manifested clinical, imaging, and operative features of true unilambdoidal craniosynostosis. These features included a thick bony ridge over the fused suture with contralateral parietal and frontal bulging and an ipsilateral occipitomastoid bulge, leading to tilting of the ipsilateral skull base and a downward/posterior displacement of the ear on the synostotic side.[3,7] These changes resulted in a trapezoidal head shape when viewed from above, which must be distinguished from more complex forms of synostosis, combinations of excessive brachycephaly with deformational posterior plagiocephaly (see Fig. 25-1), and combined ipsilateral deformational posterior and anterior plagiocephaly.[8-11] In contrast, children with deformational, nonsynostotic posterior plagiocephaly have a parallelogram-shaped head with forward displacement of the ear and frontal bossing on the side ipsilateral to the occipitoparietal flattening, accompanied by contralateral occipital

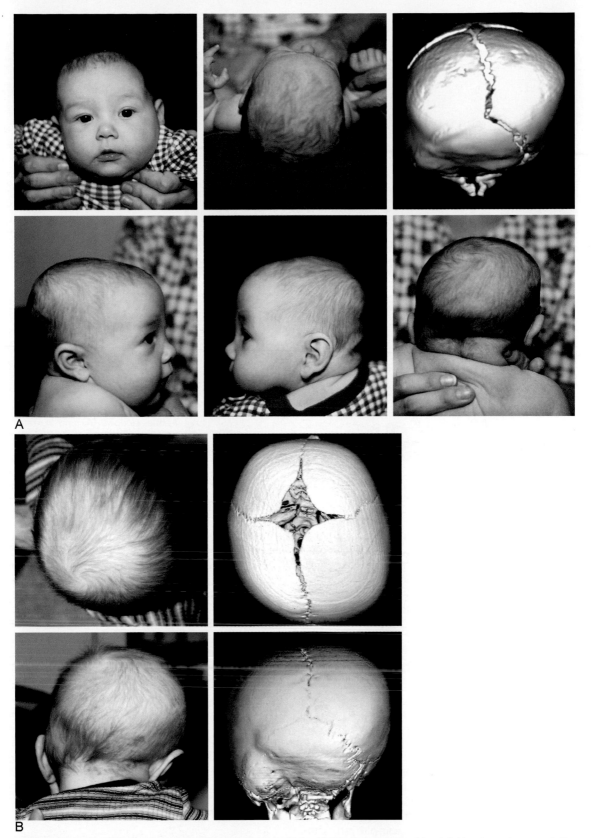

FIGURE 33-1. Two infants with left lambdoid synostosis. Note ridging of the involved lambdoid suture, downward displacement of the auricle, trapezoidal cranial asymmetry when viewed from the vertex position, downward canting of the posterior cranial base with a small posterior fossa, and peaking of the contralateral parietooccipital area. The girl shown in **A** is demonstrated radiographically in Figure 33-2, and she is shown before and after surgery in Figure 33-3.

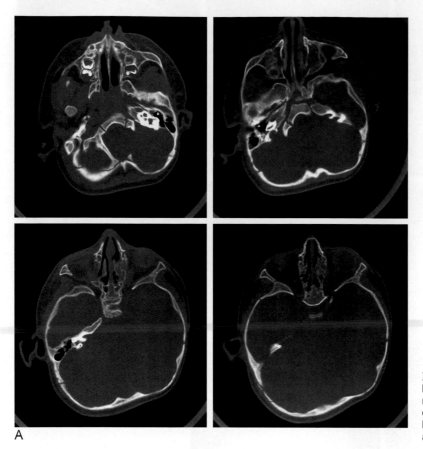

FIGURE 33-2. CT images with bone windows **(A)** and 3D reformatting **(B)** demonstrate left lambdoid synostosis with ridging, bulging of the mastoid bone, and a small posterior fossa.

*Continued*

A

bossing.[3,7] Of the 98 patients with positional head deformation, only 3 had severe, progressive deformation that required surgery; the remainder were successfully managed with changes in sleeping position or helmet therapy.[3] Occasionally, mendosal synostosis accompanies lambdoidal synostosis on the same side.[8]

## MANAGEMENT AND PROGNOSIS

Because isolated lambdoidal synostosis is usually not associated with elevations in intracranial pressure, posterior calvarectomy is performed to prevent facial scoliosis due to restricted posterior cranial expansion over the long term. Fig. 33-3 shows improvement of cranial distortion after early surgical reconstruction of the left lambdoid synostosis in the infant shown in Figs. 33-1, *A* and 33-2. Fig. 33-4 shows a 9-year-old girl with untreated left lambdoid craniosynostosis and secondarily distorted facial features. The timing for

lambdoid synostosis surgery can be later than for other types of craniosynostosis, and the response to surgery may be more variable, particularly with very late surgery. Surgery consists of removal of the synostotic lambdoid suture with reshaping of the occipital bones to allow full expansion of the skull in all directions. If associated torticollis is present, it should be treated vigorously with neck physical therapy. As shown in Fig. 25-6, the combination of positional molding with lambdoid synostosis can have an additional effect on craniofacial structures, requiring long-term treatment. Occasionally, postoperative helmet molding can help optimize results, and the possibility of lambdoid synostosis should be kept in mind when deformational plagiocephaly fails to respond to neck physical therapy and cranial orthotic therapy.

## DIFFERENTIAL DIAGNOSIS

The primary differential diagnosis is between nonsynostotic deformational posterior plagiocephaly

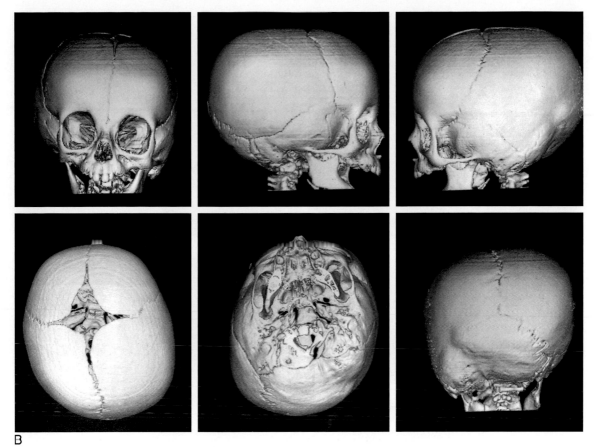

B

FIGURE 33-2. *Continued*

and unilambdoidal synostosis. Unicoronal synostosis gives rise to synostotic anterior plagiocephaly with a raised and retruded supraorbital ridge on the involved side and deviation of the nasal root toward the involved side.[9,10] Ipsilateral coronal and lambdoidal synostosis creates a strikingly trapezoidal head shape, and unicoronal synostosis with ipsilateral posterior deformation can also create a trapezoidal head shape. Both require complex and diverse treatment planning.[12] Most of the confusion in the neurosurgical and craniofacial literature prior to 1996 is about deformational posterior plagiocephaly and lambdoid synostosis; seminal papers in the plastic surgery literature have helped distinguish between these conditions.[3,4,7,9-12] Interestingly, one report of "recurrent lambdoid synostosis within two families" mentions two sets of siblings with parallelogram-shaped skulls and typical deformational posterior plagiocephaly in that histology of the lambdoid suture showed no bony ridging but rather only a fibrous zone between the

two adjacent lambdoid bone fronts.[13] Reports such as this provide reason for caution regarding the many incorrect reports of occipital plagiocephaly attributed to lambdoid synostosis that exist in the literature prior to late 1996 (i.e., large operative series of cases with obvious deformational plagiocephaly treated by lambdoid craniectomies when repositioning efforts failed to correct the asymmetry).[5,14,15]

By 1997, most craniofacial centers had become aware of these distinctions and emphasized that deformational plagiocephaly was more common in males, more frequently right-sided, and usually delayed in presentation due to persistent head turning, which is usually not true of lambdoid synostosis. Lambdoid synostosis manifests a trapezoidal head shape from birth and shows ipsilateral lambdoid ridging with occipitomastoid bossing and downward ear displacement on the involved side, as well as contralateral parietal bossing.[3,4,7,9-12] Huang et al. noted slight posterior displacement

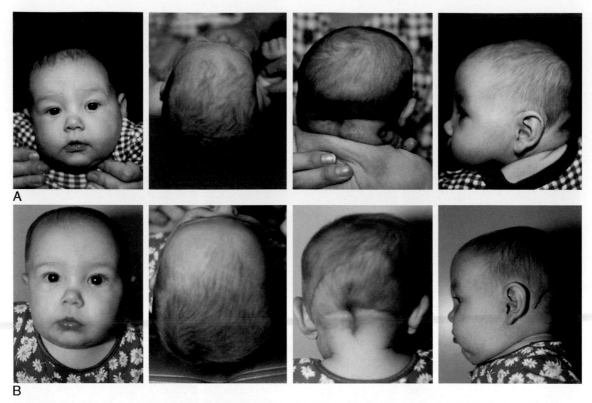

FIGURE 33-3. 3D-CT scans of a child with unilateral left lambdoid synostosis, before **(A)** and after **(B)** surgery.

of the ear on the involved side, while Menard and David noted anterior displacement on the involved side.[3,12] The cases shown in Fig. 33-1 reveal some anterior and downward displacement of the ear on the involved side, but these cases also had ipsilateral torticollis along with lambdoid synostosis. This association of torticollis with lambdoid synostosis may suggest that an unusual fetal position is a predisposition to lambdoid synostosis. Normally, the head flexes anteriorly when it descends into the birth canal; hence most cases of torticollis have ipsilateral jaw compression and canting due to this flexion; however, if the head were to retroflex instead (which is uncommon), it could compress the lambdoid suture on that side and lead to the association of lambdoid synostosis and ipsilateral torticollis, with the combined effects of torticollis-related plagiocephaly and synostosis leading to extensive craniofacial deformation (see Fig. 25-6).

Among cases of posterior plagiocephaly, unilambdoidal synostosis is quite uncommon; it accounts for only 2% to 4% of cases.[3,11] In a Seattle series from 1991 to 2001, there were 1537 cases of posterior deformational plagiocephaly, and 690 cases of craniosynostosis required surgery; 17 of the latter cases had true lambdoid synostosis (2.5%).[3] The 15% to 20% occurrence of lambdoid synostosis in earlier surgical series clearly represents overdiagnosis of posterior plagiocephaly as lambdoid synostosis before its clinical picture was fully described and documented.[14,15] The misdiagnosis of posterior deformation as unilambdoidal synostosis serves to emphasize that deformational nonsynostotic posterior plagiocephaly due to muscular torticollis should be treated promptly with neck physical therapy in early infancy so as to allow effective repositioning. When neck physical therapy and repositioning are not effective by age 6 months, helmet therapy may be required to correct head asymmetry, along with neck physical therapy for torticollis through age 12 months. Thus the primary mode of treatment for infants with torticollis-plagiocephaly deformation sequence is neck physical therapy, not surgery. If there is clinical concern regarding the possibility of lambdoid synostosis, a 3D-CT scan will usually help clarify the diagnosis.

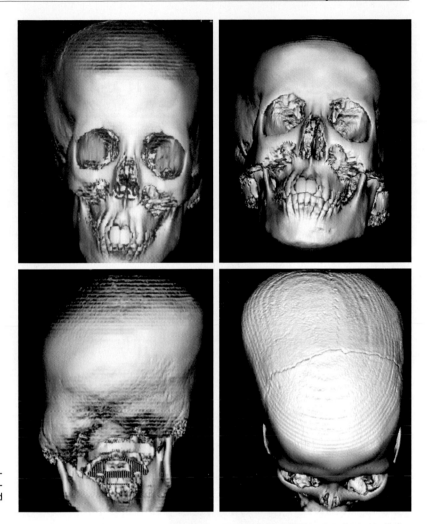

FIGURE 33-4. 3D-CT scan of a 9-year-old girl with marked craniofacial asymmetry due to untreated left lambdoid synostosis.

## References

1. Graham JM Jr: Craniofacial deformation, *Balliere Clin Paediatr* 6:293–315, 1998.
2. Cohen MM Jr, MacLean RE, eds: *Craniosynostosis: diagnosis, evaluation, and management*, ed 2, New York, 2000, Oxford University Press.
3. Huang MHS, Gruss JS, Clarren SK, et al: The differential diagnosis of posterior plagiocephaly: true lambdoid synostosis versus positional molding, *Plast Reconstr Surg* 98:765–776, 1996.
4. Dias MS, Klein DM, Backstrom JW: Occipital plagiocephaly: deformation or lambdoid synostosis, *Pediatr Neurosurg* 24:61–68, 1996.
5. Alderman B, Fernbach SK, Greene C, et al: Diagnostic practice and the estimated prevalence of craniosynostosis in Colorado, *Arch Pediatr Adolesc Med* 151:159–164, 1997.
6. Park JP, Wurster-Hill DH, Berg SZ, et al: A de-novo interstitial deletion of chromosome 6 (q22.2 p23.1), *Clin Genet* 33:65–68, 1988.
7. Ehret F, Whelan MF, Ellenbogen RG, et al: Differential diagnosis of the trapezoid-shaped head, *Cleft Palate Craniofac J* 41:13–19, 2004.
8. Tubbs RS, Wellons JC, Oakes WJ: Unilateral lambdoidal synostosis with mendosal suture involvement, *Pediatr Neurosurg* 39:55, 2003.
9. Brunteau RJ, Mulliken JB: Frontal plagiocephaly: synostotic, compensational, or deformational—discussion, *Plast Reconstr Surg* 89:21–31, 1992.
10. Cohen MM Jr: Frontal plagiocephaly: synostotic, compensational, or deformational—discussion, *Plast Reconstr Surg* 89:32–33, 1992.
11. Jones B, Hayward R, Evans R, et al: Occipital plagiocephaly: an epidemic of craniosynostosis? Craniosynostosis needs to be distinguished from more common postural asymmetry, *Br Med J* 315:693–694, 1996.
12. Menard RM, David DJ: Unilateral lambdoid synostosis: morphological characteristics, *J Craniofac Surg* 9:240–246, 1998.
13. Fryberg JS, Hwang V, Lin KY: Recurrent lambdoid synostosis within two families, *Am J Med Genet* 58:262–266, 1995.
14. Muakkassa KF, Hoffman HJ, Hinton DR, et al: Lambdoid synostosis: part 2. Review of cases managed at the Hospital for Sick Children, 1972–1982, *J Neurosurg* 61:340–347, 1984.
15. McComb JG: Treatment of functional lambdoid synostosis, *Neurosurg Clin North Am* 2:665–672, 1991.

# 34 | Multiple Sutural Craniosynostosis

## GENESIS

Constraint as the cause of multiple sutural synostosis (sagittal, metopic, coronal, and/or lambdoid) is unusual and usually results from a profound degree of prenatal head constraint. The complete restoration of normal form after early and effective surgery is much more likely when constraint is the cause of the problem (Figs. 34-1 and 34-2). Multiple sutural synostosis can also result from genetic mutations in fibroblast growth factor receptor (FGFR) genes, TWIST, or MSX2, all of which result in syndromes that may present with cloverleaf skull.[1] The cloverleaf skull shape is caused by multiple suture synostosis that involves the coronal, lambdoid, and metopic sutures with bulging of the cerebrum through the open sagittal suture or through open squamosal sutures (Figs. 34-3 and 34-4). There may also be synostosis of the sagittal and squamosal sutures with eventration through a

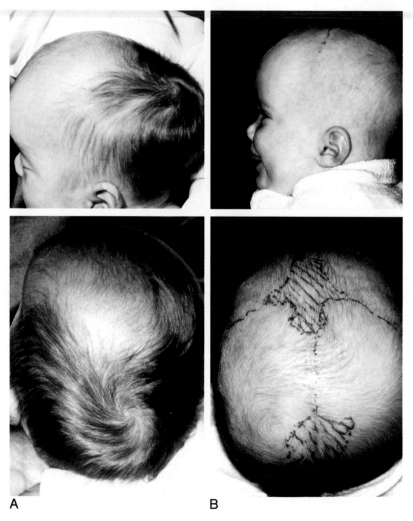

A          B

FIGURE 34-1. **A,** This infant has a cloverleaf skull appearance due to sagittal, coronal, and lambdoidal craniosynostosis. Only the metopic suture was open, and the brain growth ballooned out into this region. The coronal synostosis in addition to the bulging forehead region had distorted the mid- and upper face. A calvarectomy was performed from the supraorbital ridge to below the coronal suture, above the mastoid and the foramen magnum. The aberrant calvarium was discarded, and within several weeks a new calvarium began to form from the remaining dura mater. **B,** Two months after calvarectomy, the new calvarium had formed functional sutures at the sites of dural reflection and fontanelles, where the sutures join. At age 5 years, the patient had not required any additional surgical procedures, and she resembled her older sister in appearance.

(**A** and **B,** From Hanson JW, Sayer MP, Knopp LM, et al: Subtotal neonatal calvariectomy for severe craniosynostosis, *J Pediatr* 91:257–269, 1977.)

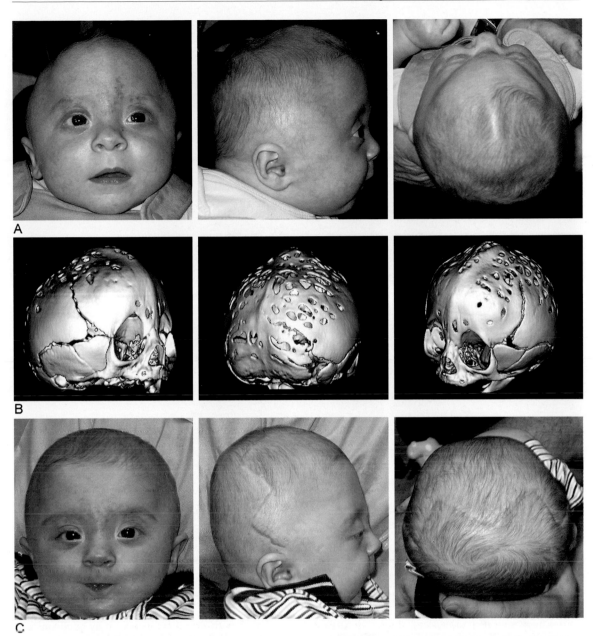

FIGURE 34-2. This neonate was born with synostosis of all midline sutures, as well as the superior coronal sutures and medial portions of the lambdoid sutures. He was part of a twin pregnancy in which prenatal ultrasounds showed that he was in a breech position, with his cranium pinched between the legs of his twin brother. The diagnosis of craniosynostosis was suspected prenatally, and the twins were delivered by cesarean section at 29 weeks of gestation. An extensive calvarectomy was performed at age 4 months. The patient is 3 months old in the preoperative photographs (**A**) and 12 months old in photographs taken after cranial orthotic therapy (**C**). His postoperative cephalic index of 103% was reduced to 92% after 5 months of orthotic therapy. **B,** Note prominent convolutional markings over the superior portions of the skull in the three-dimensional computed tomography scans. Such findings suggest increased intracranial pressure.

widely patent anterior fontanelle. One common syndrome associated with cloverleaf skull is thanatophoric dysplasia type 2, which is due to mutations in FGFR3. Type 2 Pfeiffer syndrome is usually due to mutations in FGFR2 and can result in cloverleaf skull, as can Crouzon syndrome and Apert syndrome, which are also due to mutations in FGFR2. Some rare syndromes, such as Crouzon syndrome with acanthosis nigricans (see Fig. 34-3, *B* and *C*) and Boston craniosynostosis syndrome,

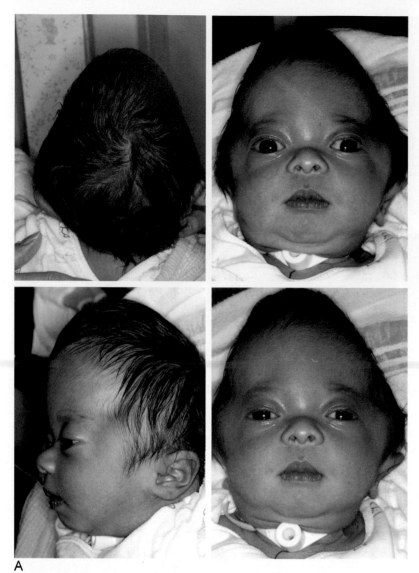

FIGURE 34-3. **A,** This patient has Crouzonoid craniosynostosis with acanthosis nigricans due to an Ala391Glu substitution in FGFR3, resulting in multiple suture synostosis and a cloverleaf skull at age 9 days. He had associated hydrocephalus and choanal atresia and required early posterior and anterior cranial reconstruction in addition to shunting for hydrocephalus and tracheostomy for choanal atresia.

*Continued*

sometimes manifest cloverleaf skull.[1] In Boston craniosynostosis syndrome, the mutant MSX2 product has enhanced affinity for binding to its deoxyribonucleic acid (DNA) target sequence, resulting in activated osteoblastic activity and aggressive cranial ossification.[2-4] In Crouzon syndrome with acanthosis nigricans (also called Crouzonoid craniosynostosis with acanthosis nigricans), a specific FGFR3 mutation (A1a391Glu) leads to early-onset acanthosis nigricans during childhood, often with associated choanal atresia and hydrocephalus. The association of choanal atresia with hydrocephalus in an individual with Crouzon syndrome–like facial features should suggest molecular analysis for this particular mutation, and the combination of hydro-

cephalus with craniosynostosis may predispose a person toward a cloverleaf skull.[5]

## FEATURES

In multiple sutural craniosynostosis, the limitations of calvarial expansion are so extreme that there is limited room for brain growth. This condition is more likely to result in elevated intracranial pressure than is single suture synostosis.[6] Besides the cloverleaf head shape caused by multiple suture synostosis, there are usually signs of increased intracranial pressure, with prominent convolutional markings and a "beaten copper" radiographic

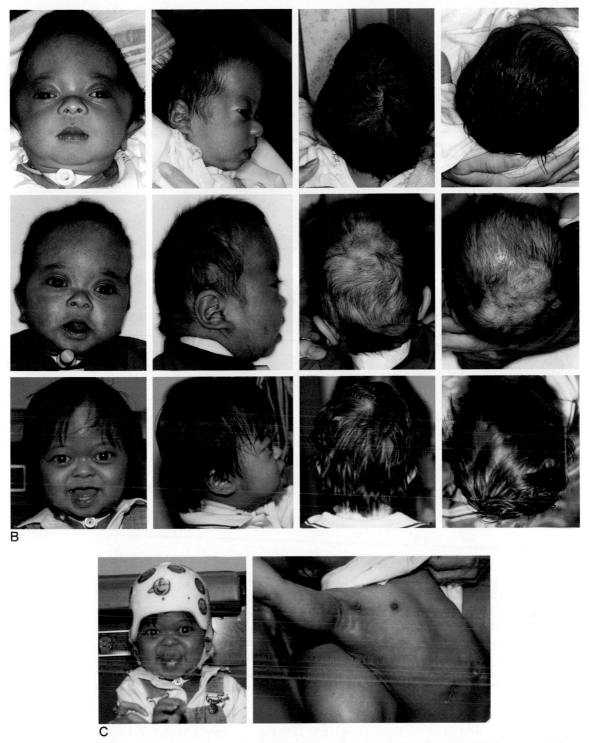

FIGURE 34-3. *Continued* **B,** The same patient after posterior remodeling and shunting for hydrocephalus at age 9 days and anterior remodeling at age 9 months. **C,** From ages 2 to 24 months, the patient received cranial orthotic therapy after both surgical procedures to channel brain growth into a symmetric cranial shape. By the end of this treatment period, striking acanthosis nigricans was apparent, leading to the diagnosis of Crouzonoid craniosynostosis with acanthosis nigricans due to an Ala391Glu substitution in FGFR3. The use of two consecutive postoperative orthotics facilitated optimal correction after each subtotal calvarectomy and prevented excessive molding after each surgery.

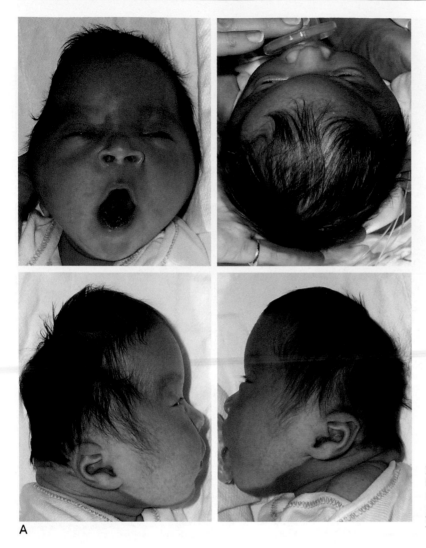

FIGURE 34-4. **A,** This patient also has multiple suture synostosis resulting in a cloverleaf skull *(top)*, but no mutation could be found in FGFR1, FGFR2, FGFR3, TWIST, MSX2, or ALX4.

*Continued*

appearance over the inner table of the skull (Fig. 34-4, *D*). Optic atrophy, proptosis, and loss of vision may occur. Combinations of sutural synostosis, such as sagittal with coronal, are also referred to as *compound craniosynostosis*.

## MANAGEMENT AND PROGNOSIS

Early extensive calvarectomy is usually merited to preserve brain function and development as well as to allow for re-formation of more normal craniofacial features. Many craniofacial surgeons prefer to begin with a posterior skull release in the early months of life (mean age, 4 months), followed by frontoorbital advancement around the end of the first year (mean age, 14 months); a ventriculoperitoneal shunt may be inserted at the time of the first procedure if associated hydrocephalus is present.[7] The use of postoperative orthotic molding can help channel brain growth into a more normal form, leading to improved postoperative results compared with those obtained via surgery alone (see Fig. 34-3, *C*).[5] When lambdoid synostosis occurs as part of a syndrome with multiple suture involvement, there is often bilateral involvement, and early posterior release may alleviate some associated increased intracranial pressure. Rarely, in some instances of syndromic coronal craniosynostosis, the combination of sagittal synostosis with underlying coronal synostosis has a corrective effect, and delayed sagittal synostosis repair can prevent the need for a second operation

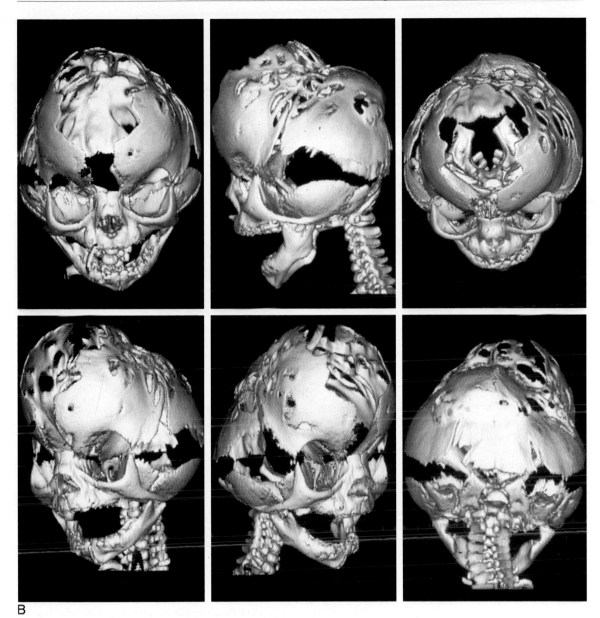

FIGURE 34-4. *Continued* **B,** Three-dimensional computed tomography scans show multiple sutural synostosis with multiple areas of cranial thinning, which would yield a "beaten copper" appearance on skull radiographs.

as effectively as a postsurgical cranial orthotic device (Fig. 34-5).

Patients with craniofacial dysostosis syndromes need to be followed carefully for hydrocephalus, which is often part of the syndrome rather than a result of the multiple suture synostosis. Restricted growth of the posterior fossa is particularly common in severe craniofacial dysostosis syndromes. Hanson et al.[8] considered the case shown in Fig. 34-1, *A* and *B* to be an early example of the efficacy of a neonatal subtotal neonatal calvarectomy at 13 days for severe nonsyndromic craniosynosto-

sis without any associated hydrocephalus. This child was clinically normal and closely resembled her older sister at age 5 years, and subsequent procedures were not needed.

## DIFFERENTIAL DIAGNOSIS

As emphasized previously, this degree of craniosynostosis may be more common in genetically determined disorders, such as Crouzon syndrome, Apert syndrome, Pfeiffer syndrome, or Saethre-Chotzen

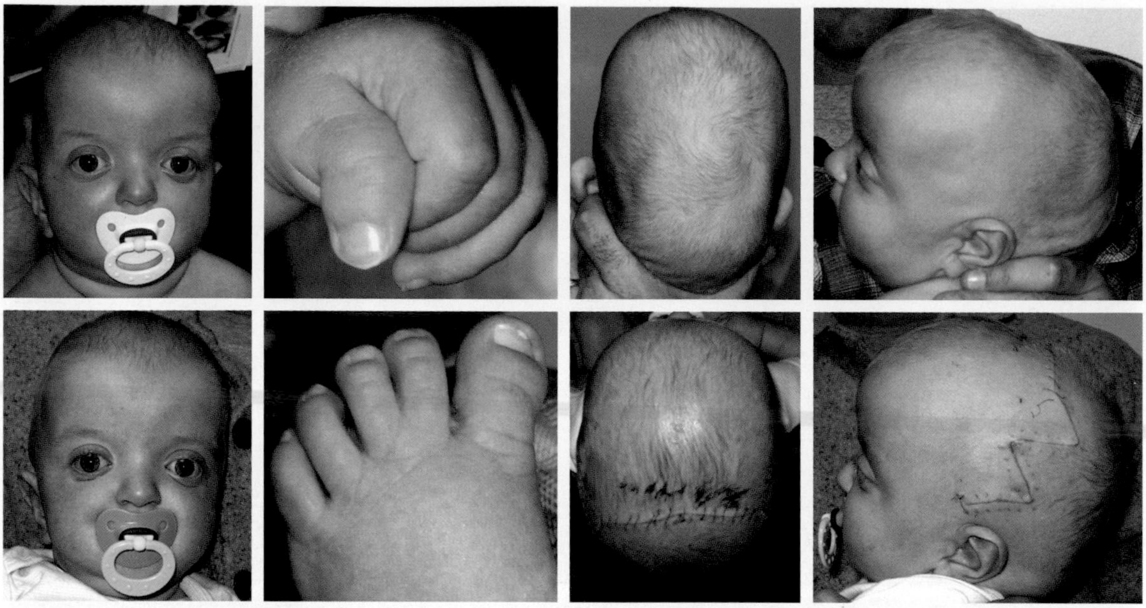

FIGURE 34-5. This boy with Pfeiffer syndrome experienced early fetal head descent and developed sagittal synostosis, which counteracted the normal tendency of his coronal sutures to fuse. Consequently, the repair of sagittal synostosis was delayed from ages 4 to 6 months. No postoperative orthotic was used, and by age 9 months his coronal synostosis had progressed.

syndrome, than in fetal head constraint. In Crouzon syndrome, sagittal and coronal synostosis occur together in 19% of patients, and involvement of the sagittal, coronal, and lambdoid sutures is even more common.[9,10] It is critically important to understand the natural history of the disorder being treated because thanatophoric dysplasia and Pfeiffer syndrome type 2 have significant early lethality, whereas other syndromes may be much more amenable to successful early treatment without a high incidence of long-term morbidity or mortality.

## References

1. In Cohen MM Jr, MacLean RE, eds: *Craniosynostosis: diagnosis, evaluation, and management*, ed 2, New York, 2000, Oxford University Press.
2. Warman ML, Mulliken JB, Hayward PG, et al: Newly recognized autosomal dominant disorder with craniosynostosis, *Am J Med Genet* 46:444–449, 1993.
3. Jabs EW, Muller U, Li X, et al: A mutation in the homeodomain of the human MSX2 gene in a family affected with autosomal dominant craniosynostosis, *Cell* 75:443–450, 1993.
4. Ma L, Golden S, Maxson R: The molecular basis of Boston-type craniosynostosis: the Pro148→His mutation in the N-terminal arm of the MSX2 homeodomain stabilized DNA binding without altering nucleotide sequence preferences, *Hum Mol Genet* 5:1915–1920, 1996.
5. Schweitzer DN, Graham JM Jr, Lachman RS, et al: Subtle radiographic findings of achondroplasia in patients with Crouzon syndrome with acanthosis nigricans due to an Ala391Glu substitution in FGFR3, *Am J Med Genet* 98:75–91, 2001.
6. Renier D, Sainte-Rose C, Marchac D, et al: Intrauterine pressure in craniostenosis, *J Neurosurg* 57:370, 1982.
7. Sgouros S, Goldin JH, Hockley AD, et al: Posterior skull surgery in craniosynostosis, *Child Nerv Syst* 12:727–733, 1996.
8. Hanson JW, Sayer MP, Knopp LM, et al: Subtotal neonatal calvariectomy for severe craniosynostosis, *J Pediatr* 91:257, 1977.
9. Lajeunie E, Le Merrer M, Bonati-Pellie C, et al: Genetic study of scaphocephaly, *Am J Med Genet* 62:282–285, 1996.
10. Mulliken JB, Gripp K, Stolle CA, et al: Molecular analysis of patients with synostotic frontal plagiocephaly (unilateral coronal synostosis), *Plast Reconstr Surg* 113:1899–1909, 2004.

# Cranial Bone Variations

# 35 Vertex Birth Molding

## GENESIS

*Vertex birth molding* describes the mechanic changes in fetal head shape due to external compression on the cranium from bony adjustments within the cranial vault that occur as the neonate in vertex presentation passes through the birth canal. Additional soft tissue swelling can significantly alter the shape of the neonatal head, and pressure against the fetal cranium can delay normal ossification in the vertex region, resulting in benign vertex craniotabes. Humans have an unusual pelvis, a large fetal head, and a complicated mechanism of labor. One major feature of human evolution is marked delay in neural development, such that our brains continue to grow slowly over a much longer period of time than do the brains of other primates. The modern human brain is only 25% of its adult size at birth and continues to grow at a rapid rate throughout the first year of life, when it reaches 50% of its adult size.[1] Human brains are 95% of adult size by age 10 years. In comparison, a chimpanzee brain is already 40% of its adult size by birth and reaches 80% of the adult volume by the end of the first year. A 1 year old *Homo erectus* brain was closer to that of apes in its growth pattern and measured 72% to 84% of adult size at that age, which implies differences in the development of cognitive abilities in *Homo erectus* compared with modern humans.[1] The early delivery of the human head appears to leave the cranium much more vulnerable to mechanic forces than in other species. The birth canal is a deep curved tube through which a mature fetal head can only pass by rotating as it descends. A number of factors influence the individual fetal cranial response to the normal forces of labor around the time of delivery, such as fetal head position and size, gestational age, maternal pelvic shape and dimensions, and the quality of uterine contractions.[2,3]

During normal vertex molding, anteroposterior compression causes the frontal and occipital bones to slide under the parietal bones along the entire length of the coronal and lambdoid sutures. This elongates the occipitofrontal diameter to its greatest possible extent so as to diminish the vertical diameter of the fetal head to its smallest dimensions (Fig. 35-1). The fetal pathologist John Ballantyne noted that during vertex molding, the occipital bone rotated in an anteroposterior direction on an "occipital hinge," with a range of motion that is much greater in a 7-month fetus than in a term infant. He also noted that an infant's head recovered to its unmolded state within 6 days after delivery.[4] Holland studied the impact of mechanic stress on the fetal head and noted that the dura mater underlying the cranial bones acted as a protective mechanism to reduce the stress transmitted to the cranial contents.[5] Decreases in dural growth-stretch tension across a suture can trigger synostosis, whereas excessive dural pressure can decrease ossification, leading to craniotabes and increased cranial flexibility. Holland described the fetal skull as a pliable shell composed of loosely jointed plates attached to a rigid cranial base, suggesting that the frontal and parietal bones bend under pressure in relation to movement at the occipital hinge.

Moloy examined the hinge action of occipital and frontal bones radiographically in stillborn infants and noted that the cranial base was capable of bending slightly to allow elevation of the occipital plates and that biparietal pressure decreased the transverse diameter enough to prevent the frontal and occipital bones from overriding the parietal bones when longitudinal pressure was applied.[6] Borell and Fernstrom used radiographs to assess molding as the fetal head passed through the birth canal, and they confirmed that vertex molding was characterized by an elevation of the vertex, an increase in the biparietal diameter, and an inward displacement of the occipital and frontal bones, which caused an overall reduction in the occipitofrontal diameter (see Fig. 35-1). They noted an association between the amount of molding and the length of labor, and they attributed normal vertex molding to pressures from the soft tissues rather than the bony pelvis.[7,8] They noted that a contracted pelvis resulted in more severe fetal head molding than seen in normal deliveries and that excessive muscular contraction in the lower uterine segment resulted in excessive vertex

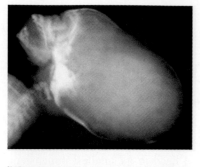

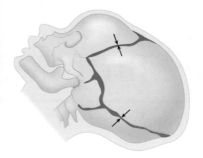

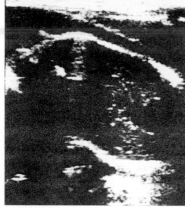

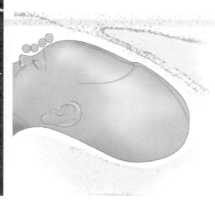

FIGURE 35-1. During normal vertex molding, anteroposterior compression causes the frontal and occipital bones to slide under the parietal bones along the entire length of the coronal and lambdoid sutures. This elongates the occipitofrontal diameter to its greatest possible extent in order to diminish the vertical diameter of the fetal head to its smallest dimensions. This is shown in the illustration and radiograph in the top frames; the bottom frames show an ultrasound view and illustration.

molding, with increased elevation of the fetal vertex (Figs. 35-2 to 35-4).

In 1980 McPherson and Kriewall[9] used engineering structural analysis techniques to investigate the biomechanics of fetal head molding. They observed that fetal cranial bone is capable of deforming under load distributions typical of normal labor, with preterm parietal bone capable of undergoing two to four times the amount of deformation than term parietal bone for the same load distribution. Although this may not result in more obvious extensive cranial molding, the transmission of pressure may be a contributing factor to the increased incidence of birth trauma and intracranial bleeds in preterm infants. In a photographic and anthropometric study of vertex molding in 319 term infants delivered vaginally, several factors influenced the degree of molding. Infants born to primiparous women, after oxytocin-stimulated labors, and via vacuum extraction showed significantly more molding. The duration of the first stage of labor did not influence the degree of molding, but a prolonged second stage in primiparous mothers was associated with more extensive molding. Infants born in the occipitoposterior and in breech presentation showed significantly less molding than those born in occipitoanterior presen-

tations. Some degree of molding does occur within the uterus prior to labor, and repetitive Braxton-Hicks contractions throughout pregnancy were also a factor that influenced the head shape of infants before the onset of labor.[10] Extreme fetal head elongation due to vertex molding from fetal cephalic fixation with persistent uterine contractions has been noted via prenatal ultrasonography as early as 30 weeks of gestation.[11]

## FEATURES

During initial cervical dilatation, pressure is greatest on the upper portion of the parietal bones, which leads to a decrease in biparietal diameter and a slight increase in the height and curvature of the vertex (see Figs. 35-1 to 35-5). At complete dilatation, the biparietal diameter decreases to its smallest dimension, with continued elevation and curvature of the vertex in addition to inward bending of both the frontal and occipital bones. As the fetus descends, pressure shifts to the lower portions of the parietal bones, causing them to rotate inward and move upward, thereby increasing the biparietal diameter as well as progressively widening the temporosquamosal and sagittal

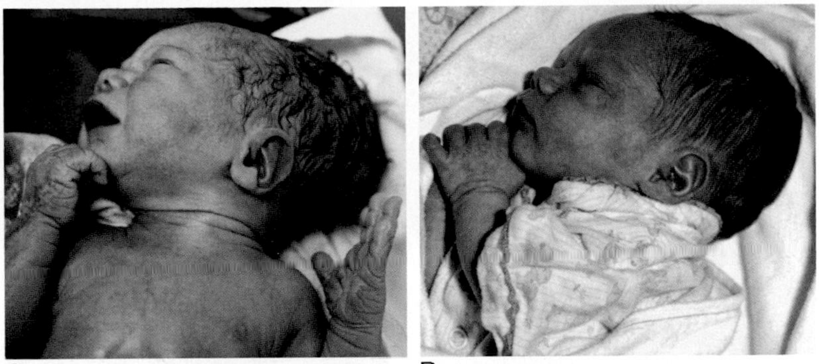

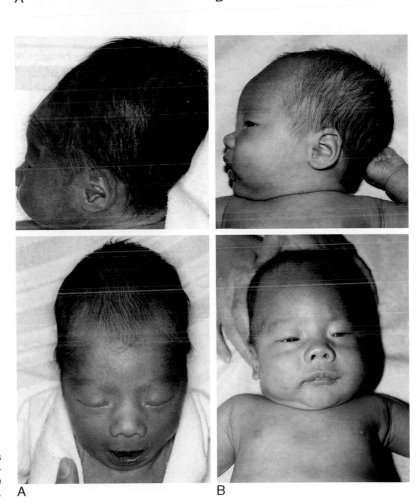

FIGURE 35-2. This small-for-gestational-age infant with rapid postnatal catch-up growth showed marked molding immediately after being born (**A**) to a small primigravida woman. By age 4 days (**B**), the molding had resolved. **A**                                    **B**

FIGURE 35-3. **A,** At birth, this infant had been in prolonged vertex. **B,** By 2 months of age, the molding had only partially resolved. **A**                                    **B**

sutures. Recovery from this molded state takes place in two phases: an acute elastic recovery before the head is actually delivered and a second, slower viscoelastic recovery during the postpartum period, which is usually completed 3 to 7 days after delivery.[9]

In the normal fetus presenting in the vertex position, there may be appreciable molding of the head at birth. This is especially likely if the infant is the first-born, if the fetal head was located deep in the uterine outlet for a prolonged time, or if the mother has a prolonged second stage of labor and/or an incompletely dilated rigid cervix. The typical vertex molded newborn head is elongated and cylindric and resumes a rounded shape within the first week of life (see Figs. 35-1

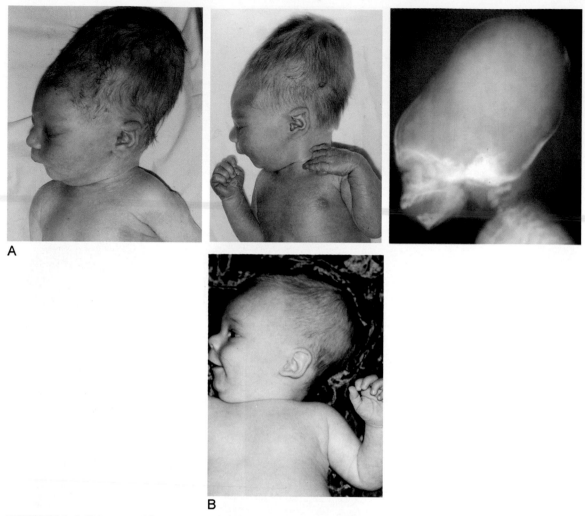

**FIGURE 35-4. A,** Extreme molding was associated with a prolonged second stage of labor due to a tight cervix that did not fully dilate prior to the delivery of this large infant. His cone-shaped vertex was palpably softened (craniotabes). **B,** The same infant at age 3 months. The craniotabes resolved, but vertex molding persists.

and 35-2).[12] The forehead tends to slope, and the parietooccipital region is prominent. Head circumference measurements may be spuriously low because of the impact of normal vertex molding. The head circumference usually shifts upward by 1 to 3 days after birth as the head remolds in relation to the true brain shape (see Fig. 35-2). Persistent vertex molding usually reflects prolonged molding during the second stage of labor due to prolonged entrapment of the fetal head.

## MANAGEMENT AND PROGNOSIS

The prognosis for spontaneous resolution of normal vertex birth molding and any accompanying traumatic components is generally excellent, and usually no treatment is necessary other than reassuring the parents that the baby is normal (see Figs. 35-2 and 35-3). With extensive vertex molding, management of the infant's resting position will usually facilitate a complete return to normal form (see Fig. 35-5).[12] It is important to observe the infant during the first week after birth to monitor resolution. During this period, the use of several procedures is worthwhile. The surface on which the baby's head rests should be relatively soft, and care should be taken to position the baby's head on the prominent vertex region during sleep. A rolled diaper or receiving blanket can be placed under the neck and shoulders in the supine resting position to provide support and maintain head position (see Fig. 35-5).[12] Another measure that may be

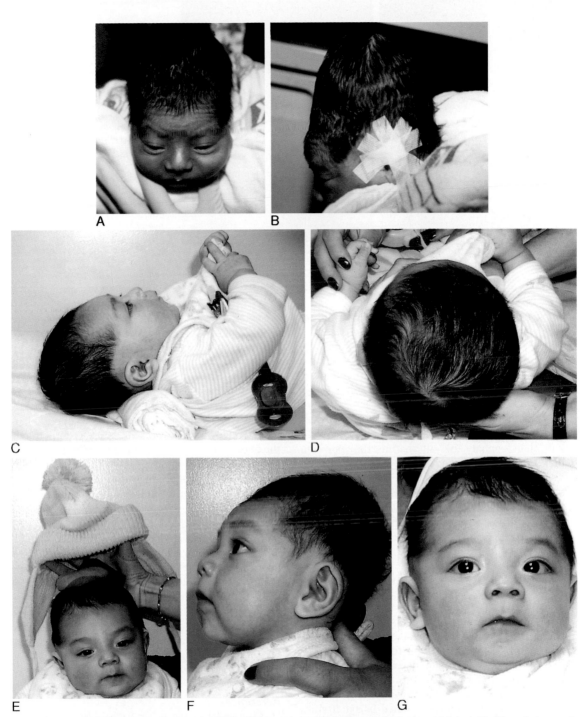

FIGURE 35-5. This male infant is shown at birth with a conic head shape and marked craniotabes (**A, B**) and at ages 2 and 3 months (**C–G**) after active management to resolve his extensive vertex molding and deformed auricle. He was positioned on his prominent vertex during sleep, with a rolled blanket under his neck and shoulders in the supine resting position to provide support and maintain head position. **E,** Another measure used when the baby was upright involved placing a 2- to 3-oz beanbag over the vertex and holding it in place with a knit cap. The weight was placed directly over the occipital prominence in an effort to collapse the cone.

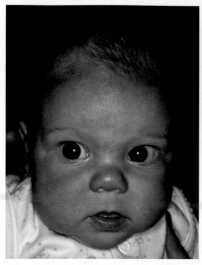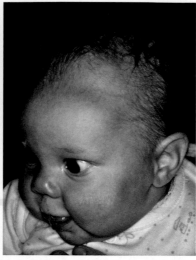

FIGURE 35-6. This infant with a prominent calvarial indentation above the frontal bones was born with her arm across her forehead. The indentation persisted during early infancy but was expected to resolve with subsequent calvarial remodeling. The frontal skull shape resembled that seen in vertex molding, but review of the birth history revealed the true cause.

used when the baby is upright in a car seat or infant swing is to place a silk or nylon stocking (sized to fit snugly but not tightly) over the baby's calvarium. This stocking can be filled with a 2- to 3-oz beanbag. The weight should be placed directly over the occipital prominence in an effort to collapse the cone. The cone-shaped cranium may foster a tendency for the infant to lie on one side of the head and face, so it is important to try to minimize postnatal plagiocephaly by alternating the side on which the baby is placed to sleep. If the baby is allowed to rest exclusively on the sides of the head, the deformation may become stabilized and the elongated, conic head shape will persist; thus, it is important to apply pressure to the vertex to help collapse the conic head shape (see Fig. 35-4).[12]

## DIFFERENTIAL DIAGNOSIS

Occasionally, vertex molding is so extensive that the possibility of craniosynostosis, encephalocele, or other causes of aberrant head shape becomes a concern. In addition, persistent fetal vertex molding can lead to permanent deformation of head shape if corrective postnatal positioning interventions are not undertaken. The differential diagnosis may include microcephaly, isolated or syndromic craniosynostosis, and various soft tissue deformities. A spuriously small occipitofrontal head circumference may give a mistaken impression of microcephaly, as may the sloping forehead. Clinical judgment of the apparent overall brain size, in addition to follow-up head circumference measurements as the calvarium returns toward a more normal shape, will usually resolve any questions in this regard. At the leading part of the parietooccipital region, edema of the skin and subcutaneous tissues may be present (the so-called *caput succedaneum*). Craniotabes may also be extensive in the vertex region (see Figs. 35-4 and 35-5). Hemorrhages may occasionally be evident in the sclera and in the retina, and a traumatic subperiosteal hemorrhage may be present, most commonly in the outer table of the parietal bone, which will give rise to a soft, fluctuant mass. With time, its borders will become elevated and craterlike as the raised periosteum begins to deposit bone at its borders. The subperiosteal hemorrhage, with a subsequent "crater rim" of bone at its outer borders, may give the impression of a depressed skull fracture, but it is actually a benign lesion. Rarely, posterior fossa hemorrhage in the term neonate can lead to severe molding with elongation of the head. Such cases are readily distinguished from benign vertex molding by abnormal neurologic examination. Finally, other calvarial deformations can result when a hand or arm is caught across the skull for a prolonged period of time (Fig. 35-6).

### References

1. Coqueugniot H, Hublin J-J, Vellon F, et al: Early brain growth in *Homo erectus* and implications for cognitive ability, *Nature* 431:299–302, 2004.
2. Compton AA: Soft tissue and pelvic dystocia, *Clin Obstet Gynecol* 30:69–76, 1987.
3. Graham JM Jr: Craniofacial deformation, *Balliere Clin Pediatr* 6:293–315, 1998.
4. Ballantyne JW: The head of the infant at birth, *Edin Med J* 36:97–111, 1890.

5. Holland E: Cranial stress in the foetus during labour and the effects of excessive stress on the intracranial contents, with an analysis of 81 cases of torn tentorium cerebelli and subdural cerebral hemorrhage, *J Obstet Gynaecol Br Emp* 29:549–571, 1922.

6. Moloy HC: Studies of head molding during labor, *Am J Obstet Gynecol* 44:762–782, 1942.

7. Borell U, Fernstrom I: X-ray diagnosis of muscular spasm in the lower part of the uterus from the degree of moulding of the fetal head, *Acta Obstet Gynecol Scand* 38:188–189, 1959.

8. Borell U, Fernstrom I: The mechanisms of labor in face and brow presentation, *Acta Obstet Gynecol Scand* 39:626–644, 1960.

9. McPherson GK, Kriewall TJ: The elastic modulus of fetal cranial bone: a first step towards an understanding of the biomechanics of fetal head molding, *J Biomechanics* 13:9–16, 1980.

10. Sorbe B, Dahlgren SS: Some important factors in the molding of the fetal head during vaginal delivery—a photographic study, *Int J Gynaecol Obstet* 21:205–212, 1983.

11. Carla SJ, Wyble L, Lense J, et al: Fetal head molding: diagnosis by ultrasound and a review of the literature, *J Perinatol* 11:105 111, 1991.

12. Graham JM Jr, Kumar A: Diagnosis and management of extensive vertex birth molding, *Clin Pediatr* 45:672–678, 2006.

# 36 Vertex Craniotabes

## GENESIS

Prolonged forceful pressure on the presenting part, usually at the vertex affecting the superior portions of the parietal bones, may result in diminished mineralization within the compressed region. The calvarium is generated from the underlying dura mater, and persistent growth-stretch tensile forces restrain cranial ossification and maintain sutural patency. Persistent cranial pressure mimics the mechanical impact of growth-stretch forces and results in temporarily restrained, localized calvarial ossification. Craniotabes is more likely to occur in first-born infants, and elicited history often shows that the fetus has experienced early fetal head descent and has been in the vertex position deep within the maternal pelvis for an unusually long period of time. Because this is usually the mother's first pregnancy, she may not be aware of anything unusual other than symptoms of urinary frequency and pressure. Mild degrees of compression-related craniotabes occur in about 2% of newborns, whereas more extensive degrees of craniotabes are less common.[1,2]

Since the theory of a compression-related pathogenesis for benign vertex craniotabes was first advanced in 1979,[1] several reports have investigated whether craniotabes might be a useful sign for the detection of subclinical rickets due to vitamin D deficiency.[3-8] Most studies failed to demonstrate any significant correlations among maternal and infant serum vitamin D, calcium, phosphorus, and alkaline phosphatase levels; craniotabes; and skeletal mineralization. However, one study showed small but statistically significant decreases in serum calcium and phosphate in mothers of infants with craniotabes compared with mothers of infants with a normal calvarium.[5] Another study showed that the mean serum 25-hydroxyvitamin D level by radioassay was significantly lower in newborns with craniotabes and in their mothers compared with control mother-infant pairs without craniotabes. Four cases of neonatal rickets were reported in infants with craniotabes who were born to mothers with florid osteomalacia due to vitamin D–deficiency rickets (causing these mothers hip and back pain and an impaired waddling gait). Both the infants and their mothers had low serum concentrations of 25-hydroxyvitamin D, elevated alkaline phosphatase, and borderline or low serum calcium and phosphorous, and they responded to treatment with vitamin D. These studies indicate that deficient maternal vitamin D intake can lead to neonatal rickets in which craniotabes may be a presenting feature, and this diagnosis should be considered in any infant without signs of fetal head compression whose mother may be at risk for nutritional deficiency; however, in these cases, the infant usually manifests generalized craniotabes and osteomalacia.

## FEATURES

The superior parietooccipital region tends to be soft to palpation by the examining fingers, and often there is a "ping-pong" sensation on finger compression. This tactile sensation resembles the indentation and snapping rebound felt when pressing on a ping-pong ball. In extreme cases, the entire top of the head can be involved (Figs. 36–1 and 36–2). The presence of a normally firm bony calvarium along the sides of the calvarium and in the mastoid regions readily differentiates this benign type of craniotabes from other forms caused by a generalized mineralization problem such as hypophosphatasia, osteogenesis imperfecta, or infantile rickets. Within the affected region of the calvarium, the sutures and fontanelles may feel wider than usual. Accentuated vertex molding and other features noted in Chapter 35 are also common associated features. The fetus with vertex craniotabes has often been more constrained than usual in late gestation and experienced prolonged vertex presentation, and there may be mild-to-moderate limitation of full movement in some joints, especially those of the lower limbs. Benign vertex craniotabes has not been reported in infants who presented in breech position, and radiolucency of the parietal bones in the vertex of the skull is considered to be a normal anatomic variant on neonatal head computed tomography scans.[9]

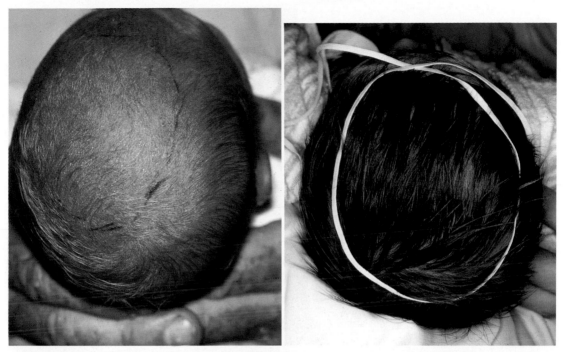

FIGURE 36-1. These newborn infants were in prolonged vertex presentation with the head engaged. Relatively forceful pressure by the examiner over the tops of the heads of the babies did not cause discomfort, this having been the normal situation for the infant in utero. Areas of soft "ping-pong" craniotabes are outlined in the vertex region.

## MANAGEMENT, PROGNOSIS, AND COUNSEL

The prognosis for postnatal recovery is excellent, and the parents should be reassured that the infant's calvarium will mineralize in a normal fashion within 1 to 2 months, that there is no risk in handling the "soft head," and that generally no special precautions or studies are merited. If the mother has vitamin D–deficient rickets and the infant has generalized craniotabes and osteomalacia, this condition generally responds promptly to vitamin D therapy over the next few months. As with other defects of skeletal mineralization, such as osteogenesis imperfecta and hypophosphatasia, care must be taken initially to avoid fractures.

## DIFFERENTIAL DIAGNOSIS

Initial concern may be generated regarding the possibility of a generalized problem of bone mineralization, such as hypophosphatasia, osteogenesis imperfecta, or rickets. The clinical examination of the entire calvarium should help resolve such concerns. The sides of the calvarium should be of normal firmness with benign vertex craniotabes,

and no other skeletal developmental problems should be present. Craniotabes may be one of the earliest signs of vitamin-D–deficient rickets; however, it usually takes several months to deplete vitamin D stores and manifest this deficiency (unless the mother is severely deficient in vitamin D and has signs of rickets herself). Vitamin D–deficient rickets is generally accompanied by metaphyseal changes at the wrist and low 25-hydroxyvitamin D concentrations (<12 ng/mL), with a variably elevated alkaline phosphatase level. The isolated compression-related type of vertex craniotabes is usually not an indication for radiographs or measurement of serum vitamin D, calcium phosphorus, or alkaline phosphatase. If there is concern about a systemic problem, then close clinical follow-up should resolve this situation without excessive laboratory or radiographic studies, because the "soft head" due to compression quickly normalizes postnatally.

Infants with osteogenesis imperfecta show generalized osteomalacia, often with blue sclera and brittle bones that fracture during delivery. The calvarium may demonstrate interspersed islands of palpable bones (wormian bones). Extensive calvarial defects consisting of absence or severe hypoplasia of the parietal bones can occur in cleidocranial dysplasia with C-terminal mutations

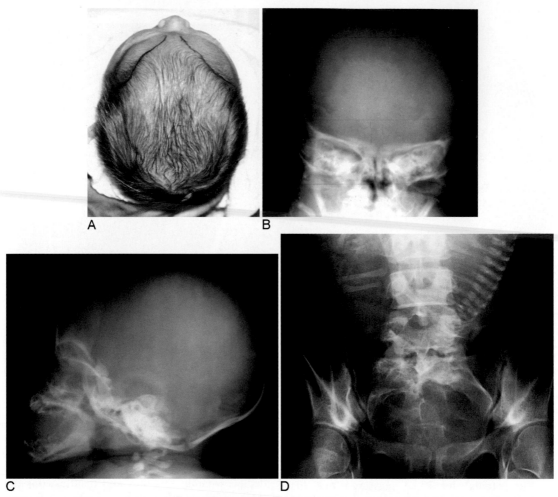

FIGURE 36-2. Vertex craniotabes **(A)**, with skull radiographs **(B** and **C)** demonstrating diminished mineralization over the vertex. The infant's primigravida mother noted early lightening and felt the baby's head rubbing against the rim of her pelvis as she walked 3 miles to and from her college classes. **D,** A pelvic radiograph of the mother taken 2 weeks before delivery, when her obstetrician documented fetal head engagement, demonstrates the position of the fetal head in the pelvis. Such early lightening in a primiparous mother is unusual.

in RUNX2 that preserve the runt domain.[10] Classically, cleidocranial dysplasia consists of large fontanelles, wide sutures, clavicular hypoplasia, supernumerary teeth, and short stature. Parietal foramina occur laterally to the midline and have well-demarcated edges, and these inherited skull ossification defects can be caused by mutations in either MSX2 or ALX4.[11] Because they are inherited in an autosomal dominant fashion, there may be an affected parent and a positive family history. The "soft head" may also convey the impression of open sutures and fontanelles, and the question of hydrocephalus or other causes of increased intracranial pressure may be raised. Such concerns may be fostered by increased transillumination in the vertex region when a strong light is held against the soft portion of the calvarium. The infant's head circumference, head shape, and general clinical status, in addition to palpation of the firm portion of the calvarium around the sides of the skull, should resolve these concerns without the need to resort to any other studies.

## References

1. Graham JM, Smith DW: Parietal craniotabes in the neonate: its origin and relevance, *J Pediatr* 95:114, 1979.
2. Fox GN, Maier MK: Neonatal craniotabes, *Am Fam Physician* 30:149–151, 1984.
3. Pettifor JM, Isdale JM, Sahakian J, et al: Diagnosis of subclinical rickets, *Arch Dis Child* 55:155–157, 1980.
4. Pettifor JM, Pentopoulos M, Moodley GP, et al: Is craniotabes a pathognomonic sign of rickets in 3-month-old infants? *S Afr Med J* 65:549–551, 1984.

5. Kokkonen J, Koivisto M, Lautala P, et al: Serum calcium and 25-OH-D in mothers of newborns with craniotabes, *J Perinat Med* 11:127–131, 1983.
6. Congdon P, Horsman A, Kirby PA, et al: Mineral content of the forearms of babies born to Asian and white mothers, *Br Med J [Clin Res]* 286:1233–1235, 1983.
7. Park W, Paust H, Kaufmann HJ, et al: Osteomalacia of the mother—rickets of the newborn, *Eur J Pediatr* 146:292–293, 1987.
8. Reif S, Katzir Y, Eisenberg Z, et al: Serum 25-hydroxyvitamin D levels in congenital craniotabes *Acta Paediatr Scand* 77:167–168, 1988.
9. Pastakia B, Herdt JR: Radiolucent "zones" in parietal bones seen on computed tomography: a normal variant, *JCAT* 8:108–109, 1984.
10. Cunningham ML, Seto ML, Hing AV, et al: Cleidocranial dysplasia with severe parietal bone dysplasia: C-terminal RUNX2 mutations, *Birth Defects Res Clin Mol Teratol* 76:78–85, 2005.
11. Mavrogiannis LA, Antonopoulou I, Baxova A, et al: Haploinsufficiency of the human homeobox gene ALX4 causes skull ossification defects, *Nat Genet* 27:17–18, 2001.

# 37 Anterior Fontanelle Bone

## GENESIS

Occasionally, the anterior fontanelle will ossify into a bony plate that may be slightly elevated in relation to the rest of the cranium. This may occur due to decreased growth-stretch tensile forces across the anterior fontanelle, and it is sometimes seen with multiple sutural synostosis. It can also occur in otherwise normal infants, in which case it is considered a normal variant.[1] The anterior fontanelle normally closes between 4 and 26 months, with 90% closing between 7 and 19 months and 42% closing before 12 months.[2,3] Delayed closure of the fonta-

nelles has been associated with a variety of pathologic conditions such as osteogenesis imperfecta, hypophosphatasia, cleidocranial dysplasia, and various other skeletal dysplasias. An ossified anterior fontanelle does not carry the same significance.

## FEATURES

Instead of the usual flat, uncalcified, diamond-shaped anterior fontanelle, there is a slightly raised, diamond-shaped plate of bone in its place (Figs. 37-1 and 37-2).

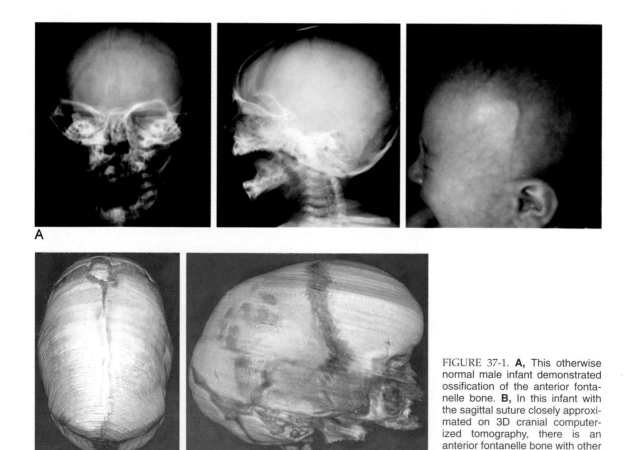

A

B

FIGURE 37-1. **A,** This otherwise normal male infant demonstrated ossification of the anterior fontanelle bone. **B,** In this infant with the sagittal suture closely approximated on 3D cranial computerized tomography, there is an anterior fontanelle bone with other sutures widely patent and an open posterior fontanelle.

230

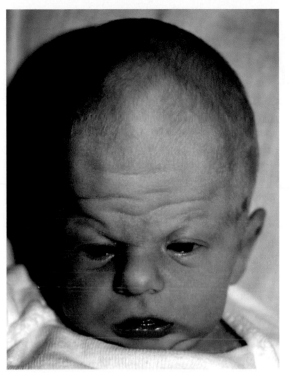

FIGURE 37-2. This child with craniotelencephalic dysplasia was born with multiple sutural synostosis and an obvious anterior fontanelle bone.

## MANAGEMENT AND PROGNOSIS

If the child is otherwise normal with no signs of craniosynostosis or osteogenesis imperfecta, then parents can be reassured that this is a normal variant (see Fig. 37-1, *A*). Occasionally the anterior fontanelle bone is associated with early closure of the sagittal suture (see Fig. 37-1, *B*). The shape of the anterior fontanelle bone often remains visible on skull radiographs throughout childhood and into adulthood, with a characteristic appearance on Towne skull radiographic projection.

## DIFFERENTIAL DIAGNOSIS

If multiple sutural synostosis is present (Fig. 37-2), it should be evident from examination of the head shape and demonstrable on radiographs and three-dimensional computed tomography scans. A careful search for associated anomalies should be undertaken to assist in identification of any underlying syndrome. Infants with osteogenesis imperfecta show generalized osteomalacia with blue sclera and brittle bones that may fracture during delivery. The calvarium may also demonstrate interspersed islands of palpable bones (wormian bones). The appearance of the fusing anterior fontanelle bone can be confused with a depressed skull fracture in the lateral radiographic projection.[4]

### References

1. Keats TE: *Atlas of normal roentgen variants that may simulate disease,* St Louis, 1992, Mosby, pp 13–15.
2. Aisenson MR: Closing of the anterior fontanelle, *Pediatrics* 6:223–225, 1949.
3. Popich GA, Smith DW: Fontanelles: range of normal size, *J Pediatr* 80:749–752, 1972.
4. Girdany BR, Blank E: Anterior fontanel bones, *Am J Roentgenol Radium Ther Nucl Med* 95:148–153, 1965.

# 38 Parietal Foramina

## GENESIS

Parietal foramina represent defects of calvarial ossification, and they manifest autosomal dominant inheritance with variable expression. They present as symmetric oval defects situated on either side of the sagittal suture and separated from each other by a narrow bridge of bone, and their size decreases with advancing age, although there is considerable intrafamilial variability. Goldsmith initially called this condition "Catlin marks" after observing the condition in 16 members of a five-generation family with the surname Catlin.[1] This condition can present as cranium bifidum in early life and develop into parietal foramina by later childhood. Cranium bifidum means literally "cleft skull," and it presents as a wide opening between the frontal and parietal bones, which normally begin their process of intramembranous ossification in the center of each bone and then spread toward the sutures. During mid-childhood, these areas ossify, leaving only symmetric openings in the frontal and parietal bones.[2] Wilkie et al.[3] described heterozygous MSX2 mutations in three unrelated families with enlarged parietal foramina, which suggests that loss of MSX2 activity results in calvarial defects. A second gene has been implicated in those families who do not link to 5q34-q35 (the location of MSX2), and mutations or deletions of ALX4 on 11p11.2 can also result in parietal foramina.[4,5] Absence or severe hypoplasia of the parietal bones can occur in cleidocranial dysplasia with mutations in RUNX2.[6] Cleidocranial dysplasia consists of large fontanelles, wide sutures, clavicular hypoplasia, supernumerary teeth, and short stature. Parietal foramina occur laterally to the midline and have well-demarcated edges.

## FEATURES

Usually, parietal foramina present as symmetric oval defects situated on each side of the sagittal suture and separated from each other by a narrow bridge of bone, and their size diminishes with age (Fig. 38-1). They are covered with scalp tissue and hair and are detected through palpation and radiography. Occasionally, brain covered by dura and intact scalp can bulge through extensive lesions, suggesting the possibility of an encephalocele, but the location of these lesions off the midline differentiates them from neural tube closure defects. Sometimes the entire sagittal suture remains widely patent from the frontal to the parietal bones (cranium bifidum), with the defect subsequently ossifying inward to resemble parietal foramina during mid-childhood or adulthood.[2] Parietal foramina may occur as an isolated trait due to mutations in or haploinsufficiency of either MSX2 or ALX4,[3-5] or it may be a component of a multiple congenital anomaly syndrome such as Saethre-Chotzen syndrome, cleidocranial dysplasia, or Rubinstein-Taybi syndrome. The combination of parietal foramina with multiple exostoses is now known to be a contiguous gene deletion of ALX4 and EXT2 on chromosome 11p11-p12 (also termed *DEFECT 11 syndrome*).

## MANAGEMENT, PROGNOSIS, AND COUNSEL

Surgery is usually unnecessary because the lesions tend to ossify inward on their own, but, occasionally, a protective helmet is used for extensive defects. Care must be exercised during delivery to avoid trauma to the brain, which underlies such extensive parietal foraminal defects.

## DIFFERENTIAL DIAGNOSIS

Location and intact scalp tissue help differentiate parietal foramina from an encephalocele. In addition, this lesion must be differentiated from scalp vertex aplasia, which is also inherited in an autosomal dominant fashion when it occurs as an isolated trait. There is usually denuded scalp over such lesions, which can include both scalp and calvarium, but their location in the midline near

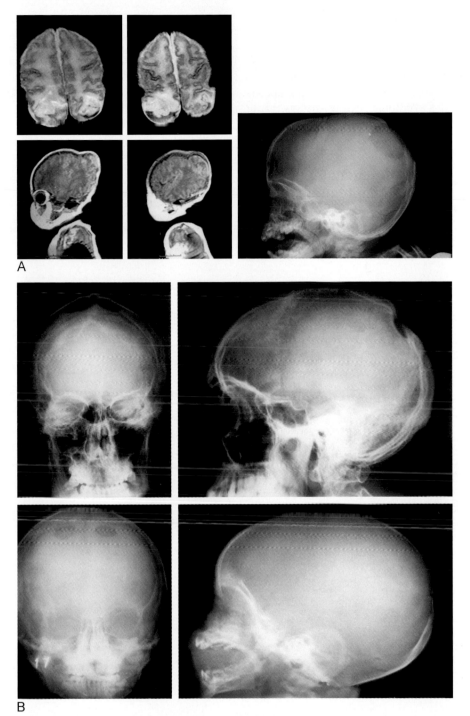

FIGURE 38-1. Familial parietal foramina. **A,** Large parietal defects at birth detected by magnetic resonance imaging *(top and center)*, with partial closure demonstrated by age 16 months on skull radiographs *(bottom)*. **B,** Parietal foramina in other members of this four-generation family with isolated parietal foramina. (Courtesy of Mark Stefan, Madigan Army Hospital, Tacoma, Wash.)

the hair whorl sets these lesions apart from parietal foramina. Scalp vertex cutis aplasia usually heals with some degree of scarring, which results in the absence of scalp hair; therefore, the scalps of both parents should be examined for these bald spots. Occasionally, areas of scalp vertex aplasia can be part of a syndrome such as trisomy 13, or they can result from vascular disruption in utero. When scalp vertex aplasia occurs with absence of digits, the possibility of Adams-Oliver syndrome needs to be considered. Finally, vertex craniotabes may present as an extensive area of incomplete calvarial ossification over the vertex in the midline, but the edges are not sharp and demarcated as in parietal foramina, and vertex craniotabes resolves quite rapidly within the first few months after birth.

## References

1. Goldsmith WM: The 'Catlin mark': the inheritance of an unusual opening in the parietal bones, *J Hered* 13:69–71, 1922.
2. Little BB, Knoll KA, Klein VR, et al: Hereditary cranium bifidum and symmetric parietal foramina are the same entity, *Am J Med Genet* 35:353–358, 1990.
3. Wilkie AOM, Tang Z, Elanko N, et al: Functional haploinsufficiency of the human homeobox gene MSX2 causes defects in skull ossification, *Nat Genet* 24:387–390, 2000.
4. Wu Y-Q, Badano JL, McCaskill C, et al: Haploinsufficiency of ALX4 as a potential cause of parietal foramina in the 11p11.2 contiguous gene-deletion syndrome, *Am J Hum Genet* 67:1327–1332, 2000.
5. Mavrogiannis LA, Antonopoulou I, Baxova A, et al: Haploinsufficiency of the human homeobox gene ALX4 causes skull ossification defects, *Nat Genet* 27:17–18, 2001.
6. Cunningham ML, Seto ML, Hing AV, et al: Cleidocranial dysplasia with severe parietal bone dysplasia: C-terminal RUNX2 mutations, *Birth Defects Res A Clin Mol Teratol* 76:78–85, 2005.

# 39 Aplasia Cutis Congenita

## Scalp Vertex Cutis Aplasia, Temporal Triangular Alopecia

### GENESIS

Aplasia cutis congenita (ACC) is a congenital, localized absence of skin that most commonly affects the scalp. It usually occurs as an isolated finding but can be associated with other abnormalities. ACC begins as multiple or solitary, sharply marginated raw areas with absence of skin (resembling ulceration); these areas mature into atrophic scars devoid of hair, usually in the scalp vertex area or midline superior occipital region.[1] Although most defects are small and superficial, approximately 20% involve absence of the skull, exposing the brain and sagittal sinus and increasing the risk for hemorrhage or infection.[2,3] When associated dura is absent, there is usually no bony regeneration.[3] The cause of these ACC lesions is heterogeneous and includes vascular disruption, trauma, teratogens, and genetic factors.[4] Because vascular disruption and placental infarcts are seen in antiphospholipid antibody syndrome, some cases of extensive ACC may be related to this maternal disease state or other genetic causes of thrombophilia during pregnancy.[5] The frequency of ACC is 1 per 3000 live births, and Frieden's classification system divides ACC into 9 subtypes (Table 39-1 and Figs. 39-1 to 39-7).[6]

### FEATURES

Lesions may be ulcerated, bullous, cicatricial, or covered with a tough, translucent membrane, and, occasionally, they extend to the bone or dura.[1] They may be circular, elongated, stellate, or triangular in shape and of variable depth.[7] Approximately 86% of the solitary lesions occur on the scalp, with most near the parietal hair whorl.[8,9] ACC type 1 manifests scalp involvement without other abnormalities (see Figs. 39-1 and 39-6), and when familial, it manifests autosomal dominant inheritance.[10,11] Less frequently, other parts of the body may be involved, with or without associated defects. When the lesions are midline and overlie the spine or midcranium, they can be associated with occult spinal dysraphism or tiny encephaloceles (ACC type 4). When there are

### TABLE 39-1 FREIDEN'S CLASSIFICATION OF APLASIA CUTIS CONGENITA

| GROUP | DEFINITION | INHERITANCE |
|---|---|---|
| 1 | Isolated scalp involvement; may be associated with single defects | AD |
| 2 | Scalp ACC with limb reduction defects (Adams-Oliver syndrome); may be associated with encephalocele | AD |
| 3 | Scalp ACC with epidermal nevus | Sporadic |
| 4 | ACC overlying occult spinal dysraphism, spina bifida, or meningoencephalocele | Sporadic |
| 5 | ACC with placental infarcts | Sporadic |
| 6 | ACC with epidermolysis bullosa | AD or AR |
| 7 | ACC localized to extremities without blistering; usually affecting pretibial areas and dorsum of hands and feet | AD or AR |
| 8 | ACC caused by teratogens (e.g., varicella, herpes, methimazole) | Sporadic |
| 9 | ACC associated with malformation syndromes (e.g., trisomy 13, deletion 4p-, deletion Xp22.1, ectodermal dysplasia, Johanson-Blizzard syndrome, Adams-Oliver syndrome) | Variable |

ACC, Aplasia cutis congenita; AD, autosomal dominant; AR, autosomal recessive.
From Frieden IJ: Aplasia cutis congenita: a clinical review and proposal for classification, *J Am Acad Dermatol* 14:646–660, 1986.

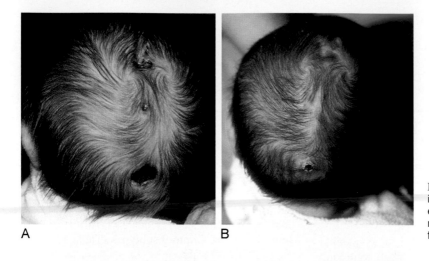

A                              B

FIGURE 39-1. Scalp ACC type 1 in an infant at birth **(A)** and several weeks later **(B)**. There were no associated anomalies, and the father had a similar scalp lesion.

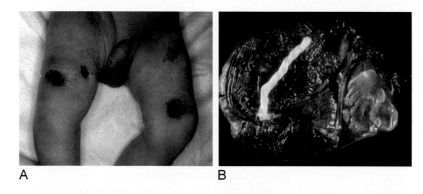

A                              B

FIGURE 39-2. ACC type 5 **(A)** in association with a deceased monozygous fetus papyraceus **(B)**. Note the lesions in the inguinal region and over the knees, which are typical for this type of ACC and should prompt a thorough placental evaluation.

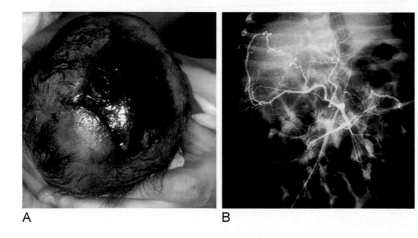

A                              B

FIGURE 39-3. Extensive scalp ACC type 5 **(A)** in association with single umbilical artery and congenital infarction of liver and gallbladder (as demonstrated by angiography) **(B)**. This type of defect should prompt an evaluation for thrombophilia and other types of vascular disruptive defects.

multiple areas of ACC involving primarily the lower extremities, particularly the flank, thighs, and knees, a careful examination of the placenta may reveal a fetus papyraceus, which occurs in 1 in 12,000 live births and affects 1 in 200 twin pregnancies (see Fig. 39-2).[12-14] Larger defects can present with complications such as hemorrhage, venous thrombosis, and (rarely) meningitis (see Fig. 39-3). With extensive ACC and other vascular disruptive defects, survival in the neonatal period can be severely compromised.[15,16] ACC can be associated with teratogenic or genetic disorders (see Figs. 39-4 to 39-7), and it is important to search for associated malformations in order to counsel

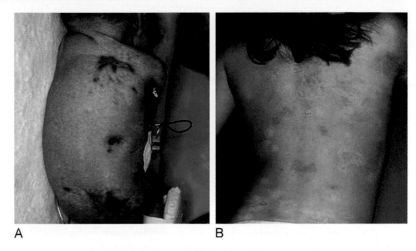

FIGURE 39-4. ACC type 8 in association with congenital herpes simplex infection. **A,** Appearance at birth. **B,** Appearance several years later, after lesions healed with scarring.

A                                B

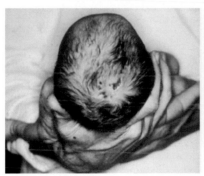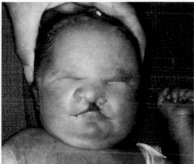

FIGURE 39-5. ACC type 9 in association with trisomy 13.

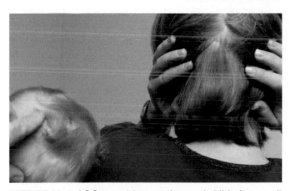

FIGURE 39-6. ACC type 1 in a mother and child after small lesions (<1 cm in diameter) healed spontaneously.

parents concerning prognosis and recurrence risks in relation to the underlying disorder. ACC associated with epidermal nevus or nevus sebaceous syndrome (or ACC type 3) is the association of a sebaceous nevus (a linear, yellow verrucose nevus) on the head and neck with variable ocular, cerebral, neurologic, skeletal, cardiac, and other abnormalities, usually occurring sporadically.[17,18]

*Epidermolysis bullosa* (EB) is a term applied to a group of hereditary skin disorders that result in the formation of blisters after minor skin trauma. The three subtypes are based on the histopathologic location of the bullae: (1) dystrophic EB with sub-epidermal bullae below the periodic acid-Schiff (PAS)–staining basement membrane, (2) junctional EB with subepidermal bullae above the PAS-staining membrane, and (3) simplex EB with intraepidermal bullae in the suprabasal area.[19] Dystrophic and simplex EB can be either autosomal recessive or dominant, but junctional EB is always autosomal recessive. EB can be associated with pyloric atresia and/or ACC and manifest autosomal recessive inheritance, and histopathology is usually of the junctional type.[19] These findings suggest that when ACC occurs with EB, it is most likely to be autosomal recessive, and some cases of junctional EB with pyloric atresia have demonstrated mutations in integrin beta 4.[19] Finally, ACC has been associated with numerous cytogenetic and genetic malformation syndromes, some of which are listed in Table 39-1 under ACC type 9 (see Fig. 39-5 and 39-7).[4,11,20-23]

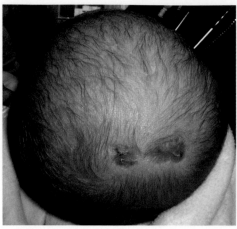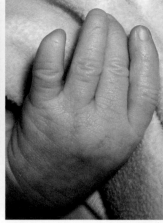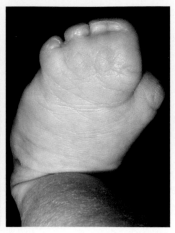

FIGURE 39-7. Adams-Oliver syndrome showing typical scalp ACC associated with digital hypoplasia/syndactyly in a hand and foot.

(From Verdyck P, Holder-Espinasse M, Van Hul W, et al: Clinical and molecular analysis of nine families with Adams-Oliver syndrome, *Eur J Hum Genet* 11:457–463, 2003.)

## MANAGEMENT, PROGNOSIS, AND COUNSEL

Wound treatment in 1-cm lesions with superficial ulceration is conservative with application of antibacterial dressings, but more extensive or deep lesions may require reconstruction of the scalp. Small hairless areas can be excised and covered with a neighboring flap from the scalp.[24] This approach works for most common scalp ACC type 1 lesions, which are most frequently round, punched-out lesions in the vertex region or, less frequently, triangular lesions in the temporal region (termed *temporal triangular alopecia*).[24,25] With extensive scalp lesions (i.e., >6 cm in diameter), it is especially important to avoid eschar formation immediately after birth by covering exposed dura with split-thickness skin grafts from adjacent healthy scalp and with moist dressings. Prompt closure is important because of the high risk of fatal hemorrhage from the sagittal sinus when the eschar becomes dry and separated, which causes the underlying dura to become damaged and tear.[3,16,26] Once the superficial defect is completely healed, the subsequent scar alopecia can be treated by tissue-expanded local flaps, pericranial flaps, or free vascularized flaps when the child is older. Also, with prompt and early closure and healthy underlying dura, cranial bone growth will occur, and the risk of fatal hemorrhage or meningitis is greatly lessened.[3,16,26] For the treatment of extensive scalp defects, some surgeons have used engineered skin consisting of an initial graft of autologous cultured fibroblasts (that lay down type IV collagen, fibronectin, and laminin), followed by a graft of cultured keratinocytes.[27] The combination of dermal and epithelial characteristics in such grafts is thought to reduce scar formation. Patients with Adams-Oliver syndrome may require extra care with split-thickness skin grafts because of abnormal vascularity in the scalp skin.[22] This syndrome is inherited in a markedly variable autosomal dominant fashion and often results in associated dural and scull defects, but, unlike parietal foramina, there have been no mutations in ALX4 or MSX2.[28] When there are extensive associated dural defects (as may occur in Adams-Oliver syndrome of ACC, type 5), autologous full-thickness cranial bone grafts may be required to close the skull defects prior to skin grafting.[3]

## DIFFERENTIAL DIAGNOSIS

Differential diagnosis is extensive and includes the initial distinction between ACC and occult spina bifida or meningoencephalocele and the determination of whether ACC is isolated or part of a broader pattern of altered morphogenesis, as delineated in Table 39-1.

### References

1. Tann HH, Tay YK: Familial aplasia cutis congenita of the scalp: a case report and review, *Ann Acad Med Singapore* 26:500–502, 1997.
2. Nichols DD, Bottini AG: Aplasia cutis congenital: case report, *J Neurosurg* 85:170–173, 1996.

3. Ploplys EA, Muzaffar AR, Gruss JS, et al: Early composite cranioplasty in infants with severe aplasia cutis congenital: a report of two cases, *Cleft Palate Craniofac J* 42: 642–647, 2005.

4. Evers ME, Steijlen PM, Hamel BC: Aplasia cutis congenita and associated disorders: an update, *Clin Genet* 47: 295–310, 1995.

5. Roll C, Hanssler L, Voit T, et al: Aplasia cutis congenita—etiological relationship to antiphospholipid syndrome? *Clin Dysmorphol* 8:215–217, 1999.

6. Frieden IJ: Aplasia cutis congenita: a clinical review and proposal for classification, *J Am Acad Dermatol* 14: 646–660, 1986.

7. Rudolph RJ, Schwartz W, Leyden JJ: Bitemporal aplasia cutis congenital, *Arch Dermatol* 110:615–618, 1974.

8. Demmel U: Clinical aspects of congenital skin defects: I. Congenital skin defects of the head of the newborn. II. Congenital defects of the trunk and extremities of the newborn. III. Causal and formal genesis of congenital skin defects of the newborn, *Eur J Pediatr* 121:21–50, 1975.

9. Stephan MJ, Smith DW, Ponzi JW: Origin of scalp vertex aplasia cutis, *J Pediatr* 101:850–853, 1982.

10. Itin P, Pletscher M: Familial aplasia cutis congenita of the scalp without other defects in 6 members of three successive generations, *Dermatologica* 177:123–125, 1988.

11. Fimiani M, Seri M, Rubegni P, et al: Autosomal dominant aplasia cutis congenita: report of a large Italian family and no hint for candidate chromosomal regions, *Arch Dermatol Res* 291:637–642, 1999.

12. Mannino FL, Jones KL, Benirschke K: Congenital skin defects and fetus papyraceus, *J Pediatr* 91:559–564, 1977.

13. Daw E: Fetus papyraceus—11 cases, *Postgrad Med J* 59:598–600, 1983.

14. Leaute-Labreze C, Depaire-Duclos F, Sarlangue J, et al: Congenital cutaneous defects as complications in surviving co-twins: aplasia cutis congenita and neonatal Volkmann ischemic contracture of the forearm, *Arch Dermatol* 143:1121–1124, 1998.

15. Lane W, Zanol K: Duodenal atresia, biliary atresia, and intestinal infarct in truncal aplasia cutis congenita, *Ped Dermatol* 17:290–292, 2000.

16. Kantor J, Yan AC, Hivnor CM, et al: Extensive aplasia cutis congenital and the risk of sagittal sinus thrombosis, *Arch Dermatol* 141:554–556, 2005.

17. Hogler W, Sidoroff A, Weber F, et al: Aplasia cutis congenita, uvula bifida, and bilateral retinal dystrophy in a girl with naevus sebaceous syndrome, *Brit J Dermatol* 140:542–543, 1999.

18. Shields JA, Shields CL, Eagle RC, et al: Ocular manifestation of the organoid nevus syndrome, *Ophthalmology* 104:549–557, 1997.

19. Maman E, Maor E, Kachko L, et al: Epidermolysis bullosa, pyloric atresia, aplasia cutis congenita: histopathological definition of an autosomal recessive disease, *Am J Med Genet* 78:127–133, 1998.

20. Zvulunov A, Kachko L, Manor E, et al: Reticulolinear aplasia cutis congenita of the face and neck: a distinctive cutaneous manifestation in several syndromes linked to Xp22, *Br J Dermatol* 138:1046–1052, 1998.

21. Edwards MJ, McDonald D, Moore P, et al: Scalp-ear-nipple syndrome: additional manifestations, *Am J Med Genet* 50:247–250, 1994.

22. Beekmans SJA, Wiebe MJ: Surgical treatment of the Adams-Oliver syndrome, *J Craniofac Surg* 12:569–572, 2001.

23. Verdyck P, Holder-Espinasse M, Van Hul W, et al: Clinical and molecular analysis of nine families with Adams-Oliver syndrome, *Eur J Hum Genet* 11:457–463, 2003.

24. Kruk-Jeromin J, Janik J, Rykala J: Aplasia cutis congenita of the scalp: report of 16 cases, *Dermatol Surg* 24: 549–553, 1998.

25. Trakimas C, Sperling LC, Skelton HG, et al: Clinical and histologic findings in temporal triangular alopecia, *J Am Acad Dermatol* 31:205–209, 1994.

26. Yang JY, Yang WG: Large scalp and skull defect in aplasia cutis congenital, *Br J Plast Surg* 53:619–622, 2000.

27. Donati V, Arena S, Capilli G, et al: Reparation of a severe case of aplasia cutis congenital with engineered skin, *Biol Neonate* 80:273–276, 2001.

28. Verdyck P, Holder-Espinasse M, Van Hul W, et al: Clinical and molecular analysis of nine families with Adams-Oliver syndrome, *Eur J Hum Genet* 11:457–463, 2003.

# 40 Cephalohematoma

## GENESIS

Cephalohematoma is a subperiosteal extracranial hemorrhage that may enlarge after delivery, sometimes taking weeks to resolve. This condition contrasts with the scalp edema of caput succedaneum, which reaches its maximal size at birth and usually resolves within a few days. Both lesions are believed to result from an injury to the cranial periosteum during labor or during a traumatic delivery, but they have also been detected as echogenic bulges on the cranium during prenatal ultrasound evaluations, which suggests that they can also arise in utero. Among 16,292 fetuses undergoing comprehensive ultrasound examinations between 1993 and 1996, 7 cephalohematomas were detected on exams performed between 23 and 38 weeks of gestation (5 occipital and 2 temporal). A diagnosis of cephalohematoma was confirmed by the neonatologist in 2 cases, and caput succedaneum was diagnosed in the remaining 5 cases. It was not possible to distinguish between cephalohematoma and caput succedaneum prenatally. None of these affected neonates were delivered by vacuum extraction or forceps or had any signs of intracranial hemorrhage or skull fracture by ultrasound, and none required any treatment. Five of these 7 cases had associated premature rupture of membranes, with oligohydramnios noted in 4 cases, suggesting oligohydramnios might have played a role.[1]

Cephalohematoma, subdural hematoma, and caput succedaneum have all been found more frequently in infants delivered by vacuum extraction than in infants delivered spontaneously.[2,3] Cephalohematoma occurs in 1% to 2% of spontaneous deliveries compared with 4% of vacuum or forceps deliveries.[4] In a prospective randomized trial of 322 cases involving continuous versus intermittent vacuum extractions, cephalohematomas were associated with the station of the presenting part, asynclitism, and increasing application-to-delivery time. None of the infants with cephalohematomas experienced any long-term complications or needed blood transfusions,[5] but fetal death and stillbirth have been reported after prenatal diagnosis of a fetal subdural hematoma following suspected or confirmed trauma.[6–9] Thus, cephalohematomas can occur prior to the onset of labor, especially with premature rupture of membranes and prolonged oligohydramnios. Maternal abdominal trauma can result in more serious subdural hematomas that can be seen by prenatal ultrasound, and this type of intracranial hemorrhage may threaten fetal survival.

Because vacuum extraction has been associated with cephalohematomas, there are concerns about whether this mode of delivery may result in more serious intracranial vascular injuries (subdural, cerebral, intraventricular, or subarachnoid hemorrhages). Among 583,340 live-born singleton infants weighing 2500 to 4000 g who were born to nulliparous women between 1992 and 1994 in California, the rate of intracranial hemorrhage was significantly higher among infants delivered by vacuum extraction, forceps, or cesarean section during labor than among infants delivered spontaneously.[10] There was an incremental increase in the rate of hemorrhage if more than one method of delivery was used. Because the rate of hemorrhage was not significantly higher among infants delivered by cesarean section before labor, much of the morbidity associated with operative vaginal delivery is thought to be due to an underlying abnormality of labor rather than the specific operative procedure. The rate of intracranial hemorrhage has decreased threefold (to less than 1%) following the substitution of plastic cups for metal cups in vacuum extractors during the 1980s.[10]

Most cephalohematomas are caused by birth trauma, and documented risk factors include fetal scalp monitors, instrumentation, and increased birth weight.[11] The mechanism of injury is related to forces that lift the scalp and pericranium off the underlying bone, thus shearing vessels and causing blood to collect in this potential space.[12] Most cephalohematomas resolve spontaneously during the first few weeks after birth, depending on their size. Complications can include an underlying skull fracture, anemia, hyperbilirubinemia, calcification, or (rarely) infection of the hematoma.

# FEATURES

Traumatic subperiosteal hemorrhages occur most frequently in the outer table of the parietal bone, giving rise to a soft fluctuant mass (Fig. 40-1). Thus, cephalohematomas occur beneath the periosteum, with no extension over a sutural margin, and definite palpable edges are usually evident. Collections of blood within the superficial subcutaneous tissues are termed *caput succedaneum*. Cephalohematomas may become apparent or enlarge after delivery, sometimes taking weeks to resolve, whereas the edema of caput succedaneum usually reaches maximal size at birth and resolves within a few days, even when it is extensive in size. Subgaleal hematomas are located between the galea aponeurotica and pericranium, and, because they are not restricted to the periosteal boundaries within cranial sutures, they can expand rapidly to involve the entire scalp and cause life-threatening volume loss, whereas cephalohematomas tend to remain localized.[11] Most cephalohematomas resorb within the first week, and if the clot has not resorbed by the fourth week, the clot may form fibrous tissue, with calcification beginning at the periphery of the hematoma.[12] With time the borders of a cephalohematoma may become elevated and craterlike as the raised periosteum begins to deposit bone at its borders. Calcified cephalohematomas usually resolve slowly over the next few years during the normal process of cranial bone remodeling with calvarial growth, but some lesions may persist and require further management (Figs. 40-2 and 40-3).

# MANAGEMENT AND PROGNOSIS

Cephalohematomas are benign lesions that begin as soft fluctuant masses within the periosteum of the parietal bones. Parents should be reassured that most cephalohematomas resolve during the first month of postnatal life. In rare cases, extensive cephalohematomas may slowly calcify during the first year of life. Rarely, cephalohematomas can become infected, usually in the setting of a predisposing factor such as trauma or a systemic infection that results in sepsis or meningitis.[13-15] An increase in the size of the cephalohematoma after 48 hours, failure to resorb, or signs of an infected wound (an enlarging, fluctuant, erythematous lesion with demineralization of the underlying bone) should prompt incision and drainage with culture for identification of the infectious agent. The most common organism (in about half the cases) is *Escherichia coli*, but a wide variety of other organisms have been reported, and it is important to determine the type of organism and its sensitivities to antibiotics. Early-onset infection of cephalohematoma occurs within the first 2 weeks, usually due to bacteremic seeding from a systemic infection; delay in diagnosis or drainage can prove fatal. Late-onset cases occur after 3 weeks and are usually associated with cellulitis over the lesion and osteomyelitis in the underlying bone. In both early- and late-onset cases, the mainstay of treatment is incision and drainage with long-term antibiotic treatment, especially when osteomyelitis is present.[14-16] If an extensive

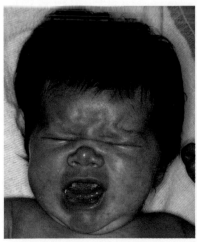
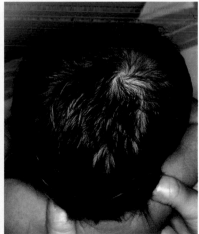

FIGURE 40-1. Right facial droop from traumatic right lower facial palsy with associated traumatic right parietal cephalohematoma. These lesions occur most frequently in the right superior parietal region.

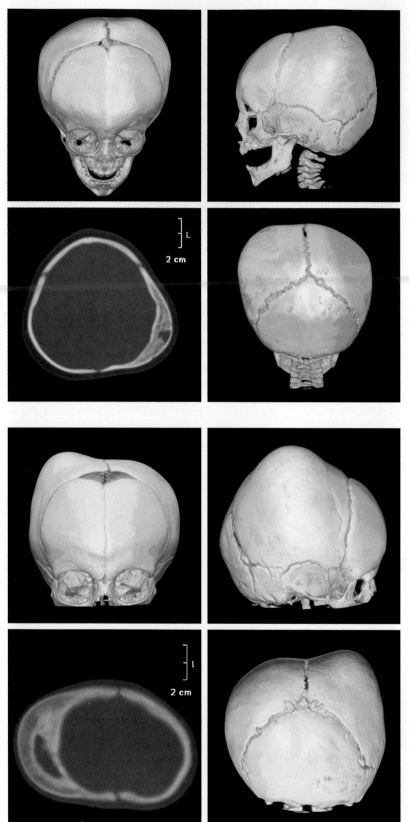

FIGURE 40-2. Persistent left calcified cephalohematoma at age 7 months, shown by three-dimensional computed tomography scan with a cross-sectional image through the lesion.

(Courtesy of Dr. Michael Cunningham and Darcy King, Division of Craniofacial Medicine, Department of Pediatrics, University of Washington Medical School, Seattle, Wash.)

FIGURE 40-3. Persistent right calcified cephalohematoma at age 11 months, shown by three-dimensional computed tomography scan with a cross-sectional image through the lesion. This lesion was surgically reconstructed.

(Courtesy of Dr. Michael Cunningham and Darcy King, Division of Craniofacial Medicine, Department of Pediatrics, University of Washington Medical School, Seattle, Wash.)

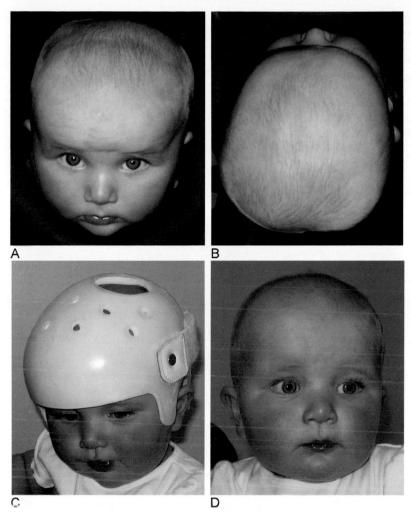

FIGURE 40-4. **A,** This girl was seen at 6 months with torticollis-plagiocephaly deformation sequence resulting in right occipital flattening and a 1.2-cm diagonal difference. After a vacuum-suction delivery, she had a 4 × 6-cm calcified cephalohematoma in the right superior parietal bone, which did not change in size for 5 months after birth. **B,** When viewed from above, the calcified cephalohematoma obscured the view of her occipital flattening, which was sufficient to merit orthotic therapy. She wore a cranial orthotic with an off-centered opening in the top **(C)** so as to apply pressure to the calcified cephalohematoma, which resolved over the next 4 months, as did the plagiocephaly **(D).**

cephalohematoma fails to resorb after 1 month, some clinicians advocate aspiration of the lesion to prevent formation of fibrous tissue and calcification. This should only be done using sterile technique with variation in the needle trajectory to prevent formation of a straight tract through which hematoma fluid can leak or infection can be introduced.[16] In two infants with extensive calcified cephalohematomas evident at ages 3 to 4 months, the use of a cranial orthotic led to prompt resolution of the lesion during the next 3 to 5 months (Fig. 40-4).[11]

## DIFFERENTIAL DIAGNOSIS

At the cranial vertex, edema of the skin and subcutaneous tissues may occur, the so-called *caput succedaneum.* Caput succedaneum can cross suture lines and is maximal in size at birth; it resolves in just a few days. The subperiosteal hemorrhage associated with a cephalohematoma may manifest a subsequent "crater rim" of bone at its outer borders, which sometimes gives the impression of a depressed skull fracture, but a cephalohematoma is a benign lesion. Epidural hematoma is extremely rare in the neonate and usually due to postnatal head trauma resulting from a fall and skull fracture; however, it can also be associated with an overlying cephalohematoma. When a skull fracture is suspected beneath a cephalohematoma, a computed tomography scan will clarify the clinical picture, and a craniotomy can be performed to relieve pressure on the brain through the prompt evacuation of the epidural hematoma that may result from tearing of a meningeal artery or venous bleeding.[17]

## References

1. Petrikovsky BM, Schneider E, Smith-Levitin M, et al: Cephalohematoma and caput succedaneum: do they always occur in labor? *Am J Obstet Gynecol* 179:906–908, 1998.
2. Fall O, Ryden G, Finnstrom K, et al: Forceps or vacuum extraction? A comparison of effects on the newborn infants, *Acta Obstet Gynecol Scand* 65:75–80, 1986.
3. Teng FY, Sayre JW: Vacuum extraction: does duration predict scalp injury? *Obstet Gynecol* 89:281–285, 1997.
4. Broekhuizen FF, Washington JM, Johnson F: Vacuum extraction versus forceps delivery: indications and complications, 1979–1984, *Obstet Gynecol* 69:338–342, 1987.
5. Bofill JA, Rust OA, Devidas M, et al: Neonatal cephalohematoma from vacuum extraction, *J Reprod Med* 42:565–569, 1997.
6. Demir RH, Gleisher N, Myers S: A traumatic antepartum subdural hematoma causing fetal death, *Am J Obstet Gynecol* 160:619–620, 1989.
7. Gunn TR, Becroft DMO: Unexplained intracranial haemorrhage in utero: the battered fetus? *Aust N Z J Obstet Gynaecol* 24:17–22, 1984.
8. Winter TC, Mack LA, Cyr DR: Prenatal sonographic diagnosis of scalp edema/cephalohematoma mimicking an encephalohematoma mimicking an encephalocele, *Am J Roentgenol* 161:1247–1248, 1993.
9. Grylack L: Prenatal sonographic diagnosis of cephalohematoma due to pre-labor trauma, *Pediatr Radiol* 12:145–147, 1982.
10. Towner D, Castro MA, Eby-Wilkens E, et al: Effect of mode of delivery in nulliparous women on neonatal intracranial injury, *N Engl J Med* 341:1709–1714, 1999.
11. Petersen JD, Becker DV, Fundakowski CE, et al: A novel management for calcifying cephalohematoma, *Plast Reconstr Surg* 113:1404–1409, 2004.
12. Kaufman HH, Hochberg J, Anderson RP, et al: Treatment of calcified cephalohematoma, *Neurosurgery* 32:1037–1040, 1993.
13. Kao HC, Huang YC, Lin TY: Infected cephalohematoma associated with sepsis and skull osteomyelitis: report of one case, *Am J Perinatol* 16:459–462, 1999.
14. Goodwin MD, Persing JA, Duncan CC, et al: Spontaneously infected cephalohematoma: case report and review of the literature, *J Craniofac Surg* 11:371–375, 2000.
15. Dahl KM, Barry J, DeBlesi RL: *Escherichia hermannii* infection of a cephalohematoma: case report, review of the literature, and description of a novel invasive pathogen, *Clin Infect Dis* 35:e96–e98, 2002.
16. Firlik KS, Adelon PD: Large chronic cephalohematoma without calcification, *Pediatr Neurosurg* 30:39–42, 1999.
17. Lieu AS, Sun ZM, Howng SL: Bilateral epidural hematoma in a neonate, *Kaohsiung J Med Sci* 12:434–436, 1996.

# 41 Wormian Bones

## GENESIS

Wormian bones are accessory bones that occur within cranial suture lines, and, although they do not cause any impairment themselves, their significance is variable. In one study, the majority of children with an "excessive" number of wormian bones had some abnormality of the central nervous system.[1] Reported abnormalities ranged from gross malformations to minimal brain dysfunction, although this study may have been biased because it used a hospital-based population. Thus, some individuals with many wormian bones may have other anomalies and/or central nervous system dysfunction. The name *wormian bones* is derived from a Danish anatomist named Olaus Worm who described these small irregular ossicles located within cranial sutures in a letter to Thomas Bartholin in 1643.[1,2] They occur most commonly in the lambdoid sutures and within fontanelles, and the pathogenesis of wormian bones is thought to be related to variations in dural growth stretch along open sutures and within fontanelles, causing ossification defects. Such sutural bones persist and are not incorporated into the adjacent bone during mineralization and maturation. Although the prevalence of wormian bones in the general population varies from 8% to 15%, the true prevalence is around 14%.[1,2] Males are more often affected than females, and differences among ethnic groups have been noted, with the highest incidence in Chinese individuals (80%).[2] Ethnic variation in wormian bones may suggest a possible genetic influence, but environmental influences could also play a role.

A positive correlation has been noted between the frequency of lambdoid wormian bones and the degree of deformation observed in primitive cultures that practice frontooccipital head binding, which suggests that these bones form in relation to changes in pressure along the lambdoid sutures.[3,4] Note that the term "Inca bone" was initially used as a synonym for *wormian bones* in deformed Peruvian skulls, which were mistakenly considered to be a racial trait.[2] In rabbits with premature coronal synostosis, wormian bones appeared in the coronal and sagittal sutures after the onset of cranial growth alterations induced by premature coronal synostosis, which suggests that wormian bones form in relation to external factors.[5] Nondeformed crania have more wormian bones than circumferentially deformed crania but have fewer wormian bones than anteroposteriorly deformed crania.[6] This may relate to variations in tension across the sutures, a hypothesis tested by O'Loughlin, who demonstrated that the frequency and location of wormian bones vary depending on the type and degree of cranial deformation, with posteriorly placed wormian bones appearing in greater numbers in deformed crania and with sagittal synostosis.[7] The increased frequency of wormian bones noted in Chinese infants might be related to their traditional supine infant sleeping position and the resultant pressure against their occiput. If so, an increased frequency of wormian bones may soon be noted in other cultures that have adopted the supine sleep positioning to prevent sudden infant death syndrome (SIDS), and it might be expected that more wormian bones will be associated with a higher cephalic index.

## FEATURES

Wormian bones are accessory bones that occur within cranial suture lines or fontanelles.[1,2] They occur singly or in large numbers and are diagnosed radiographically. They appear as intramembranous ossifications, and, in the fetus, they are composed of a single layer of compact bone on the dural side.[3] Although they can occur within any suture, they are rare in coronal or sagittal sutures and appear most frequently in the lambdoid sutures and other posterior sutures. Wormian bones are usually normal variants that can be detected prenatally. Given the large number of associated syndromes for which they are an associated finding, the prenatal detection of wormian bones should prompt a search for other associated anomalies involving the brain and for metabolic abnormalities affecting skull ossification.[3,9]

## MANAGEMENT AND PROGNOSIS

Wormian bones require no management other than the recognition of their significance as possibly being associated with an underlying disorder that may require diagnosis and management.[8] Wormian bones are commonly seen in osteogenesis imperfecta (Fig. 41-1) and other disorders that result in defective cranial bone mineralization, such as cleidocranial dysplasia (Fig. 41-2), hypophosphatasia, pycnodysostosis, Hajdu-Cheney syndrome (Fig. 41-3), and Grant syndrome. Such infants also become quite brachycephalic as a consequence of occipital pressure from postnatal supine positioning with soft cranial bones, which may increase the propensity to form wormian bones.[9] Wormian bone are also associated with premature aging disorders such as progeria, acrogeria, and mandibular dysplasia, as well as with Menkes' syndrome.

## DIFFERENTIAL DIAGNOSIS

Wormian bones could be mistaken for a skull fracture, but experienced radiographic interpretation should resolve this error.

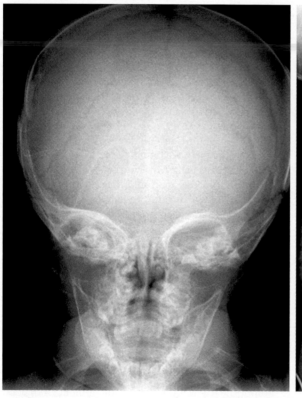
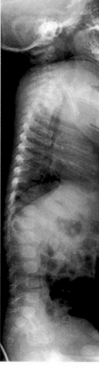

FIGURE 41-1. This child with osteogenesis type IV due to defective collagen type 1 has marked osteopenia of the skull and spine with multiple wormian bones, as well as a history of multiple fractures with minimal trauma.

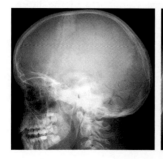
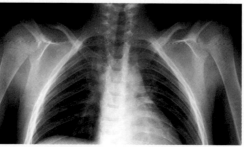

FIGURE 41-2. This child with cleidocranial dysplasia has multiple wormian bones and clavicular hypoplasia, with delayed eruption of teeth and delayed closure of the anterior fontanelle due to a mutation in CBFA1 (RUNX2).

# 42 Breech Presentation Deformation

## GENESIS

The frequency of singleton breech presentation at term is 3.1% and rises to 6.2% when multiple births are included.[1, 4] Breech presentation is an important cause of deformation, and fully one third of all deformations occur in babies who have been in breech presentation (Fig. 42-1).[2] Because 2% of newborns have deformations, this indicates that 0.6% of neonates have one or more deformations due to breech presentation; therefore, this topic will be given extensive coverage. Among infants born with deformations, 32% were in breech presentation (versus 5% to 6% of normally formed infants), and 23% of malformed infants were also in breech presentation.[3] Among 142 infants with spina bifida, 38% were in breech presentation, and 68% of these infants had lower-extremity weakness or paralysis. Among those infants with paralyzed legs, 93% manifested breech presentation; thus, breech presentation becomes more likely with fetal inability to power the legs.[4] Numerous fetal and maternal factors can lead to breech presentation and thereby increase the risk for adverse outcomes. Some of these factors include prematurity (25% breech), twinning (34% breech), oligohydramnios due to chronic leakage (64% breech), uterine malformations, placenta previa, maternal hypertension, and fetal malformations.

Breech presentation is more common in the primigravida, especially the older primigravida, presumably because of the shape of the uterus and the reduced space for fetal and uterine growth. The spatial restrictions associated with twinning also increase the likelihood of breech presentation, especially for the second-born. The prematurely born baby is also less likely to have shifted into the vertex birth position, and prematurity is more common with multiple births. Unless there is oligohydramnios or twinning, the premature fetus in breech presentation generally does not have associated deformations because there has not been sufficient constraint to cause molding. Furthermore, breech presentation can be considered normal with prematurity because at 32 weeks of gestation, 25% of all fetuses are

in breech presentation; after this time, the majority of fetuses shift into vertex presentation.[3] Any situation that causes oligohydramnios, whether it be chronic leakage of amniotic fluid or lack of urine flow into the amniotic space, will restrict movement and greatly increase the chance of the fetus being in breech presentation. Alterations in the size and shape of the uterine cavity may also increase the frequency of breech presentation. This may be secondary to uterine structural anomalies or myomas. The implantation and placement of the placenta may also be a factor, as 66% of placentas in breech delivery implant in the cornual-fundal region (versus 4% of vertex presentations), whereas in 76% of vertex presentations, the placenta implants on the midwall of the uterus (versus 4% of breech presentations).[3]

Although the best mode of delivery for infants in breech presentation is controversial, most studies suggest that the risk for neonatal morbidity and mortality is increased when infants in breech presentation are delivered vaginally as opposed

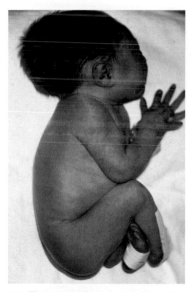

FIGURE 42-1. This term infant was delivered from a complete breech presentation and is shown in her position of comfort with a breech head, prominent occipital shelf, and equinovarus foot deformations.

to via cesarean section.[3,5-8] Traumatic injuries following vaginal delivery of breech infants can include fractures and dislocations, brachial plexus injuries, facial nerve injuries, cerebral hemorrhages, bruising with hyperbilirubinemia, cervical cord injuries, cord prolapse, birth asphyxia, and testicular trauma.[2-5] In most large series, these types of injuries occur less frequently with cesarean delivery, but in some recent series using modern delivery methods, the rate of such injuries is similar in planned vaginal breech delivery compared with elective cesarean section. This has led some authors to suggest that with a normal pelvis and normal term birth weight, assisted vaginal breech delivery by an experienced obstetrician may be as safe as cesarean section delivery, which increases the risk of maternal morbidity in most large studies.[9-11] Because of the risk of cervical cord injuries with vaginal delivery, most studies have relegated breech infants with hyperextended heads for automatic cesarean section.[5] Trials of vaginal delivery have succeeded in 60% to 70% of patients, without significant differences in outcome measures for primiparas versus multiparas or for frank versus non-frank breech presentations.[9,11] In North America, 70% to 80% of all women with breech presentation deliver by cesarean section (with similar trends observed in other parts of the world), so obstetric resident training experience with vaginal breech deliveries may be insufficient to guarantee sufficient expertise.[12]

Breech presentation shows a familial tendency, and 22% of multiparous women delivering a breech infant had previously experienced a breech delivery.[4] If the first infant in a family is breech-born, there is a 9.4% chance the second child will be breech-born; whereas if the first child is vertex, there is only a 2.4% chance the second will be breech (this being the background risk for breech delivery).[13] Women with recurring breech presentation have a lower risk of adverse perinatal outcome, possibly due to increased attention to perinatal care.[8] The familial tendency toward breech deliveries may be related to inherited uterine structural characteristics, or it may be a consequence of a genetic neuromuscular or fetal malformation syndrome such as myotonic dystrophy. Presumably, the lower risk of adverse perinatal outcome relates to detection of maternal anatomic abnormalities (or fetal genetic abnormalities) that might result in closer follow-up during subsequent pregnancies.

In about 70% of fetuses in breech presentation, the legs are extended in front of the abdomen (Fig. 42-2).[4] Once the movements of the fetus

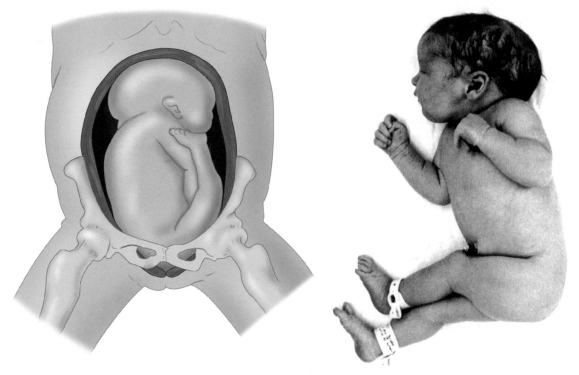

FIGURE 42-2. Frank breech presentation in a term infant. Note his extended legs with flexed thighs and shoulders thrust up beneath the occipital shelf in his position of comfort.

become limited by extension of the legs in front of the abdomen, the fetus has less chance of extricating itself from the breech presentation,[13] and Dunn has used the analogy of the "folding body press" wrestling hold.[4] Once a wrestler has an opponent in a position with the legs in front of the abdomen, there is little the opponent can do to escape. Breech presentation with the hips flexed and knees extended is termed *frank breech* (see Figs. 42-2 and 42-3, *A* and *D*). When the hips and knees are flexed, it is called *complete breech* (Fig. 42-3, *C*), and when the hips and knees are extended, it is referred to as to *the footling breech*, as depicted in Fig. 42-3, *B*. With modern methods of delivery, the particular type of breech presentation appears to have no significant effect on adverse outcomes associated with the mode of delivery, despite that cord prolapse occurs much less frequently with frank breech presentation (0.4%) versus complete breech (4%–10.5%) or footling breech presentation (15%–28.5%).[11]

## FEATURES

Prolonged breech position in late fetal life gives rise to increased uterine fundal pressure and molding of the fetal head, which may become retroflexed. This type of constraint results in anteroposterior elongation of the head (dolichocephaly) with a prominent occipital shelf, the so-called "breech head" (Fig. 42-4).[14] The shoulders are often thrust under the lower auricle, and the mandible may be distorted. The legs may be caught in front of the fetus, which tends to dislocate the hips and, occasionally, causes genu recurvatum of the knee and often calcaneovalgus position of the feet. In the frank breech position, with the legs flexed across the abdomen, the feet are likely to be compressed into a calcaneovalgus position, whereas in the complete breech position with the knees flexed, equinovarus foot deformation may develop. The genital region, as the presenting part, may be molded and edematous (Fig. 42-5). Dunn noted that 32% of all deformations in the neonate were related to breech presentation.[1] In his series of more than 6000 babies, 100% of genu recurvatum cases related to breech presentation, as did 50% of hip dislocation cases and 20% to 25% each for cases of mandibular asymmetry, torticollis, and talipes equinovarus (Fig. 42-6). Traction to the brachial plexus or phrenic nerve during difficult deliveries or vaginal breech deliveries may occur, and 75% of cases of diaphragmatic paralysis caused by birth injury have associated brachial plexus palsy.[15-18]

## Craniofacial

The head is elongated into a dolichocephalic form, often with a prominent occipital shelf. There may be redundant folds of skin in the posterior neck as a result of compression due to retroflexion of the head (Fig. 42-7). The lambdoid sutures may appear to be overlapping because of the fetal head constraint. The lower auricle may be forced upward into the location where the shoulder has been, and the manubrial region of the mandible may have a "hollow" appearance. The shoulder compression is often asymmetric; hence, there may be asymmetry of the mandible with an upward "tilt" on the more compressed side. Torticollis may occur secondary to asymmetric stretching or frank tearing of the sternocleidomastoid muscle or due to clavicular fracture during a traumatic breech vaginal delivery, and 20% of torticollis cases occur in babies who were in breech presentation.[2,3] A study of 224 term infants in breech presentation compared with 3107 term infants in vertex presentation revealed the following anomalies to be associated with breech presentation: frontal bossing, prominent occiput, upward-slanting palpebral fissures, low-set ears, torticollis, and congenital hip dislocation.[19] Dolichocephaly was confirmed by caliper measurements on 100 term infants in breech presentation and compared with 100 term infants in vertex presentation. Third-trimester biparietal diameters were smaller than expected in the breech infants, and the birth cephalic index was less than 76%.[20]

## Limbs

All gradations of hip dislocation occur in breech presentation, which is considered to be the consequence of the constrained position in utero forcing the hip from its usual socket. The legs have generally been hyperflexed in front of the fetus, and this is often the "position of comfort" in the early neonatal period (see Figs. 42-2 and 42-3). As a consequence, it may be difficult to fully extend and abduct the hips into the position that is usually used to detect dislocation of the hips. Full movement at the knees may also be somewhat limited. Frank breech presentation is the most common cause of genu recurvatum. The extended leg position may lead to calcaneovalgus foot deformity, whereas the flexed leg position more commonly leads to an equinovarus foot deformity. Traction to the brachial plexus, especially the upper plexus, occurs during delivery when the angle between the neck and shoulder is suddenly and forcibly increased with the arms in an adducted position. This can also

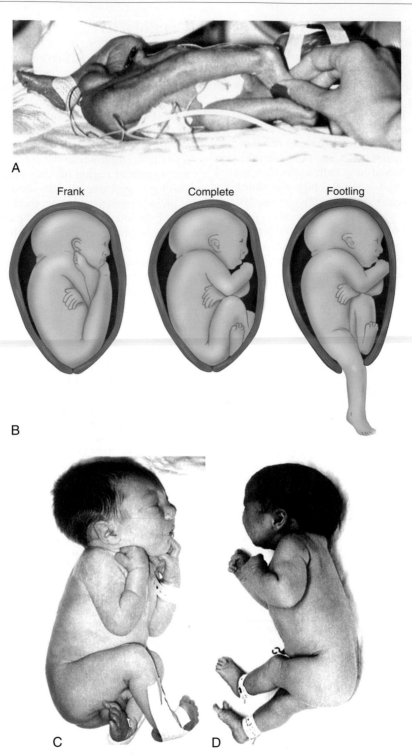

FIGURE 42-3. **A,** This infant was born prematurely from a frank breech presentation with genu recurvatum as a consequence. **B,** Diagrams of types of breech presentation. **C,** This infant had been in complete breech presentation with flexed thighs and knees. Taping treated the equinovarus foot deformations, and a breech head is clearly evident. **D,** This infant with extended knees and flexed thighs had been in prolonged frank breech presentation with dislocated hips and a breech head. Note the characteristic position of comfort. When the thighs were extended, the result was great discomfort.

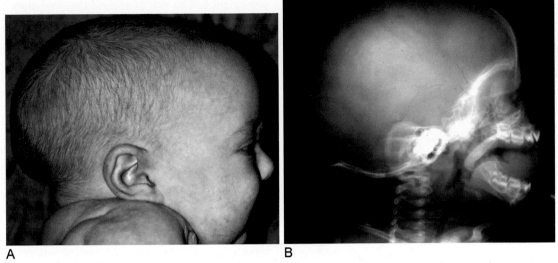

FIGURE 42-4. **A,** This dolichocephalic breech head demonstrates the tendency for the lower auricle to be uplifted by pressure from the shoulder in utero. **B,** The prominent occipital shelf is evident on a lateral skull radiograph.

FIGURE 42-5. **A,** This infant exhibits breech head and overfolded superior helix. **B,** The edematous swelling on the labia majora and hemorrhagic edematous swelling of the labia minora and external vagina are secondary to prolonged constraint of this presenting part in the frank breech presentation. Look carefully for the ring-like zone around the buttocks and genitalia, which appears to represent the site of cervix indentation on the presenting part.

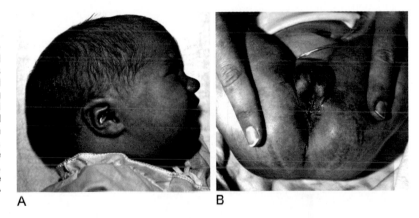

occur during breech deliveries when the adducted arm is pulled forcefully downward to free the after-coming head, which accounts for 9% to 24% of brachial plexus palsies.[15-17] The lower plexus is most susceptible to injury when traction is exerted on an abducted arm, such as occurs during breech deliveries when traction is applied to the trunk or legs while the after-coming arm is fixed in abduction.[14] When traction is particularly rapid and forceful, then diffuse multifocal injury occurs, including avulsion of the roots from the cord in the most severe injuries. Fractures of the femur, humerus, and clavicle are more common in breech babies, as is bruising with secondary hyperbilirubinemia.[3,5]

## Genitalia

The buttocks and genitalia tend to be the leading parts at delivery and may show edema and/or bruising (see Fig. 42-5). Hydrocele of the testicle is also frequent.

## OTHER COMPLICATIONS OF BREECH PRESENTATION

It is important to emphasize that some of the complications presented in this section result primarily from vaginal delivery of a baby in breech

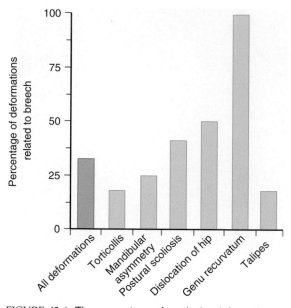

FIGURE 42-6. The percentage of particular deformations related to breech presentation in Dunn's study of more than 6000 newborn infants.

(From Dunn PM: Fifth European Congress of Perinatology, Uppsala, Sweden, 1976, p 79.)

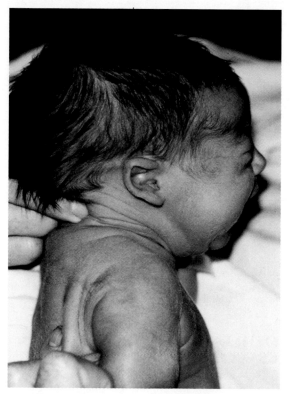

FIGURE 42-7. Breech head with overfolded superior helix and marked skin redundancy over the back from marked compression due to prolonged oligohydramnios.

presentation. The risk of vaginal delivery must be weighed in each case against the risk of cesarean section. Because more cesarean sections are being performed for breech presentation, especially in the primigravida, the frequency of serious complications has decreased. Previously, perinatal mortality was 13% for breech presentation, and prematurely born infants, twins, and babies with malformations accounted for much of this mortality rate.[3] It is important to appreciate that the premature baby is more likely to be in the breech position in early gestation. However, it is also important to realize that the breech position *itself* is frequently associated with premature labor. The overall frequency of breech presentation in premature deliveries between 28 and 36 weeks of gestation was 24%.[3] For the term singleton infant in breech presentation without malformation, the perinatal mortality was 1%.[3] The breech fetus is more likely to have the head become entrapped during the second stage of labor, which tends to increase the frequency of tentorial tears and intracranial bleeding, asphyxia (five- to six-fold greater risk), and trauma relating to the attempt to "pull" out the infant during a vaginal delivery.[3] Serious consequences include trauma to the cervicothoracic nerve roots, brachial plexus, and/or compression of the vertebral artery with cerebral ischemia.

In a meta-analysis of 24 studies of singleton term breech deliveries published between 1966 and 1992, perinatal mortality was corrected to exclude antepartum stillbirths and infants with major congenital anomalies. The corrected perinatal mortality rate ranged from 0 to 48 per 1000 births among the 24 reports and was higher among infants in the planned vaginal delivery group than in the planned cesarean group (odds ratio [OR] = 3.86; confidence interval [CI] = 2.22–6.69).[5] The main causes of death were head entrapment, cerebral injury and hemorrhage, cord prolapse, and severe asphyxia. Cord prolapse occurred in as many as 7.4% of women who had a trial of labor, depending on the type of breech presentation (0%–2% for frank breech, 5%–10.5% for complete breech, 8% to 16% for double footling breech, and 10% to 28.5% for single footling breech), with cord prolapse twice as common in multiparas (6%) than in nulliparas (3%).[5] Low 5-minute Apgar scores (i.e., less than 7) occurred more frequently in the planned vaginal delivery group (OR = 1.95; 95% CI = 1.45–2.61), and the incidence of birth trauma was 0.3% to 6% among the 24 studies (OR = 3.96; 95% CI = 2.76–5.67). If all the retrospective studies were excluded, the OR for traumatic birth injuries in the prospective studies was 5.16 (95% CI = 2.63–10.13), and long-term infant morbidity occurred more frequently in the planned vaginal delivery group (OR = 2.88; 95% CI = 1.04–7.97).[5] Cerebral palsy was noted in 16 of 26 affected children and was associated with perinatal factors such as hyperextended head, cord prolapse, or difficult delivery.[5] Overall maternal morbidity was lower among women in the planned vaginal delivery group (OR = 0.61; 95% CI = 0.47–0.80).[5]

Among 371,692 singleton live births in breech presentation between 1989 and 1991 in the United States, cesarean delivery had significantly lower neonatal mortality for all birth weight groups when compared with primary vaginal births, despite a higher prevalence of fetal malformations in the cesarean group.[1] In the group with birth weights >2500 g, neonatal mortality in the primary vaginal birth group was 5.3 per 1000 versus 3.2 per 1000 in the cesarean group.[1] In a study of 15,818 non-malformed term singleton Swedish infants delivered from breech presentation between 1987 and 1993, infants delivered vaginally were at higher risk for infant mortality (OR = 2.5) and birth injury (OR = 12.2).[7] Infants delivered by emergency cesarean section were at increased risk for neonatal seizures (OR – 4.1), and infants delivered vaginally or by emergency cesarean section were at increased risk for low 5-minute Apgar scores. Maternal morbidity was highest among women who delivered by emergency cesarean section (2.8%) when compared with elective cesarean section (1.7%) and vaginal delivery (1.8%).[7] Among 39,353 Norwegian breech presentation births delivered between 1967 and 1994, the perinatal loss rate was 5.6% (versus 1.3% for nonbreech presentations), and if antenatal stillbirths were excluded, the rates were 3.9% for breech versus 0.76% for vertex, suggesting that live breech infants were five times more likely to die during the perinatal period than non-breech infants.[8] Relative risk (RR) for perinatal death was higher for vaginal delivery than for cesarean delivery (RR = 5.4; 95% CI = 4.7–6.2). Studies that reported no significant differences in neonatal morbidity and mortality for vaginal versus cesarean deliveries of infants in breech presentation generally involved smaller numbers (705 or 268 consecutive breech presentations) at one or two institutions.[9,11]

Of gravest concern is the vaginal delivery of a breech fetus with a hyperextended head (ultrasound-measured angle of less than 90 degrees between the cervical vertebrae and the tangent plane of the occipital bone), which occurs in 11% to 15% of breech fetuses and was associated with cervical cord damage in 8 of 11 cases delivered vaginally versus 0 of 20 fetuses delivered by cesarean section.[21] Abroms et al[22] reported a 21% incidence of cervical cord transection among 88 neonates born with hyperextension of the head associated with breech and transverse presentations. All neonates with cord transection were delivered vaginally, whereas none of the neonates delivered by cesarean section suffered permanent spinal cord transection. These results have been confirmed in other studies demonstrating a 22% risk of long-term neurologic sequellae in association with hyperextension of the fetal head[23] and a high risk of spinal cord injury that may be prevented by elective cesarean delivery.[23-28] The acute symptoms of cervical cord transection are usually respiratory problems, a weak cry, poor muscle tone, poor feeding, and often death with high cervical lesions.

In vaginal breech deliveries, the mechanism of injury is usually longitudinal distraction, which leaves the vertebral column intact and occurs most frequently in the lower cervical or upper thoracic region, resulting in symptoms of diaphragmatic breathing and hypotonia with hyperreflexia that is worse in the lower extremities, with or without associated brachial plexus and phrenic nerve injury.[29,31] Thus, plain radiographs are not helpful, but spinal ultrasound and magnetic resonance imaging can localize and define the extent of the lesion (Fig. 42-8).[29-31] Survivors are usually severely debilitated with spastic diplegia or quadriplegia. Lesser degrees of cord damage at C5 to C6 may produce hand and forearm weakness with flexor weakness and wrist drop. Less commonly, the damage occurs at the C8 to T1 cord level, yielding extensor weakness with the fingers and hands flexed. About 50% of infants with Erb's and Klumpke's pareses recover, usually by 3 to 5 months of age. Compression of the vertebral artery may occur, which yields secondary problems in the medullary area of the brain. A number of cerebral palsy cases in the past may have been related to problems engendered by vaginal breech delivery; however, one recent paper attributes the higher risk of cerebral palsy in breech versus vertex presentations (OR = 1.56; 95% CI – 0.9–2.4) to a higher rate of breech infants who are small for gestational age.[32] Breech presentation infants were more commonly classified as diplegic (77.8%) than were vertex presentation infants (42.3%).[32]

Another complication that may be secondary to vaginal breech delivery is traumatic transection of the pituitary stalk during delivery, with consequent hypopituitarism.[33-35] Among patients with ectopia of the posterior pituitary, absence or hypoplasia of the pituitary stalk, and hypoplasia of the anterior pituitary, there is a strong association with vaginal breech delivery and multiple pituitary hormone deficiency.[34,35] A traumatic cause could only

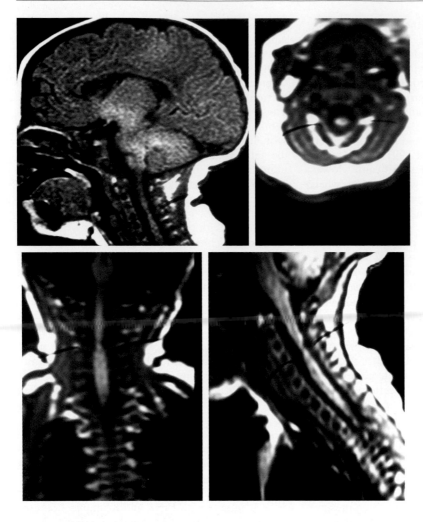

FIGURE 42-8. Cord transection caused by vaginal delivery of a fetus in breech presentation. The slash marks indicate cervical cord constriction caused by the injury.

explain 32% of such cases, and other cases had associated congenital midline brain anomalies.[35] One paper suggested that vaginal breech delivery of patients with this syndrome resulted in multiple pituitary hormone deficiencies, whereas cesarean section or normal vertex delivery was followed only by idiopathic growth hormone deficiency.[34]

## MANAGEMENT, PROGNOSIS, AND COUNSEL

In the prevention and management of breech presentation, three factors must be considered. First is the prevention of deformities and complications due to vaginal delivery by moving the fetus into the vertex position before the time of delivery via a method referred to as *external cephalic version*. Second is the avoidance of complications related to vaginal delivery of the breech fetus by using cesarean section delivery, particularly when

the fetal head is hyperextended. Third is the management of any deformations and complications after delivery of the breech fetus.

## External Cephalic Version

External cephalic version is the external manipulation of the fetus from the breech or transverse position into the vertex position (Fig. 42-9). Current opinion holds that in late pregnancy, external cephalic version should be offered to mothers with a singleton breech presentation, using tocolytics in nulliparous women to relax the uterus.[10] This procedure is successful in 40% of nulliparous women and 60% of multiparous women when performed after 38 weeks.[10] In a retrospective study of 157 breech deliveries and 1325 vertex deliveries followed by ultrasound examinations during the second and third trimesters (without use of version techniques), fetuses in breech presentation at

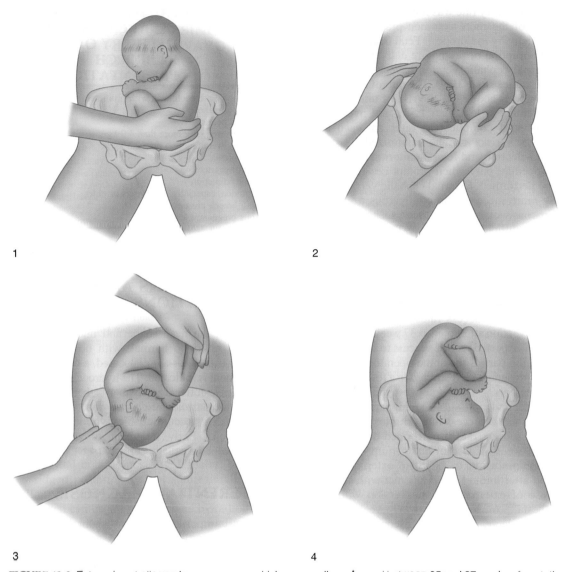

FIGURE 42-9. External cephalic version maneuvers, which are usually performed between 35 and 37 weeks of gestation, convert a breech presentation to a cephalic presentation.

25 weeks or later were at high risk for malpresentation at delivery, with 71% of breech presentations at 25 to 29 weeks and 83% of breech presentations at 32 to 34 weeks persisting until delivery.[36] After the 33rd week, there is little likelihood of a vertex presentation changing to breech, and 90% of fetuses in both breech and vertex presentation have assumed their final presentation.[36]

During the past two decades, the cesarean section rate for singleton term breech presentations has approached 90% in many centers, contributing substantially to the rising rate of cesarean delivery.[12] External cephalic version has been advocated as an alternative to breech delivery and

cesarean birth and is safe and cost effective.[35,37] In a review of 12 U.S. studies on 1339 patients undergoing external version at 35 weeks or later and using similar protocols (patient selection, tocolysis, ultrasound scanning, cardiotocographic monitoring, and Rh immunoglobulin protection), 63.3% had a vaginal delivery and 36.7% had cesarean births, whereas 83.2% of controls had cesarean delivery; thus, the cesarean delivery rate was reduced by more than half.[37] Among five European studies in which external version was attempted on 541 patients at 33 weeks or later, the success rate and proportion of vertex vaginal deliveries was about 10% lower than in the United States, but the

25. Daw E: Management of the hyperextended fetal head, *Am J Obstet Gynecol* 124:113–115, 1976.
26. Weinstein D, Margalioth EJ, Navot EJ, et al: Neonatal fetal death following cesarean section secondary to hyper-extension of the fetal head, *Acta Obstet Gynecol Scand* 62:629–631, 1983.
27. Bhagwanani SG, Price HV, Laurence HV, et al: Risks and prevention of cervical cord injury in the management of breech presentation with hyperextension of the fetal head, *Am J Obstet Gynecol* 115:1159–1161, 1973.
28. Ballas S, Toaff R, Jaffa AJ: Deflexion of the fetal head in breech presentation: incidence, management and outcome, *Obstet Gynecol* 52:653–655, 1978.
29. Morota N, Sakamoto K, Kobayashi N: Traumatic cervical syringomyelia related to birth injury, *Child Nerv Syst* 8:234–236, 1992.
30. Rossitch E, Oakes WJ: Perinatal spinal cord injury: clinical, radiographic and pathologic features, *Pediatr Neurosurg* 18:149–152, 1992.
31. de Vries E, Robben SGF, ven den Anker JN: Radiologic imaging of severe cervical spinal cord birth trauma, *Eur J Pediatr* 154:230–232, 1995.
32. Krebs L, Topp M, Langhoff-Roos J: The relation of breech presentation at term to cerebral palsy, *Br J Obstet Gynaecol* 106:943–947, 1999.
33. Fujita K, Matsuo N, Mori O, et al: The association of hypopituitarism with small pituitary, invisible pituitary stalk, type 1 Arnold-Chiari malformation, and syringomyelia in seven patients born in breech position: a further proof of birth injury theory on the pathogenesis of "idiopathic hypopituitarism," *Eur J Pediatr* 151:266–270, 1992.
34. Maghnie M, Larizza D, Triulzi F, et al: Hypopituitarism and stalk agenesis: a congenital syndrome worsened by breech delivery? *Horm Res* 35:104–108, 1991.
35. Triulzi F, Scotti G, di Natale B, et al: Evidence of a congenital midline brain anomaly in pituitary dwarfs: a magnetic resonance imaging study in 101 patients, *Pediatrics* 93:409–416, 1994.
36. Tadmor OP, Rabinowitz R, Alon L, et al: Can breech presentation at birth be predicted from ultrasound examinations during the second or third trimesters? *Int J Gynecol Obstet* 46:11–14, 1994.
37. Zhang J, Bowes WA, Forney JA: Efficacy of external cephalic version: a review, *Obstet Gynecol* 82:306–312, 1993.
38. Thunedborg P, Fischer-Rasmussen W, Tollund L: The benefit of external cephalic version with tocolysis as a routine procedure in late pregnancy, *Eur J Obstet Gynecol Reprod Biol* 42:23–27, 1991.
39. Kornman MT, Kimball KT, Reeves KO: Preterm external cephalic version in an outpatient environment, *Am J Obstet Gynecol* 172:1734–1741, 1995.
40. Benifla JL, Goffinet F, Darai E, et al: Antepartum transabdominal amnioinfusion to facilitate external cephalic version after initial failure, *Obstet Gynecol* 84:1041–1042, 1994.
41. Dugoff L, Stamm CA, Jones OW, et al: The effect of spinal anesthesia on the success rate of external cephalic version: a randomized trial, *Obstet Gynecol* 93:345–349, 1999.
42. Shalev E, Battino S, Giladi Y, et al: External cephalic version at term—using tocolysis, *Acta Obstet Gynecol Scand* 72:455–457, 1993.
43. Schachter M, Kogan S, Blickstein I: External cephalic version after previous cesarean section—a clinical dilemma, *Int J Gynecol Obstet* 45:17–20, 1994.
44. Braun FHT, Jones KL, Smith DW: Breech presentation as an indicator of fetal abnormality, *J Pediatr* 86:419–421, 1975.

# 43 Transverse Lie Deformation

## GENESIS

Transverse lie occurs in 2.5 per 1000 deliveries and is associated with multiparity (90%), prematurity (13%), placenta previa (11%), polyhydramnios (8%), uterine anomalies (8%), and uterine myomas (3%), especially when myomas are located in the lower uterine segment. Predisposing factors such as uterine structural anomalies, prematurity, and placenta previa are found in 66% of primiparas, but only 33% of multiparas manifest these factors.[1] Thus, multiparity is the most common factor, and women delivering transverse-lying infants tend to be older than those delivering vertex-presenting infants; the other factors such as low-lying placenta, uterine anomalies, myomas, or prematurity occur more frequently in primigravidas. Laxity of abdominal musculature in multiparous women is considered the predominant factor accounting for the liability toward transverse lie in these women. The occurrence of polyhydramnios may relate to the inability of the fetus to swallow amniotic fluid because the mouth is pushed up against the side of the uterus.

version followed by induction of labor has been recommended for multiparous women, but transverse lie in a primigravida should not be treated the same as in a multigravida in whom laxity of the abdomen has been the major cause for a transverse lie.[3] In a comparative study of expectant management versus external version, only 7.9% of 254 patients with an unstable lie were primiparous, and only 1 of these 11 women had spontaneous version (versus 34% of the multiparous women). When managed by version, 4 (44%) primiparous women required emergency cesarean sections, whereas 94% of the multiparous women had successful vaginal deliveries.[4] Thus, the rarity of transverse lie among primiparous women implies that it is likely to be accounted for by some type of underlying pathology, such as the predisposing factors listed previously. The proven value of external cephalic version in term breech deliveries and in multiparous women with a transverse lie should not be extended to primiparous women with a transverse lie, who may have

## FEATURES

Full frontal constraint may flatten the face, limit mandibular growth, and cause a retroflexed head with a prominent occipital shelf. There may be associated torticollis and/or scoliosis, as well as other associated deformations (Figs. 43-1 to 43-3).

## MANAGEMENT

Management of transverse lie at term consists of expectant management, external cephalic version, or elective cesarean section.[2,3] With expectant management, the spontaneous conversion rate to a longitudinal lie before labor is as high as 83%.[2] This must be weighed against the increased risks of cord prolapse and birth trauma/asphyxia with persistent transverse lie and against the risks of cesarean section. For this reason, external

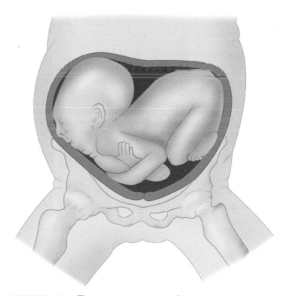

FIGURE 43-1. Transverse presentation.

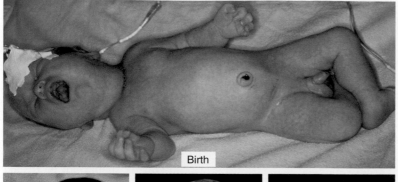

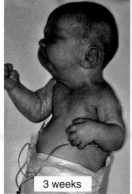 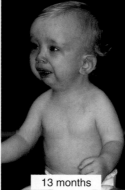 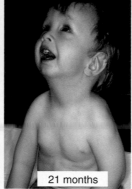

Birth

3 weeks

13 months

21 months

FIGURE 43-2. This infant was born at 36 weeks of gestation, having been in prolonged transverse lie since 17 weeks of gestation due to oligohydramnios that resulted from slow leakage of amniotic fluid. Despite prolonged physical therapy, the severe compression of facial structures persisted through 21 months. (See Fig. 23-1 for follow-up at age 30 months, when persistent jaw growth deficiency was still evident.)

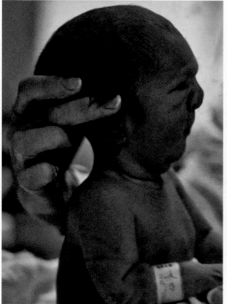 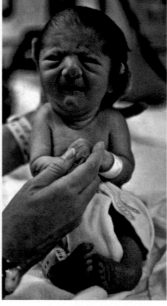

FIGURE 43-3. Flattening of the face with redundant "compression" skin folds in addition to equinovarus foot deformities in an infant who had been in prolonged transverse presentation, apparently with the head retroflexed and the face forced against the wall of the uterus. The infant's appearance progressively improved and returned to normal form.
(Courtesy of John Carey, University of Utah Medical School, Salt Lake City, Utah.)

some kind of underlying pathology inhibiting the normal process of version. Unresolved transverse lie is usually an indication for cesarean section using a transverse lower uterine segment incision, as neglected transverse lie can result in uterine rupture and other complications.[5,6] Some authors have advocated the use of intravenous nitroglycerine to induce uterine atonia and facilitate internal podalic version in cases of twins in which the second twin is in transverse lie.[7]

## DIFFERENTIAL DIAGNOSIS

The remarkable facial compression in babies born from a transverse lie can cause unusual facial features that may resemble a malformation syndrome or craniosynostosis.

*References*

1. Gemer O, Segal S: Incidence and contribution of predisposing factors to transverse lie presentation, *Int J Gynecol Obstet* 44:219–221, 1994.
2. Phelan JP, Boucher M, Mueller E, et al: The nonlaboring transverse lie: a management dilemma, *J Reprod Med* 31:184–186, 1986.
3. Lau WC, Fung HYM, Lau TK, et al: A benign polyploid adenomyoma: an unusual cause of persistent fetal transverse lie, *Eur J Obstet Gynecol Reprod Biol* 74:23–25, 1997.
4. Edwards RL, Nicholson HO: The management of the unstable lie in late pregnancy, *J Obstet Gynaecol Br Commonw* 76:719–720, 1969.
5. Segal S, Gemer O, Sassoon E: Transverse lower uterine segment incision in cesarean sections for transverse lie, *Arch Gynecol Obstet* 255:171–172, 1994.
6. Gemer O, Kopmar A, Sassoon E, et al: Neglected transverse lie with uterine rupture, *Arch Gynecol Obstet* 252:159–160, 1993.
7. Dufour P, Vinatier D, Vanderstichele S, et al: Intravenous nitroglycerine for internal podalic version of the second twin in transverse lie, *Obstet Gynecol* 92:416–419, 1998.

# 44 Face and Brow Presentation Deformation

## GENESIS

In face and brow presentations, the face is the compressed presenting part, usually with extension of the head (Fig. 44-1). Face presentation occurs in 1 to 2 per 1250 deliveries, and persistent brow presentation is less common.[1-3] Brow presentation occurs in 1 per 1444 deliveries.[3] Face presentation is more common in multiparas (81%) and is variably associated with large infants weighing more than 4000 g (42%), small infants weighing less than 2300 g (16%), and cephalopelvic disproportion.[1-3] High parity, low birth weight, and cephalopelvic disproportion have also been proposed as etiologic factors in brow presentation, with associated cephalopelvic disproportion attributed to the presenting diameters of the fetal head being greater in brow presentation than in face or vertex presentations.[3] There may actually be selection for mothers with a smaller pelvis because the fetus within a larger pelvis may convert to face or vertex before being recognized as a brow presentation. About half to two thirds of all brow presentations spontaneously convert to either face (30%) or vertex presentations (20%) if given an adequate trial of labor.[3]

When a brow converts to a face presentation, the occiput usually lodges in the maternal sacrum, and additional force on the head converts it to mentum anterior.[4] In converting from brow to vertex, the brow engages transversely and rotates to face the pubic bones, and then the head flexes to become occipitoposterior; thus, many occipitoposterior presentations may have entered the pelvis as brow presentations.[4] In the era before prenatal diagnosis, the fetal mortality for face presentations was around 10%, with many deaths attributed to either attempted version, extraction, or conversion maneuvers (which are contraindicated with face or brow presentations) or to anencephaly.[1] When corrected to exclude anomalous infants, the mortality rate for face presentations delivered spontaneously or by low forceps is less than 2%.[3] Among all the proposing factors previously listed, high parity appears to be the most important.[3] Because increased extensor muscle tone cannot cause extension of a fetal head that is fixed in the pelvis, face presentation in a primigravida woman with an engaged presenting part is less likely to occur during the last 2 to 3 weeks of pregnancy. On the other hand, the fetal head is often not engaged prior to the onset of labor in multiparous women, such that face presentation occurs more frequently.[3]

## FEATURES

### Face Presentation

In face presentation, the fetal head is hyperextended so that the occiput touches the back, and the presenting part is the fetal face between the orbital ridges and the chin (see Fig. 44-1).[3] Most cases of face presentation (97%) are diagnosed by vaginal examination during labor and delivery, with 59% of face presentations mentum anterior, 15% mentum transverse, and 27% mentum posterior.[3] The growth of the fetal mandible and nose

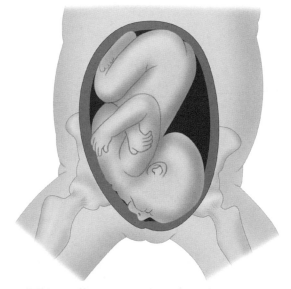

FIGURE 44-1. Face presentation with mentum transverse, emphasizing the mechanism for jaw compression and prominence of the occipital shelf.

266

may be restrained, and the position of comfort for the baby after birth is often with the neck retroflexed (Figs. 44-2 and 44-3). As a consequence of compression of the chin and anterior neck with retroflexion, redundant folds of skin in the anterior upper neck may be present (see Figs. 44-3 to 44-5), with persistent retrognathia and a prominent occipital shelf (see Figs. 44-3 and 44-4). In some instances, the prolonged facial compression causes feeding difficulties with difficulty in swallowing. There may also be jaw subluxation and a palpable/audible click as the jaw moves in and out of its socket (similar to that detected with a subluxable hip). The infant pictured in Fig. 44-4, A was one such case. In another case, an infant with 24 hours of labor as a persistent mentum posterior presentation experienced significant laryngotracheal trauma, resulting in respiratory obstruction from compression against the maternal sacrum.[5]

## Brow Presentation

In brow presentation, the fetal head is midway between flexion and hyperextension, and the presenting part is the brow between the orbital ridges and the anterior fontanelle.[3] Most cases of brow presentation are diagnosed during labor and delivery, with cephalopelvic disproportion associated with many persistent brow presentations and resulting in prolonged dysfunctional labors. With

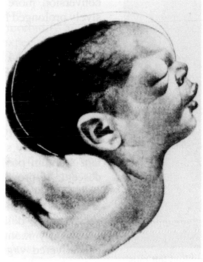
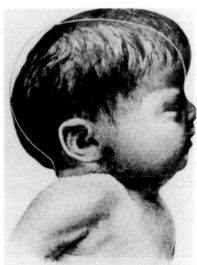

FIGURE 44-2. Examples of face and brow presentation. The white lines indicate the normal calvarial contour. (From von Ruess AR: *The disease of the newborn*, New York, 1921, William Wood.)

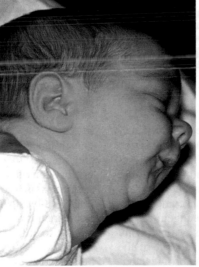
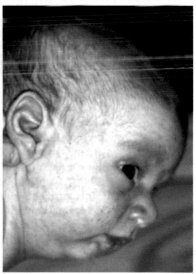

FIGURE 44-3. Newborn infant of a small primigravida mother. **A,** This infant was in prolonged face presentation for at least the last 2 months of gestation, leading to the extended head and restricted nasal and mandibular growth, as well as the compressive overgrowth of skin in the anterior neck. **B,** By 6 weeks of age, the catchup growth of the nose and mandible is evident, and the head had settled into a more normal alignment.

A                                        B

6. Jennings PN: Brow presentation and vaginal delivery, *Aust NZ J Obstet Gynecol* 8:219–224, 1968.
7. Levy DL: Persistent brow presentation: a new approach to management, *South Med J* 69:191–192, 1976.
8. Westgren M, Svenningsen NW: Face presentation in modern obstetrics—a study with special reference to fetal long-term morbidity, *Z Geburtsh U Perinat* 188:87–89, 1984.
9. Duff P: Diagnosis and management of face presentation, *Obstet Gynecol* 57:105–112, 1981.
10. Watson WJ, Read JA: Electronic fetal monitoring in face presentation at term, *Military Med* 152:324–325, 1987.
11. Schwartz Z, Dgani R, Lancet M, et al: Face presentation, *Aust N Z J Obstet Gynecol* 26:172–176, 1986.
12. Neuman M, Beller U, Lavie O, et al: Intrapartum bimanual reversal of face presentation: preliminary report, *Obstet Gynecol* 84:146–148, 1994.
13. Herabutya Y, Supakarapongkul W, Chaturachinda K: Face presentation in Ramathi Hospital: a 12-year study, *J Med Assoc Thai* 67(Suppl 2):31–35, 1984.
14. Prevedourakis CN: Face presentation: an analysis of 163 cases, *Am J Obstet Gynecol* 94:1092–1097, 1966.

# Whole-Body Deformation or Disruption

# 45 Small Uterine Cavity Deformation

## BICORNUATE OR MYOMATOUS UTERUS

### GENESIS

Several different types of problems may limit the size and/or shape of the uterus and thus enhance the likelihood of fetal deformation.[1] Examples include a malformed uterus due to failure of the müllerian ducts to completely fuse during embryogenesis, resulting in either symmetric or asymmetric structural anomalies of the uterus such as didelphic uterus with duplicated cervix, bicornuate uterus, septate uterus, and arcuate uterus (Fig. 45-1). Estimates of Müllerian duct anomaly frequency vary widely based on the mode of ascertainment (hysterosalpingography [HSG] and magnetic resonance imaging [MRI] are more sensitive than ultrasound) and certain selection biases (reproductive tracts are more commonly investigated in women with miscarriage and infertility, and anomalies are more prevalent in women with these problems). Among 167 women who underwent laparoscopic sterilization (and therefore were assumed to represent a normal reproductive population), 1.2% were found to have a bicornuate uterus, and 3.6% had a septate uterus, yielding a total prevalence of uterine malformations of 5.4%; the prevalence was significantly higher among oligomenorrheic women with reduced fertility.[2] Other estimates for the frequency of uterine anomalies range from 1% to 10% based on ascertainment by laparoscopy or MRI.[3,4] A prospective ultrasound study of the prevalence of Müllerian duct anomalies in 2065 consecutive menstruating girls and adult women (ages 8 to 93 years) yielded a rate of approximately 1 in 250 women.[5]

It is estimated that at least 1% to 2% of women have a clinically significant malformation of the uterus and that the general risk of a deformation problem for a fetus in a malformed uterus is about 30%.[1] Such deformations can include craniofacial deformations, overlapping sutures, joint contractures, limb deformations or disruptions, edema and/or grooves, and thoracic constriction resulting in pulmonary hypoplasia.[1,6-8] This would imply that 3 to 6 infants per 1000 may have a deformation problem secondary to gestation within a malformed uterus. Vascular disruption within the fetal limb can also occur with severe uterine constriction.[9] Rarely, a large uterine fibroid can also result in fetal deformation and/or disruption,[9,10] and sometimes a small fibroma will enlarge rapidly under the

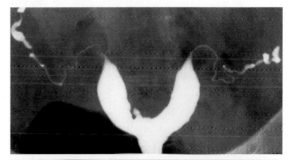
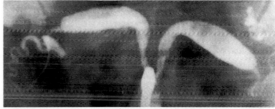
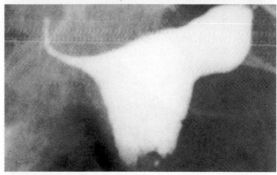

FIGURE 45-1. Three examples of bicornuate uterus shown by HSG, each of which was responsible for a deformational problem in the offspring.

influence of increased levels of estrogen during late gestation.

## FEATURES

All gradations of deformation of craniofacial structures, limbs, and thorax may occur, including overall constraint of fetal growth (Figs. 45-2 to 45-5). A deep groove in the thorax and left arm in one fetus was attributed to compression from the septum of a bicornuate uterus, while another fetus had marked molding of the head, which was trapped in the left uterine horn.[6] Prolonged constraint within a bicornuate uterus has resulted in multiple joint contractures from fetal immobility.[7] Another report documented prenatal detection of calvarial asymmetry in a 27-week fetus in vertex presentation due to pressure on the fetal head by a baseball-sized leiomyoma in the posterior uterine wall. At birth, there was a 3- × 4-cm depression of the left parietal bone with atrophy of the right sternocleidomastoid muscle. By 6 months, growth and development were normal,

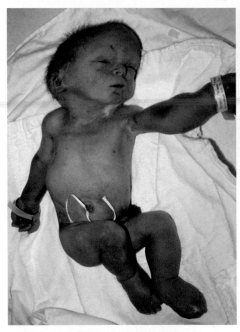

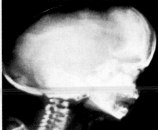

FIGURE 45-2. Severely deformed newborn infant delivered from a bicornuate uterus who died of respiratory insufficiency due to constraint-induced lung hypoplasia. The proximal constraint of limb has resulted in distal lymphedema, and the head has been molded out of alignment in such a manner as to give the impression of low-placed ears. The mother had a history of five previous miscarriages.

(From Miller ME, Dunn PM, Smith DW: Uterine malformation and fetal deformation, *J Pediatr* 94:387, 1979.)

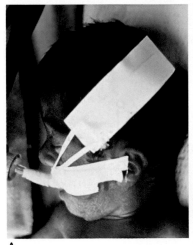

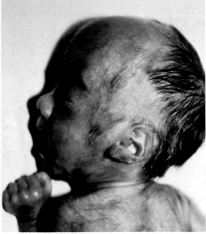

A                    B

FIGURE 45-3. **A,** Infant born prematurely born at 34 weeks with compressed craniofacies that initially had raised questions regarding coronal craniostenosis. **B,** Within 3 weeks, the face had grown forward and the question of craniostenosis was resolved.

(Courtesy of Kenneth Lyons Jones, University of California, San Diego, Calif. From Miller ME, Dunn PM, Smith DW: Uterine malformation and fetal deformation, *J Pediatr* 94:387, 1979.)

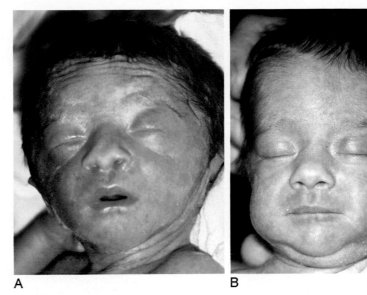

FIGURE 45-4. **A,** This infant was born at 34 weeks from a bicornuate uterus (same infant as in Fig. 45-1, *B*), demonstrating a compressed face and nose with redundant skin. **B,** Follow-up at age 32 days showed a complete return toward normal form.

**A**                    **B**

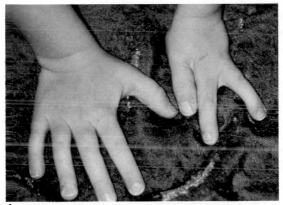

**A**

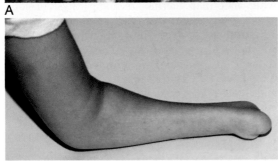

**B**

FIGURE 45-5. **A,** Ulnar longitudinal ray defect of the left hand in an infant born to a mother with a bicornuate uterus (same infant as in Fig. 45-1, *A*). **B,** Terminal transverse hemimelia of the left arm in a child born to a woman with a bicornuate uterus.

(From Graham JM Jr, Miller ME, Stephan MJ, et al: Limb reduction anomalies and early in-utero limb compression, *J Pediatr* 96:1052, 1980.)

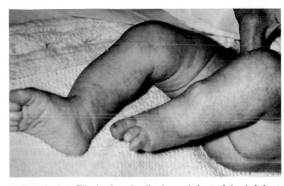

FIGURE 45-6. Fibular longitudinal ray defect of the left foot with a short, bent lower leg in an infant born to a woman with a large uterine leiomyoma.

the calvarial depression had partially resolved, and the torticollis was improved.[8] There is a significantly increased incidence of caudal dysplasia in pregnancies associated with uterine leiomyomata, possibly due to fetal leg compression (Figs. 45-6 and 45-7).[10] Constraint of thoracic growth may be sufficient to impair lung growth and maturation and cause pulmonary hypoplasia. Familial Müllerian duct anomalies can occur, often in association with renal and urinary tract anomalies; therefore, a previous family history of Müllerian and/or renal anomalies should prompt further investigation.[11-15]

The small uterine cavity may also result in miscarriage, stillbirth, prematurity, and fetal deformation and/or vascular disruption. Insufficient uterine

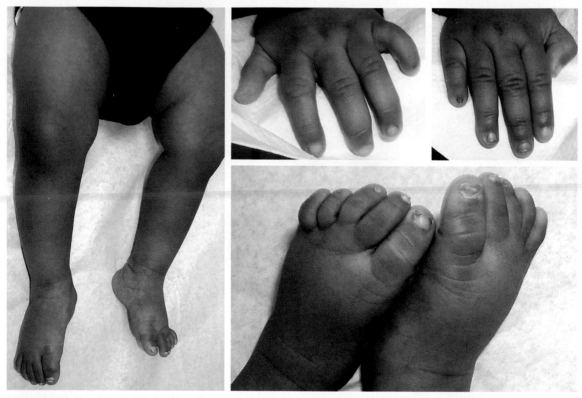

FIGURE 45-7. Hypoplastic left leg and distal digital hypoplasia in an infant delivered by cesarean section due to extensive uterine leiomyomata, which were so enlarged that they had to be surgically resected so that the baby could be delivered.

space for fetal growth should be considered as one possible explanation when a history of multiple miscarriages, stillbirths, prematurity, cervical incompetence, abdominal pregnancy, and/or serious deformation problems is obtained.[16-20] Such findings may lead to the detection of a uterine malformation, as these problems are more frequent among oligomenorrheic women with reduced fertility.[2]

In a case-control study of 38 infants (32 liveborn and 6 stillborn) born to mothers with a bicornuate uterus, the risk for congenital defects was about four times higher than in women with a normal uterus.[21] Five defects were significantly more common: nasal hypoplasia, omphalocele, limb deficiencies (hypoplasia or absence of metacarpals, metatarsals, phalanges), teratoma, and acardiaanencephaly. Other defects were common but did not reach statistical significance: microcephaly, microtia, esophageal atresia, syndactyly, limb contractures, scoliosis, and micrognathia. Among the 38 cases born to women with a bicornuate uterus, 13 of 38 (34.2%) had deformations (limb contractures, scoliosis, nasal hypoplasia, micrognathia, and clubfoot), which is similar to the 30% risk

suggested previously.[1] Vaginal bleeding was significantly more common than in mothers with a normal uterus (54.1% versus 14.1%), and vaginal bleeding has previously been associated with limb reduction defects.[9,10,21] In a study of 322 women with abnormal uterine bleeding, hysteroscopy detected asymptomatic Müllerian anomalies in 10% of these women. The women with Müllerian anomalies had a significantly higher incidence of spontaneous abortion and lower cumulative live birth rates,[19,20] which suggests that some fetuses with severe defects may have been lost earlier in gestation in this case-control study of liveborn and stillborn infants.[21]

## MANAGEMENT, PROGNOSIS, AND COUNSEL

Surgical improvement of the uterine size, if indicated and possible, may greatly improve the chances of rearing a normal fetus to a term birth.[20] Large uterine fibroids may also merit consideration of surgical intervention. Among 62 women with uterine malformations, 5 had unexplained infertility of over 2 years' duration, and the remaining 57 had a total of 127 pregnancies between 1971 and 1988. There was a 36% rate of abortion, 22% infants were delivered prematurely, and 42% were delivered at term. Breech presentation occurred in 46% of 127 pregnancies and 63% of 81 cases in which pregnancy continued beyond 28 weeks required cesarean section. Perinatal mortality was 37%, and the fetal survival rate was 61%.[16] Among 1200 women with repeated reproductive loss, 188 (15.7%) had a congenital uterine anomaly detected by HSG, and none of their 233 presurgical pregnancies lasted to term. After metroplasty, more than 84% of their pregnancies were successfully maintained, versus a 94.4% rate of spontaneous loss before 12 weeks of gestation in 47 women with uterine anomalies and no surgery.[18] Another similar study demonstrated uterine anomalies in 49% of 81 patients investigated for recurrent pregnancy wastage, with 27% breech or transverse presentation, only 25% delivering at term, and prematurely born infants often small for gestational age.[19] There was also an excess of bleeding during pregnancy and premature rupture of membranes, with dystocia from malpresentation being the major indication for cesarean section.

Surgical correction, if possible, can improve outcomes,[20] but it is important to be certain that the fertility and obstetric problems stem from purely uterine causes before surgical correction is attempted. Cervical incompetence is common with Müllerian abnormalities (28%–30% with a bicornuate uterus; the rate is even higher with a septate uterus).[16] Septate uterus was associated with the highest rate of recurrent spontaneous abortions, possibly due to placental ischemia caused by scant vasculature within the septum, as well as its poorly developed endometrium, combined with the spatial restrictions imposed by the septum. Abdominal metroplasty completely ameliorated fetal survival in six cases with a septate uterus, and more recent technological renovations have allowed transcervical lysis of the uterine septum via hysteroscopic techniques instead of abdominal metroplasty.[20] Fetal survival until delivery depends on the type of uterine malformation (65% for arcuate uterus, 45% for unicornuate and didelphys uterus, and 40% for bicornuate and septate uterus).[21] Unicornuate uterus is difficult to repair, but occasionally the noncommunicating rudimentary horn can be resected between pregnancies, as it is not associated with an excess of infertility. Fortunately, unicornuate uterine malformations have the second-highest rate of fetal survival (66%), after bicornuate uterus.[15] The relatively poor decidua and

endometrium in the noncommunicating horn of a unicornuate uterus predisposes to placenta percreta, and there was uterine rupture (at a mean gestational age of 24 weeks) in 8 of 17 cases of pregnancies in noncommunicating uterine horns, with only 7 of 17 such infants surviving.[17] Some of these fetuses became abdominal pregnancies after rupture of the rudimentary uterine horn (sometimes heralded by the onset of shoulder pain, indicating the presence of intraperitoneal blood or fluid rising to the diaphragmatic surface).[17] The diagnosis of Müllerian anomalies in the gravid uterus is notoriously difficult, and midtrimester fetal ultrasounds can miss such anomalies; however, use of a combination of ultrasound and HSG in nonpregnant patients is highly accurate in the diagnosis of Müllerian abnormalities.[17,20]

Uterine myomata occur in 2% to 15% of pregnancies depending on maternal age, and although most myomas remain small and asymptomatic, 10% to 40% of affected pregnancies will have myoma-related complications.[23-25] These problems include an increased risk for fetal loss, increases in the size of the myomata, prematurity, intrauterine growth retardation, abruptio placentae, fetal malpresentation, increased rates of cesarean section delivery, postpartum hemorrhage, and puerperal sepsis, in addition to the problems outlined previously; therefore there have been attempts to remove myomata surgically or via uterine artery embolization.[26-28] Uterine fibroids have been reported in 27% of pregnant women, and 50% of infertile women become pregnant after myomectomy.[26] Among 84 patients who underwent surgical removal of myomas before in vitro fertilization, 28 (33%) became pregnant, resulting in 21 live births (25%). Among 84 patients who underwent in vitro fertilization without previous surgery, only 13 became pregnant (15%), resulting in 10 live births (12%); these data confirm the beneficial effect of removing fibroids before undergoing in vitro fertilization.[26] Among 26 pregnancies in women who underwent uterine artery embolization to treat symptomatic fibroids, their rate of fetal loss and other prenatal complications was no greater than their background risk, and there were no neonatal complications; however, there was an increase in delivery by cesarean section (88%).[27] Attempts to remove myomata during pregnancy because of persisting symptoms (which could be counteracted by conservative measures) are rare.[25] In one such case, a twin whose placenta was over the myoma that was surgically removed at 12 weeks of gestational age was born with growth deficiency, hydrocephalus, clubfeet, hypoplasia of the nails and terminal phalanges, and placental hemorrhage, thrombosis, and

## Limbs

The hands and feet may be edematous with positional deformation, and there is often stiffness of the joints, with flexion contractures of the elbows, knees, and feet (Fig. 46-6).[23] Hip dislocation may occur, especially with breech presentation. In surviving infants, these limb defects respond readily to physical therapy.

## Thorax and Lungs

The chest circumference is decreased, and radiographs reveal a bell-shaped chest with small lung fields, an elevated diaphragm, and pneumothoraces from high-pressure ventilation. Thoracic growth is restrained; this was initially hypothesized to cause the lungs to remain small and underdeveloped,[1] but it is actually inhibition of breathing movements (essential for lung growth) and/or abnormal fluid dynamics within the lungs themselves that result in decreased intraluminal fluid pressures and cause poor lung growth.[19] Lung growth often does not progress beyond the 4- to 5-month level of development, leading to hypoplasia (Fig. 46-7), and because the lungs lack surfactant, they remain incapable of aerobic expansion and/or oxygen exchange. This respiratory insufficiency is the most common cause of demise in the immediate postnatal period, and peak inspiratory pressures of greater than 30 cm $H_2O$ are required, often resulting

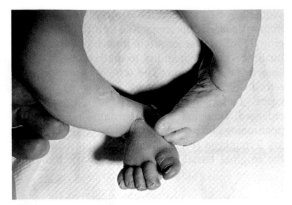

FIGURE 46-6. Renal agenesis with severe oligohydramnios and foot deformations at term delivery.

in pneumothoraces and interstitial emphysema (Fig. 46-8). Many infants die from hypoxemia, but some survive with pulmonary hypertension and pulmonary interstitial emphysema.[18,19,22]

## Skin

The skin tends to be redundant, which is presumably the result of overgrowth related to external constraint.[24] This gives rise to accentuated inner canthal and infraorbital skin folds, which contribute to the "Potter" facies and sometimes yield the false impression of a webbed neck (see Fig. 46-5).

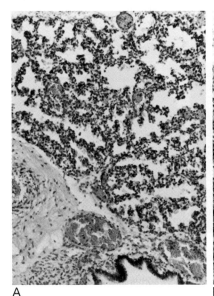
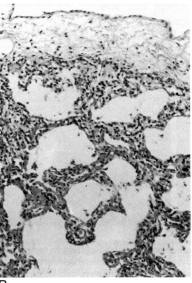

A

B

FIGURE 46-7. Lung hypoplasia secondary to severe oligohydramnios, yielding non-expansile lung with limited aerobic exchange (A) in contrast to a normal lung (B).
(From Thomas IT, Smith DW: Oligohydramnios, cause of the non-renal features of Potter's syndrome, *J Pediatr* 84:811, 1974.)

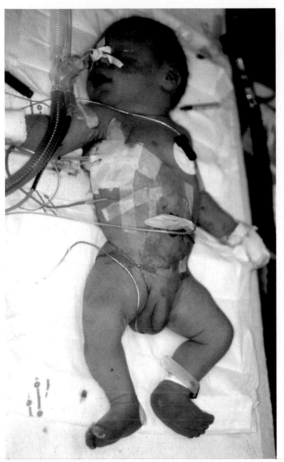

FIGURE 46-8. Renal agenesis in a newborn with lethal pulmonary hypoplasia and pneumothoraces as a consequence of attempted ventilation and resuscitation.

## Other

Concretions of amnion cells may build up on the relatively dry surface of the placenta, a feature termed *amnion nodosa*. The umbilical cord is usually short.[25]

## MANAGEMENT, PROGNOSIS, AND COUNSEL

If the oligohydramnios is due to renal agenesis or another type of severe renal problem, attempts to artificially oxygenate the neonate are of little or no value. However, if the deficit of amniotic fluid is due to chronic leakage of amniotic fluid, then survival hinges on the severity of oligohydramnios, the gestational age at which rupture occurs, and the duration of oligohydramnios, all of which determine the extent of pulmonary hypoplasia.[11] The importance of gestational age at premature rupture of membranes is related to the histologic development of the lungs, which can be divided into 3 stages: (1) the pseudoglandular stage (5 to 17 weeks; all major lung elements are formed with the exception of those related to gas exchange); (2) canalicular stage (16 to 25 weeks; terminal bronchioles give rise to respiratory bronchioles and then to thin-walled terminal sacs); and (3) terminal sac stage (24 weeks to birth; an increase in the number of terminal sacs rapidly increases the gas exchange area). If oligohydramnios is limited to the terminal sac stage, it does not affect lung growth, but when oligohydramnios occurs during the canalicular stage, the result is a cumulative reduction in lung size.[17] Thus, the risk for pulmonary hypoplasia diminishes when oligohydramnios occurs after 24 weeks of gestation.[18-27] The duration of severe oligohydramnios and the gestational age at which oligohydramnios had its onset are independent risk factors. Severe oligohydramnios lasting longer than 14 days with rupture of membranes before 25 weeks has a mortality rate of more than 90%.[21] Rupture at an early gestational age with severe oligohydramnios predisposes to joint contractures, and the risk for deformation relates to the duration of oligohydramnios.[23] If such an infant survives, there is usually catch-up growth within a few months after birth, with a restitution toward normal form with physical therapy.

For the obstetrician, management efforts are balanced between expectant management versus risks from prematurity if delivery is expedited, with attempts to prevent acute complications such as infection, cord prolapse, and placental abruption. When rupture occurs before 24 weeks, there is great risk for pulmonary hypoplasia, and prompt delivery is generally untenable. With rupture after 24 weeks, it is unlikely that prolongation of the pregnancy beyond this time will further increase the risk of pulmonary hypoplasia, but it can affect the development of skeletal deformation; therefore delivery within 2 weeks of rupture seems feasible once the risk of complications from prematurity becomes low.[27] Other measures include attempts to increase the amount of amniotic fluid via maternal bed rest and/or instillation of antibiotics and saline into the amniotic cavity to restore amniotic fluid volume.[28,29] Transabdominal amnioinfusion has been attempted for diagnostic and therapeutic purposes in women with second-trimester oligohydramnios. By instilling normal saline with indigo carmine dye, premature rupture of membranes was documented by the vaginal appearance of dye in 22 of 71 (31%) of patients with severe oligohydramnios. Of these 71 patients, 28 (39%) had anomalies diagnosed or confirmed after amnioinfusion, and 17 (24%) had a diagnosis of intrauterine growth retardation.[28,29] Thus, transabdominal amnioinfusion can be useful for diagnostic purposes in severe oligohydramnios, and transvaginal infusion may be useful for relief of fetal variable decelerations, with no apparent increased risk for maternal or neonatal infection but also no demonstrable clinical benefit.[29]

The recurrence risk for oligohydramnios sequence relates to the basic problem that gave rise to the oligohydramnios. Thus, with chronic leakage of fluid, the recurrence risk would be very low unless the early rupture of amniotic membranes is due to inherited Ehlers-Danlos syndrome (because classic Ehlers-Danlos syndrome is associated with early amnion rupture and is inherited in an autosomal dominant fashion). With defects such as obstructive uropathy or renal agenesis, the recurrence risk may be higher. Renal agenesis may recur and be associated with an increased risk for renal anomalies in first-degree relatives.[30] With infantile polycystic kidney disease, the risk may be as high as 25% due to autosomal recessive inheritance, and fetal autopsy studies are essential to make this diagnosis.[13] Prenatal diagnosis should be offered for subsequent pregnancies when oligohydramnios is due to a fetal malformation problem.

## DIFFERENTIAL DIAGNOSIS

Oligohydramnios sequence may be caused by failure to produce amniotic fluid due to renal or urinary tract malformations, which may be isolated defects or part of a syndrome.[13,23] Some of these problems have a genetic or chromosomal basis, which may become evident from autopsy studies and is important information from a genetic counseling perspective with respect to natural history and recurrence risk.[13,23] The recurrence risk for premature rupture of membranes depends on whether it is associated with an underlying connective tissue disorder such as Ehlers-Danlos syndrome. Most of the time, premature rupture of membranes is a sporadic occurrence, but this should not be assumed without further evaluation.

### References

1. Thomas IT, Smith DW: Oligohydramnios, cause of the non-renal features of Potter's syndrome, including pulmonary hypoplasia, *J Pediatr* 84:811–814, 1974.
2. Czeizel A, Vitez M, Kodaj I, et al: Study of isolated apparent amniogenic limb deficiency in Hungary, 1975–1984, *Am J Med Genet* 46:372–378, 1993.
3. Czeizel A, Vitez M, Kodaj I, et al: Causal study of isolated ulnar-fibular deficiency in Hungary, 1975–1984, *Am J Med Genet* 46:427–433, 1993.
4. Higgenbottom MC, Jones KL, Hall BD, et al: The amniotic band disruption complex; timing of amniotic rupture and variable spectrum of consequent defects, *J Pediatr* 95:544–549, 1979.
5. Miller ME, Graham JM Jr, Higgenbottom MC, et al: Compression-related defects from early amnion rupture: evidence for mechanical teratogenesis, *J Pediatr* 98:292–297, 1981.
6. Kalousek DK, Bamforth S: Amnion rupture sequence in previable fetuses, *Am J Med Genet* 31:63–73, 1988.
7. Moore TR: Clinical assessment of amniotic fluid, *Clin Obstet Gynecol* 40:303–313, 1997.
8. Grubb DK, Paul RH: Amniotic fluid index and prolonged antepartum fetal heart rate decelerations, *Obstet Gynecol* 79:558–560, 1992.
9. Crowley O, O'Herlihy C, Boylan P: The value of ultrasound measurement of amniotic fluid volume in the management of prolonged pregnancies, *Br J Obstet Gynecol* 91:444–448, 1984.
10. Golan A, Lin G, Evron S, et al: Oligohydramnios: maternal complication and fetal outcome in 145 cases, *Obstet Gynecol Invest* 37:91–95, 1994.
11. Matsuda Y, Kouno S: Fetal and neonatal outcomes in twin-oligohydramnios-polyhydramnios sequence including cerebral palsy, *Fetal Diag Ther* 17:268–271, 2002.
12. Chiang M-C, Lein R, Chau A-S, et al: Clinical consequences of twin-twin transfusion, *Eur J Pediatr* 162:68–71, 2003.
13. Newbould MJ, Barson AJ: Oligohydramnios sequence: the spectrum of renal malformations, *Br J Obstet Gynecol* 101:598–604, 1994.
14. Palacios J, Rodriguea JI: Extrinsic fetal akinesia and skeletal development: a study in oligohydramnios sequence, *Teratology* 42:1–5, 1990.
15. Chamberlain MB, Manning FA, Morrison L, et al: Ultrasound evaluation of amniotic fluid. II. The relationship of increase amniotic fluid volume to perinatal outcome, *Am J Obstet Gynecol* 150:250–254, 1984.
16. Brace RA, Wolf EJ: Normal amniotic fluid volume changes throughout pregnancy, *Am J Obstet Gynecol* 161:382–388, 1989.
17. Brace RA: Physiology of amniotic fluid volume regulation, *Clin Obstet Gynecol* 40:280–289, 1997.
18. Rotschild A, Ling EW, Puterman ML, et al: Neonatal outcome after prolonged preterm rupture of the membrane, *Am J Obstet Gynecol* 162:46–52, 1990.
19. Richards DS: Complications of prolonged PROM and oligohydramnios, *Clin Obstet Gynecol* 41:817–826, 1998.
20. Rib DM, Sherer DM, Woods JR: Maternal and neonatal outcome associated with prolonged premature rupture of membranes below 26 weeks' gestation, *Am J Perinatol* 10:369–373, 1993.
21. Nimrod C, Varela-Gittins F, Machin G, et al: The effect of very prolonged membrane rupture on fetal development, *Am J Obstet Gynecol* 148:540–543, 1984.
22. Thibeault DW, Beatty EC, Hall RT, et al: Neonatal pulmonary hypoplasia with premature rupture of fetal membranes and oligohydramnios, *J Pediatr* 107:273–277, 1985.
23. Christianson C, Huff D, McPherson E: Limb deformations in oligohydramnios sequence: effects of gestational age and duration of oligohydramnios, *Am J Med Genet* 86:430–433, 1999.
24. Smith DW: Commentary: redundant skin folds in the infant—their origin and relevance, *J Pediatr* 94:1021–1022, 1979.

25. Miller ME, Higginbottom MC, Smith DW: Short umbilical cord: its origin and relevance, *Pediatrics* 67:618–621, 1981.

26. Moessinger AC, Collins MH, Blanc WA, et al: Oligohydramnios-induced lung hypoplasia: the influence of timing and duration in gestation, *Pediatr Res* 20:951–954, 1986.

27. Kilbride HW, Yeast J, Thiebault DW: Defining limits of survival: lethal pulmonary hypoplasia after midtrimester premature rupture of membranes, *Am J Obstet Gynecol* 175:675–681, 1996.

28. Fisk NM, Ronderos-Dumit D, Soliani A, et al: Diagnostic and therapeutic transabdominal amnioinfusion in oligohydramnios, *Obstet Gynecol* 78:270–278, 1991.

29. Kilpatrick SJ: Therapeutic interventions for oligohydramnios: amnioinfusion and maternal hydration, *Clin Obstet Gynecol* 40:328–336, 1997.

30. Morse RP, Rawnsley BE, Crow HC, et al: Bilateral renal agenesis in three consecutive siblings, *Prenat Diagn* 7:573–579, 1987.

# 47 Fetal Akinesia Sequence

## GENESIS

Fetal movement is essential to normal joint morphogenesis. Joints develop secondarily within the condensed mesenchyme of the developing bones, and chronic lack of movement leads to joint contractures.[1-4] Fetal akinesia is associated with a specific combination of clinical findings that is sometimes called the *Pena-Shokeir phenotype* because these signs were first described as part of Pena-Shokeir syndrome.[2] These findings include fetal growth retardation, congenital contractures with underdeveloped limbs, polyhydramnios, pulmonary hypoplasia, short umbilical cord, and craniofacial alterations such as micrognathia, occasional cleft palate, hypertelorism, and short neck (Fig. 47-1). Hall emphasized the causal heterogeneity of this condition,[3] and Moessinger[4] demonstrated that rat fetuses paralyzed by daily transuterine injections of curare from day 18 of gestation until term on day 21 demonstrated a consistent pattern of abnormalities that he termed the *fetal akinesia deformation sequence* (FADS). In a dramatic human example, the mother of an infant born with multiple joint contractures (arthrogryposis) had received tubocurarine for 19 days in early pregnancy for the treatment of tetanus.[5] This phenotype represents an etiologically heterogeneous deformation sequence that can result from neuropathy, myopathy, restrictive dermopathy, teratogens, and intrauterine constraint due to prolonged oligohydramnios, which results in extrinsic fetal immobilization. Pena-Shokeir syndrome was first described in 1974 as an autosomal recessive type of fetal akinesia (see the affected brothers in Fig. 47-1), and, since that time, multiple cases have been reported with a wide variety of associated findings, which suggest causal heterogeneity and warrant the use of the more general term FADS.[2]

To provide appropriate care and counseling, it is most important to distinguish extrinsic factors that limit fetal movement (e.g., oligohydramnios or fetal crowding) from intrinsic factors due to neuromuscular abnormalities (Fig. 47-2). Both types of problems can lead to abnormalities of fetal presentation, hence the association between breech presentation and fetal abnormalities.[6] Fetal

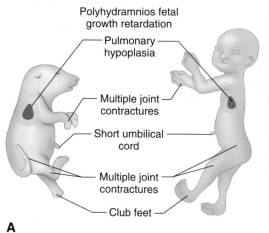
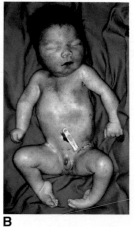
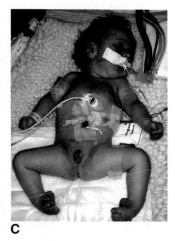

Polyhydramnios fetal growth retardation

Pulmonary hypoplasia

Multiple joint contractures

Short umbilical cord

Multiple joint contractures

Club feet

**A**  **B**  **C**

FIGURE 47-1. **A,** The fetal akinesia deformation sequence is a causally heterogeneous phenotype that can occur with a variety of congenital neuropathies and myopathies. **B** and **C,** These two newborn siblings with type I Pena-Shokeir syndrome were born with polyhydramnios, lethal pulmonary hypoplasia, and joint contractures. Attempts to diagnose recurrences during the second trimester were unsuccessful because the affected fetuses were still moving at this time, but polyhydramnios and limited fetal movement were evident during the third trimester. (**A,** From Moessinger AC: Fetal akinesia deformation sequence. An animal model, *Pediatrics* 72:857, 1983.)

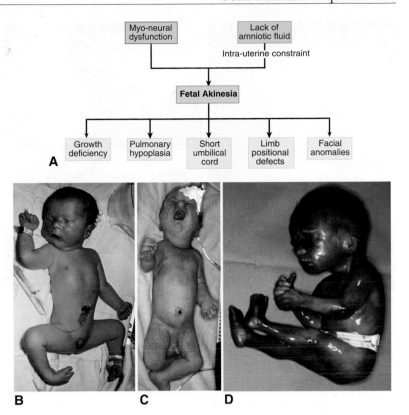

FIGURE 47-2. **A,** This diagram demonstrates the etiologically heterogeneous phenotype that results from fetal akinesia. **B,** This infant was born with myotonic dystrophy to a mother with the same condition. He had multiple joint contractures with thin bones and respiratory insufficiency. **C,** This infant was immobilized in a transverse lie after amnion rupture at 26 weeks. **D,** This fetus had bilateral renal agenesis resulting in oligohydramnios.

immobilization during late gestation can also give rise to transient joint limitation in normal newborns. In a morphometric study of 13 newborns with fetal akinesia due to oligohydramnios deformation sequence, normal growth of long bones and jaws distinguished fetuses with extrinsic fetal akinesia (5 with renal agenesis and 8 with obstructive uropathy) from those with intrinsic fetal akinesia due to congenital neuromuscular diseases, which resulted in slender, brittle, hypoplastic long bones and micrognathia.[7] There is ample evidence in both experimental animals and humans that fetal akinesia due to a variety of causes can lead to multiple joint contractures and other manifestations of fetal akinesia sequence.[1-10]

The fetal akinesia phenotype occurs in Pena-Shokeir syndrome (see Fig. 47-1), an autosomal recessive disorder,[2,11,12] and also in a number of other genetic fetal malformation syndromes.[8] Myotonic dystrophy can produce this phenotype[13] (Fig. 47-2, *B*), and similar effects have been noted in infants born to mothers with myasthenia gravis due to transplacental transfer of immunoglobulins, which are thought to create a neuromuscular blockade in the fetus (Fig. 47-3).[14-16] The manifestations and severity of fetal akinesia sequence may depend on the timing, duration, and degree of fetal akinesia, with multiple pterygia and increased nuchal

translucency resulting from early prolonged fetal akinesia (Fig. 47-4).

Duration of fetal akinesia may be determined through an analysis of the individual features. Prolonged neuromuscular akinesia limits bone growth, which affects subperiosteal growth in bone breadth much more severely then linear growth. This leads to the development of thin bones that may be susceptible to fractures.[17] The size of a muscle relates to the magnitude and frequency of forces it brings to bear across a joint, and with diminished function, muscles tend to atrophy. Thus, prolonged fetal akinesia results in low birth weight. Absence of flexion creases implies that the joint has never functioned, and, because most joints flex by the early second trimester, this implies early cessation of fetal movement. Polyhydramnios is a relatively late manifestation of the fetal akinesia sequence, which is usually associated with micrognathia due to diminished fetal swallowing. Fetal lung movements are necessary for normal pulmonary growth and maturation, thus, deficient diaphragmatic function can lead to pulmonary hypoplasia. The importance of fetal respiratory movements in normal lung morphogenesis was highlighted by a case report that described an infant with pulmonary hypoplasia due to phrenic nerve agenesis and diaphragmatic amyoplasia.[18] In an experimental fetal

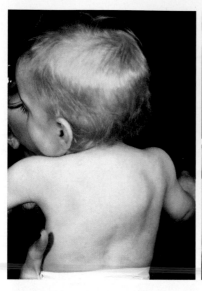
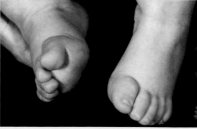
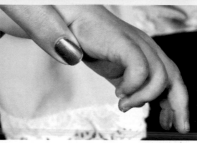

FIGURE 47-3. This female infant was born to a mother with myasthenia gravis. Both the infant and a subsequent sibling were born with hypotonia, multiple joint contractures, and severe scoliosis. (Courtesy of Mark Stephan, Madigan Army Hospital, Tacoma, Wash.)

rabbit model, destruction of the fetal cervical spinal cord in the C4–C6 region caused complete atrophy of the diaphragm in addition to cutting off motor pathways from the respiratory center. Higher lesions at C1–C3 preserved the phrenic nerve supply and hence allowed normal diaphragmatic growth but prevented any coordinated fetal respiratory activity. Each operation, when performed at 23 days of gestation during the late pseudoglandular phase of lung development, resulted in severe lung hypoplasia.[19] Consequently, with severe fetal akinesia that inhibits fetal swallowing and fetal lung movements, the fetus is usually born with micrognathia, polyhydramnios, and respiratory insufficiency from pulmonary hypoplasia.

The association of a shortened umbilical cord implies that fetal akinesia began during or prior to mid-gestation. Umbilical cord growth is influenced by tensile forces and depends on both fetal motion and the amount of space available for fetal movement.[20] This has been demonstrated in both humans and rats.[20-22] Oligohydramnios can severely limit fetal movement during the last half of gestation, and there is overlap between the oligohydramnios sequence and the fetal akinesia sequence, but oligohydramnios does not limit fetal long bone growth to the same extent seen with neuromuscular akinesia, which also results in thin, fragile bones.[7,17] Compression of skin in the oligohydramnios sequence leads to skin redundancy, whereas fetal akinesia is associated with thin, tight skin with few flexion creases.

Restrictive dermopathy is a rare, lethal, autosomal recessive disorder characterized by thin, shiny, rigid skin, and characteristic facial features (e.g., large anterior fontanelle; hypertelorism; a short, narrow, upturned nose; blepharophimosis with swollen lids

and exophthalmos; a small, open, O-shaped mouth; and micrognathia), whereby rigidity of the skin causes secondary generalized flexion contractures and restricted respiratory movements.[22-24] This condition results from autosomal recessive mutations in Laminin A/C *(LMNA)* or in a metalloproteinase gene involved in prelamin A post-translational processing *(FACE1)*, and it is another cause of the fetal akinesia phenotype. Similar skin findings been seen in type II Gaucher disease associated with icthyosis.[8]

When foot deformations are associated with polyhydramnios, this usually implies an intrinsic neuromuscular abnormality, whereas foot deformations associated with oligohydramnios suggest extrinsic constraint. In a study of 30 fetuses with FADS, detailed neuropathologic studies that included the brain, spinal cord, and muscles allowed a specific diagnosis to be made in 16 cases (53%).[25] Of these 16 cases, 9 had central nervous system abnormalities, 1 had spinal cord abnormality (spinal muscular atrophy I), 3 had a primary myopathy (nemaline myopathy and myotonic dystrophy), and 3 had a recognizable syndrome. In 10 other cases, neuromuscular pathology was evident but no specific diagnosis could be established. Only 4 patients had normal neuromuscular findings with no apparent etiology for the FADS. Most importantly, recurrences in subsequent pregnancies were noted among all three groups (specific diagnosis, nonspecific neuromuscular pathology, and normal neuromuscular pathology).[25]

## FEATURES

As described previously, the etiology of FADS is heterogeneous, and the severity of the phenotype

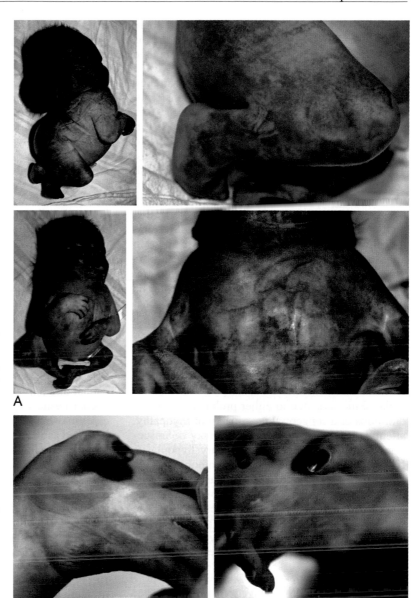

FIGURE 47-4. **A,** This fetus was recognized by prenatal ultrasound as having virtually no fetal movement and a large nuchal cystic hygroma. The hands were clenched, with no finger creases on examination. Amniocentesis revealed a normal karyotype, and multiple pterygia were noted postnatally. This illustrates the severe consequences of prolonged fetal akinesia in a fetus with lethal multiple pterygium syndrome and nuchal cystic hygroma. Muscle pathology demonstrated neurogenic atrophy. Some cases of lethal multiple pterygium syndromes have inactivating mutations in an embryonal acetylcholine rooeptor -subunit gene *(CHRNG)*. **B,** Absent flexion creases in the fetus with lethal multiple pterygium syndrome and nuchal cystic hygroma.

varies from severe, generalized, early-onset disorders to milder defects that present later in pregnancy.[25] The features of FADS often include breech head and features of Pena-Shokeir syndrome,[2] an autosomal recessive disorder that occurs in 1 in 12,000 births and has an extremely heterogeneous pathogenesis, hence the use of the term Pena-Shokeir phenotype as an alternative to FADS; however, the latter terminology is the preferred designation because Pena-Shokeir syndrome should be considered as only one subtype of FADS. Findings include fetal growth retardation, congenital contractures with underdeveloped limbs, polyhydramnios, pulmonary hypoplasia, short umbilical cord, and craniofacial alterations such as micrognathia, occasional cleft palate, hypertelorism, and short neck. The finding of prenatal-onset growth deficiency with polyhydramnios may suggest a neuromuscular cause, and fetal pathology can help establish a more specific diagnosis in many cases.[25] Polyhydramnios may result in premature delivery with severe respiratory distress due to pulmonary hypoplasia. A variety of congenital neuropathies and myopathies

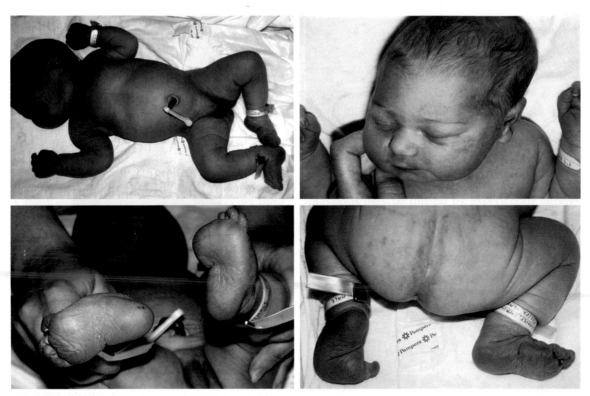

FIGURE 48-4. This infant was an abdominal pregnancy, with her head under the stomach and feet under the gallbladder. (Courtesy of Dr. Will Cochran, Beth Israel Hospital and Harvard Medical School, Boston, Mass.)

deficiency; the combined rate for both malformations and deformations is 21.4%.[16] The type of limb deficiency seen with abdominal pregnancy appears to be due to vascular disruption rather than a result of limb malformation, and, in some cases, it may be attributed to the severity of early fetal compression.[16]

## MANAGEMENT

When extrauterine pregnancy occurs, the embryo/fetus seldom survives, and oligohydramnios is frequent. If survival does occur, there is likely to be severe constraint of fetal development, and survival is greatly improved if the amniotic sac remains intact.[14] The overall mortality rate for the embryo/fetus is 75% to 95%,[17] with death usually resulting from pulmonary hypoplasia due to oligohydramnios and possibly fetal thoracic compression.[18] In a 1993 literature review concerning abdominal pregnancies, the maternal mortality rate dropped from 18.2% to 4.5% during the preceding 20 years, and the survival rate for infants of 30 weeks' gestation was 63%.[16] During surgery for an abdominal

pregnancy, the fetus should be removed and the cord clamped close to the placenta with minimal manipulation. Placental manipulation can lead to significant blood loss because there is no normal cleavage plane and no intrinsic mechanism similar to uterine contractility to control bleeding.[19] There is a 53.8% risk of peritonitis, intra-abdominal abscess, sepsis, or other febrile morbidity with advanced abdominal pregnancies, and a reported colonization of the gestational cavity with group B *Streptococcus* has been attributed to a ruptured tubal ectopic pregnancy that seeded the abdominal cavity with vaginal flora. Thus, preoperative prophylactic antibiotics and intraoperative cultures of the abdominal cavity and gestational sac have been suggested.[19] Most ovarian pregnancies (92%) fail to survive beyond the first trimester, and they present earlier than abdominal pregnancies because of the vascularity of the ovary and associated maternal hemorrhage.[11] Whereas the traditional treatment of advanced abdominal pregnancy was with laparotomy, the use of improved diagnostic techniques, such as transvaginal ultrasonography, have enabled new, minimally invasive laparoscopic techniques, selective embolization of vessels that supply the placenta, and medical management of the placenta with methotrexate.[20,21]

# DIFFERENTIAL DIAGNOSIS

Differential diagnosis includes pelvic sepsis, food poisoning, and ruptured ectopic pregnancy.[5] Ovarian pregnancies are rare events (about 10 times less common than abdominal pregnancies), and they must be distinguished from tubal ectopic pregnancy and hemorrhagic ovarian cyst.[11] Careful ultrasound assessment is indicated for every hemodynamically stable patient with a suspected ectopic pregnancy, and failure to respond to induction is a classic clue that the pregnancy might be extrauterine. If the pregnancy is not visualized in the uterus or tubes, then unusual locations such as the cervix, cornua, ovaries, and pouch of Douglas should be checked, as the rarer forms of ectopic pregnancy are generally more dangerous than tubal ectopic pregnancies. Unexplained abdominal ascites in a patient with a positive pregnancy test and no intrauterine gestational sac may be associated with abdominal pregnancy.[22] An ectopic pregnancy that implanted on the diaphragm and resulted in spontaneous hemothorax due to trophoblastic invasion of the pleura has also been reported.[23] Nontubal ectopic pregnancies account for less than 5% of all ectopic pregnancies but result in approximately 20% of the fatalities; therefore, additional measures such as laparoscopy and other imaging modalities (e.g., magnetic resonance imaging) may aid in diagnosis and management.[19,23] The most commonly reported anatomic locations of primary peritoneal implantations are the pouch of Douglas and the posterior uterine wall, but other reported locations have included the liver, spleen, intestines, retroperitoneum, diaphragm, broad ligament, omentum, ovary, and within a cesarean scar.[21-25] The key to early and successful diagnosis and management appears to be strong clinical suspicion and, simply put, "knowing where to look."

## References

1. Bouyer J, Coste J, Fernandez H, et al: Sites of ectopic pregnancy: a 10-year population-based study of 1800 cases, *Hum Reprod* 17:3224–3230, 2002.
2. Pisarska MD, Carson S: Incidence and risk factors for ectopic pregnancy, *Clin Obstet Gynecol* 42:2–8, 1999.
3. Kitade M, Takeuchi H, Kikuchi I, et al: A case of simultaneous tubal-splenic pregnancy after assisted reproductive technology, *Fertil Steril* 83:e19–e21, 2005.
4. Atrash HK, Friede A, Hogue CJ: Abdominal pregnancy in the United States: frequency and maternal mortality, *Obstet Gynecol* 69:333–337, 1987.
5. Ombelet W, Vandermerwe JV, Assche FA: Advanced extrauterine pregnancy: description of 38 cases with literature survey, *Obstet Gynecol* 59:386–397, 1988.
6. Martin JN, McCaul JF IV: Emergent management of abdominal pregnancy, *Clin Obstet Gynecol* 33:438–447, 1990.
7. Connor GF: Case of the month, *Crit Rev Comput Tomogr* 45:11–16, 2004.
8. Dubinsky TJ, Guerra F, Gormaz G, et al: Fetal survival in abdominal pregnancy: a review of 11 cases, *J Clin Ultrasound* 24:513–517, 1996.
9. Dover RW, Powell MC: Management of a primary abdominal pregnancy, *Am J Obstet Gynecol* 172:1603–1604, 1995.
10. Audain L, Brown WE, Smith DM, et al: Cocaine use as a risk factor for abdominal pregnancy, *J Natl Med Assoc* 90:277–283, 1998.
11. Nisenblat V, Leibovitz Z, Tal J, et al: Primary ovarian ectopic pregnancy misdiagnosed as first-trimester missed abortion, *J Ultrasound Med* 24:539–543, 2005.
12. Lee W, Voet RL, Poliak J: Combined intrauterine and ovarian pregnancy: a case report, *J Reprod Med* 30:563, 1985.
13. Hallet JG: Abdominal pregnancy: a study of twenty-one consecutive cases, *Am J Obstet Gynecol* 152:444–449, 1985.
14. Tan KL, Goon SM, Wee JH: The pediatric aspects of advanced abdominal pregnancy, *J Obstet Gynaec Br Commonw* 76:1021–1028, 1969.
15. Uglow MG, Clarke NM: Congenital dislocation of the hip in extrauterine pregnancy, *J Bone Joint Surg Br* 78:751–753, 1996.
16. Stevens CA: Malformations and deformations in abdominal pregnancy, *Am J Med Genet* 47:1189–1195, 1993.
17. Delke I, Veridanio NP, Tancer ML: Abdominal pregnancy: review of current management and addition of 10 cases, *Obstet Gynecol* 60:200–204, 1982.
18. Bell JB, Gerdes JS, Bhutani VK, et al: Chronic lung disorder following abdominal pregnancy, *Am J Dis Child* 141:1111–1113, 1987.
19. Bergstrom R, Mueller G, Yankowitz J: A case illustrating the continued dilemmas in treating abdominal pregnancy and a potential explanation for the high rate of postsurgical febrile morbidity, *Gynecol Obstet Invest* 46:268–270, 1998.
20. Rahamon J, Berkowitz R, Mitty H, et al: Minimally invasive management of an advanced abdominal pregnancy, *Obstet Gynecol* 103:1064–1068, 2004.
21. Graesslin O, Dedecker F, Quereux C, et al: Conservative treatment of ectopic pregnancy in a cesarean scar, *Obstet Gynecol* 105:869–871, 2005.
22. Ross JA, Hacket E, Lawton F, et al: Massive ascites due to abdominal pregnancy, *Hum Reprod* 12:390–391, 1997.
23. Fishman DA, Padilla LA, Joob A, et al: Ectopic pregnancy causing hemothorax managed by thoracscopy and actinomycin D, *Obstet Gynecol* 91:837–838, 1998.
24. Deshpande N, Mathers A, Acharya U: Broad ligament twin pregnancy following in-vitro fertilization, *Hum Reprod* 14:852–854, 1999.
25. Valley MT, Pierce JG, Daniel TB, et al: Cesarean scar pregnancy: imaging and treatment with conservative surgery, *Obstet Gynecol* 91:838–840, 1998.

# 49 Early Embryonic Compression or Disruption

## Tubal Ectopic Pregnancy, Early Uterine Compression, Early Amnion Rupture

## GENESIS

Constraint that occurs during the latter period of gestation can cause molded deformations with good prospects for spontaneous or assisted return to normal form; however, when constraint occurs during early morphogenesis, it can have more severe and lasting impacts on form. The types of defects that can be produced by such compression during this early period of organogenesis (i.e., within the first trimester) fall into three categories: molded deformations, incomplete morphogenesis, and disruptions of morphogenesis (Table 49-1). All three types of defects were produced experimentally by Poswillo after early amniotic sac puncture in rat embryos at 15.5 days' gestation.[1] At this stage of gestation, the rat embryo is at a period of development equivalent to that of the 6- to 7-week human embryo, and mesenchymal condensations have formed bones within the developing limbs, but the fingers are not fully separated (Fig. 49-1). The lip has fused, but the palatal shelves have not yet closed (Table 49-2). Amniotic bands were only present in 19% of the rat fetuses in Poswillo's study, and there were no defects in control animals.[1] Treated animals showed a small jaw that was caused by compression of the mandible against the sternum. In all but one rat fetus, this caused the tongue to be thrust between the posterior palatal shelves, thereby preventing closure of the palatal shelves (similar to what is seen in Pierre Robin sequence). Poswillo found that 29% of these rat fetuses with Robin sequence defects induced by oligohydramnios and compression also had limb defects.[1] Defects such as cleft palate and syndactyly were also interpreted as incomplete morphogenesis secondary to compression. Limb reduction defects involving the radius, femur, and other long bones were interpreted as resulting from vascular disruption due to focal hemorrhage and necrosis.

Vascular disruption is the most common cause of limb deficiency. In a hospital-based surveillance program of 161,252 infants born in the years 1972 to 1974 and 1979 to 1994, the overall prevalence of limb reduction defects was 0.69 per 1000 live births, with 34% of these defects attributed to vascular disruption (a prevalence of 0.22 per 1000 live births).[2] Kennedy and Persaud demonstrated that early amnion puncture, particularly on day 15 in the rat, leads to edema and hemorrhage, thereby causing tissue damage and resorption within the distal limbs, and these researchers showed that lower limbs are more affected than upper limbs (Figs. 49-2 and 49-3).[3] Webster et al demonstrated that a broad variety of uterine manipulations in pregnant mice during a similar early stage of

## TABLE 49-1. TYPES OF DEFECTS PRODUCED BY CONSTRAINT IN EARLY GESTATION

| DEFECT | DESCRIPTION |
| --- | --- |
| Molded deformations | Similar to those produced in late fetal life but often more severe; more difficult to return to normal form because of early onset |
| Incomplete morphogenesis | Constraint may limit or prevent full completion of a normal stage in morphogenesis |
| Disruption of morphogenesis | Constraint may cause edema, hemorrhage, and focal necrosis with loss of previously formed tissue |

296

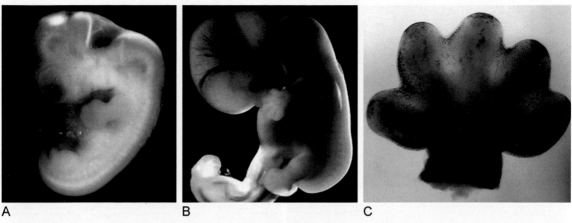

FIGURE 49-1. Human embryo at 32 to 36 days of development **(A)**, with the hand plate formed but no separation of the finger rays. By day 11 **(D)**, the process of apoptosis removes soft tissue between the digits **(C)**. Around this time constraint of the developing limb has been found in animal studies to cause edema, hemorrhage, and resorptive necrosis with loss of previous limb tissues. The process of separation of the digits may also be impaired, yielding syndactyly.

**TABLE 49-2. DEFECTS IN RAT FETUSES AFTER AMNION PUNCTURE AT 15.5 DAYS***

| DEFECT | PREVALENCE |
| --- | --- |
| Molded deformations | 100% |
| Micrognathia | 100% |
| Talipes | 5% |
| Incomplete morphogenesis | 97% |
| Failure of palatal closure | 97% |
| Syndactyly | 9% |
| Disruption of morphogenesis | 12% |
| Absent radius, femur | 6% |
| Phocomelia | 6% |

From Poswillo D: Observations of fetal posture and causal mechanisms of congenital deformity of the palate, mandible and limbs, *J Dent Res* 45:583, 1966.
*15.5 days in the rat fetus is similar to 42 to 45 days in the human fetus.

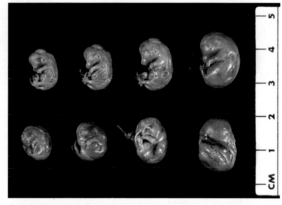

FIGURE 49-2. After early amnion puncture on day 15, rat fetuses are compressed in a cephalocaudal fashion with the developing mandible thrust against the sternum. From left to right, rat embryos are shown at 12, 24, 36, and 48 hours after amniotic puncture *(bottom row)*; a control fetus of the same gestational age is shown in the top row.
(Courtesy of T.V.N. Persauds, Department of Anatomy, University of Manitoba, Winnipeg, MP, Canada.)

gestation can result in hemorrhagic disruption of various fetal structures.[4]

The combination of early embryonic compression with vascular disruption that results in extensive extremity and body wall defects in humans has been termed *limb-body wall complex* (Fig. 49-4).[5-10] This defect occurs with a birth prevalence of 0.26 per 10,000 births, with half of the cases being stillborn, and there is a strong association with very low birth weight, short gestational age, and younger maternal age.[10] The spectrum of defects can include variable combinations of body wall defects with evisceration of thoracic and/or abdominal organs, limb deficiency, neural tube defects, and facial clefts, with or without amniotic bands and renal agenesis. Lower limbs are more severely and consistently affected than upper limbs, with distal structures more involved than proximal structures, similar to what is seen in rats subjected to early amnion puncture on day 15, which suggests a vascular pathogenesis.[10]

Infants with limb reduction defects due to early exposure to misoprostol or chorion villus sampling (CVS) have asymmetric digit loss, constriction rings, and syndactyly, as a result of vascular disruption in limb structures that had formed normally (Fig. 49-5). These defects can resemble

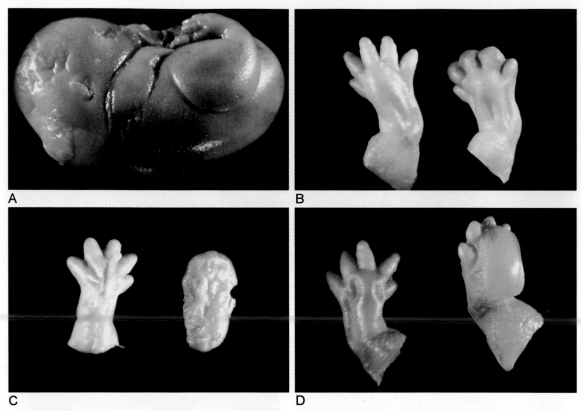

FIGURE 49-3. The limb compression leads to edema and hemorrhage, thereby causing tissue damage and resorption within the distal limbs, with lower limbs more affected than upper limbs. **A,** The rat fetus is shown 48 hours after amnion puncture on day 15 with edema, compression, and banding around a digit on the right foot. Individual paws are shown 36 hours after puncture with adactyly **(B)** and 48 hours after puncture with blebs **(C, D)**. Control paws of the same gestational age are shown on the left in **B** to **D**.
  (Courtesy of T.V.N. Persauds, Department of Anatomy, University of Manitoba, Winnipeg, MP, Canada.)

amniotic band disruption.[2] The underlying mechanism of such vascular disruption is embryonic hypotension and hypoxia followed by endothelial cell damage, hemorrhage, and necrosis with tissue loss.[4] Such defects are more likely to involve distal structures in the upper body (hands and tongue) than proximal structures or the lower body, with middle digital rays more affected than medial or lateral rays (see Fig. 49-5).[2,11-13] This milder spectrum of defects after early CVS may relate to milder insults and later timing than the spectrum of defects seen with body wall complex, but the pathogenesis is similar. The frequency of terminal transverse limb reduction defects is significantly higher after CVS than in nonexposed pregnancies, with earlier procedures resulting in more severe types of defects.[14,15] Absence of the distal portion of the third finger, with tapering and stiff joints, appears to be a distinctive feature of exposure to CVS.[15]

Misoprostol, a synthetic analog of prostaglandin E1, increases the amplitude and frequency of uterine contractions and stimulates uterine bleeding. When used illegally to induce abortions during the first trimester, it has been associated with limb reduction defects and Möbius sequence.[16-19] Other unsuccessful attempts to induce abortion during the first trimester have resulted in similar defects as well as other vascular disruption defects, such as arthrogryposis, amyoplasia, gastroschisis, bowel atresia, and scalp defects. Other types of defects may occur due to incomplete morphogenesis or compression, such as scoliosis, facial clefts, heart defects, cortical gyral abnormalities, camptodactyly, and syndactyly.[20-23] Similar defects have resulted after severe abdominal trauma in early pregnancy[24-28] and also after high maternal fever in early pregnancy.[29] These defects have also been reproduced experimentally through early amnion puncture, uterine manipulations, or hyperthermia in pregnant rats and mice.[1,5,21]

Matsunaga and Shiota recognized early spatial limitation as a significant factor in constraint-

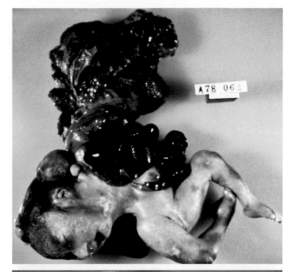

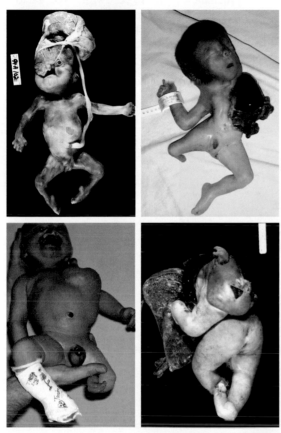

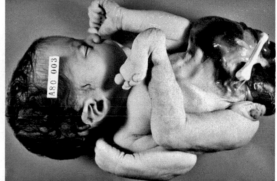

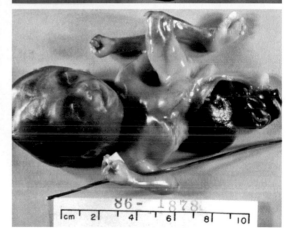

FIGURE 49-4. Examples of very early amnion rupture in lethally affected fetuses with facial clefts, amniotic disruption of limbs and facial structures, and limb-body wall defects.

(From Graham JM Jr, Miller ME, Stephan MJ, et al: Limb reduction anomalies and early in-utero limb compression, *J Pediatr* 96:1052, 1980.)

induced malformations, noting that 11.6% of 43 embryos and fetuses recovered from ectopic tubal pregnancies had structural defects, as did 6.2% of 97 fetuses from myomatous pregnancies, in contrast to a 3.3% incidence of structural defects among 3474 normally implanted therapeutic abortuses from non-myomatous uteri.[30] Amelia was present in 2 of the 5 fetuses with structural defects who implanted in a fallopian tube (Fig. 49-6), which is consistent with the notion that early fetal

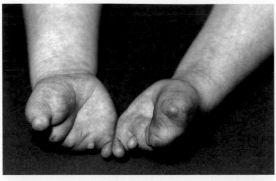

FIGURE 49-5. Disruptive loss of fingers in the hand (affecting central digits more severely) as a consequence of CVS performed at 7 to 8 weeks of gestation.

disruption leads to more severe limb reduction defects.[30]

*Ectopic pregnancy*, defined as the implantation of a fertilized ovum outside the uterus, occurs most commonly in the fallopian tube (see Fig. 49-6), with 70% implanting in the ampulla, 12% in the isthmus, 11% in the fimbrial end, 2% in the interstitial region, and 3% ovarian.[31] The incidence of ectopic pregnancies increased from 4.5 per 1000 pregnancies in 1970 to 19.7 per 1000 pregnancies in 1992, with risk factors including tubal damage or sterilization, use of an intrauterine device, infertility, previous genital infections, multiple sexual partners, and cigarette smoking.[31,32]

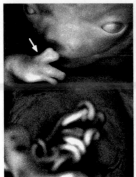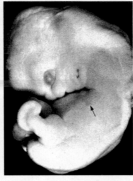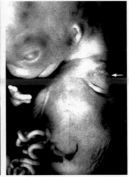

A

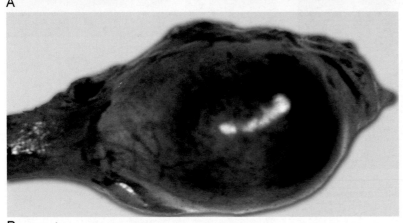

B

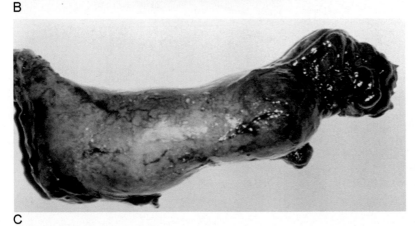

C

FIGURE 49-6. Embryos recovered from resected fallopian tubes showing amelia and syndactyly **(A)**. Ectopic pregnancies occur most commonly in the fallopian tube (95.5% of all ectopic pregnancies). These examples of tubal pregnancies demonstrate fimbrial implantation **(B)** (11% of all ectopic pregnancies) and isthmus implantation **(C)** (12% of all ectopic pregnancies).

## FEATURES

Among patients with body wall complex, with or without amniotic bands, observed defects have included scoliosis, joint contractures, Robin sequence, syndactyly, body wall defects with evisceration of thoracic and/or abdominal organs, limb deficiency, neural tube defects, facial clefts, with or without amniotic bands.[5-10] These defects are of a type that cannot be readily explained by amniotic band constriction alone, and lower limbs are more severely and consistently affected than upper limbs, with distal structures more involved than proximal structures, which suggests a vascular pathogenesis for many of these defects. Defects associated with CVS include terminal transverse limb reduction defects (with or without nubbing), amniotic band-like anomalies of the hands (e.g., digital fusion, syndactyly, constriction rings, loss of distal digits, tapered fingers with stiff joints; digits 2 to 4 are especially affected), hypoglossia, cranial nerve dysfunction, hemangiomas, intestinal atresia, clubfoot, and gastroschisis.[11-15,33-35] Defects associated with unsuccessful attempts at pregnancy termination or early abdominal trauma include arthrogryposis, amyoplasia, gastroschisis, bowel atresia, scalp defects, limb defects, Möbius sequence, scoliosis, facial clefts, heart defects, cortical gyral abnormalities, hydrocephaly, porencephaly, camptodactyly, and syndactyly.[16-28] Limb defects of all three types described in Table 49-2 have been noted in individuals who have been reared in constrictive environments, such as a fallopian tube, bicornuate uterus, or a uterus with large fibroids (see Chapter 45).[6,7,30] Unilateral limb defects of the type shown in Fig. 49-7 are typical of those seen with early limb compression.

## MANAGEMENT, PROGNOSIS, AND COUNSEL

Corrective surgery to improve limb function is indicated. In some cases of terminal transverse limb reduction defects, the use of prostheses can be beneficial. In most cases, infants learn to use the limbs they are born with much more readily than those who experience traumatic amputations after birth.

## DIFFERENTIAL DIAGNOSIS

Occasionally, distal limb reduction defects occur with scalp vertex aplasia due to the genetic disorder, Adams-Oliver syndrome (see Fig. 39-7). Death of

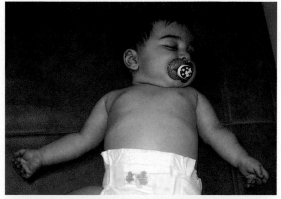
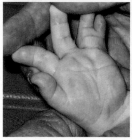
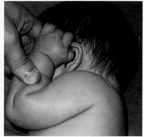

FIGURE 49-7. This infant with hypoplasia and compression-related dimpling of his left arm has hypoplasia with syndactyly of digits 4 and 5 of the left hand, which suggests early compression of the left arm and shoulder.

one monozygotic co-twin can result in vascular disruption defect in the surviving co-twin.[36] It should be kept in mind that arthrogryposis has many other causes that are much more common than failed obstetric termination procedures. Such procedures are usually recorded in the medical records (unless they are performed illegally); thus, with a careful history and pathologic examination of the products of conception, there should be little confusion as to the pathogenesis of such defects. Terminal transverse hemimelia has been associated with familial defects in anticoagulation,[37] and this can be investigated in the affected child and his or her mother by performing a thrombophilia evaluation. If defects are found, further treatment during subsequent pregnancies may be merited.

### References

1. Poswillo D: Observations of fetal posture and causal mechanisms of congenital deformity of the palate, mandible and limbs, *J Dent Res* 45:584–596, 1966.
2. McGuirk CK, Westgate MN, Holmes LB: Limb deficiencies in newborn infants, *Pediatrics* 108:e64, 2001.
3. Kennedy LA, Persaud TVN: Pathogenesis of developmental defects induced in the rat by amniotic sac puncture, *Acta Anat* 97:23–35, 1977.
4. Webster WS, Lipson AH, Brown-Woodman PDC: Uterine trauma and limb defects, *Teratology* 35:253–260, 1987.

5. Pagon RA, Stephens TD, McGillivray BC, et al: Body wall defects with reduction limb anomalies: report of fifteen cases, *BDOAS* 15(5A):171–185, 1979.

6. Graham JM Jr, Miller ME, Stephan MJ, et al: Limb reduction anomalies and early in-utero limb compression, *J Pediatr* 96:1052–1056, 1980.

7. Graham JM Jr: Causes of limb reduction defects: the contribution of fetal constraint and/or vascular disruption, *Clin Perinatol* 13:575–591, 1986.

8. Van Allen MI, Curry C, Gallagher L: Limb body wall complex: I, *Pathogenesis.* Am J Med Genet 28:529–548, 1987.

9. Van Allen MI, Curry C, Walden CE, et al: Limb body wall complex: II, *Limb and spine defects Am J Med Genet* 28:549–565, 1987.

10. Martinez-Frias ML: Clinical and epidemiological characteristics of infants with body wall complex with and without limb deficiency, *Am J Med Genet* 73:170–175, 1997.

11. Burton BK, Schulz CJ, Burd LI: Limb anomalies associated with chorionic villus sampling, *Lancet* 79:726–730, 1992.

12. Los FJ, Brandenburg H, Niermeijer MF: Vascular disruptive syndromes after exposure to misoprostol or chorionic villus sampling, *Lancet* 353:843–844, 1999.

13. Light TR, Ogden JA: Congenital constriction band syndrome: pathophysiology and treatment, *Yale J Biol Med* 66:143–155, 1993.

14. Brumback BA, Holmes LB, Ryan LM: Adverse effects of chorionic villus sampling: a meta-analysis, *Stat Med* 18:2163–2175, 1999.

15. Golden CM, Ryan LM, Holmes LB: Chorionic villus sampling: a distinctive teratogenic effect on fingers? *Birth Defects Res (Part A)* 67:557–562, 2003.

16. Gonzalez CH, Vargas FR, Perez ABA, et al: Limb deficiency with or without Mobius sequence in seven Brazilian children associated with misoprostol use in the first trimester of pregnancy, *Am J Med Genet* 47:59–64, 1993.

17. Pastuszak AL, Schuler L, Speck-Martins CE, et al: Use of misoprostol during pregnancy and Mobius syndrome in infants, *N Engl J Med* 338:1881–1885, 1998.

18. Oriolli IM, Castilla EE: Epidemiological assessment of misoprostol teratogenicity, *Br J Obstet Gynaecol* 107:519–523, 2000.

19. Vargus FR, Schuler-Faccini L, Brunoni D, et al: Prenatal exposure to misoprostol and vascular disruption defects: a case-control study, *Am J Med Genet* 95:302–306, 2000.

20. Reid CO, Hall JG, Anderson C, et al: Association of amyoplasia with gastroschisis, bowel atresia and defects of the muscular layer of the trunk, *Am J Med Genet* 78:451–457, 1986.

21. Lipson AH, Webster WS, Brown-Woodman PD, et al: Moebius syndrome: animal model, human correlations,

and evidence for a brainstem vascular etiology, *Teratology* 40:339–350, 1989.

22. Holmes LB: Possible fetal effects of cervical dilatation and uterine curettage during the first trimester of pregnancy, *J Pediatr* 126:131–134, 1995.

23. Hall JG: Arthrogryposis (AMC) associated with unsuccessful attempts at termination of pregnancy, *Am J Med Genet* 63:293–300, 1996.

24. Meyer H, Cummins H: Severe maternal trauma in early pregnancy: congenital amputations in infant at term, *Am J Obstet Gynecol* 40:150–160, 1941.

25. Steigner M, Stewart RE, Setoguchi Y: Combined limb deficiencies and cranial nerve dysfunction: report of 6 cases, *BDOAS* 11:133–141, 1975.

26. Ossipoff V, Hall BD: Etiologic factors in the amniotic band syndrome in a study of 24 patients, *BDOAS* 13:117–132, 1977.

27. Traboulsi EI, Maumene IH: Extraocular muscle aplasia in Moebius syndrome, *J Pediatr Ophthalmol* 23:120–122, 1986.

28. Viljoen DL: Porencephaly and terminal transverse limb defects following severe maternal trauma in early pregnancy, *Clin Dysmorphol* 4:75–78, 1995.

29. Martinez-Frias ML, Garcia-Mazario MJ, Feito-Caldas C, et al: High maternal fever during gestation and severe limb disruptions, *Am J Med Genet* 98:201–203, 2001.

30. Matsunaga E, Shiota K: Ectopic pregnancy and myoma uteri: teratogenic effects and maternal characteristics, *Teratology* 21:61–69, 1980.

31. Bouyer J, Coste J, Fernandez H, et al: Sites of ectopic pregnancy: a 10-year population-based study of 1800 cases, *Hum Reprod* 17:3224–3230, 2002.

32. Pisarska MD, Carson S: Incidence and risk factors for ectopic pregnancy, *Clin Obstet Gynecol* 42:2–8, 1999.

33. Firth HV, Boyd PA, Chamberlain P, et al: Severe limb abnormalities after chorionic villus sampling at 56-66 days' gestation, *Lancet* 337:762–763, 1991.

34. Mahoney MJ: Limb abnormalities and chorionic villus sampling, *Lancet* 337:1422–1423, 1991.

35. Stoler JM, McGuirk CK, Lieberman E, et al: Malformations reported in chorionic villus sampling exposed children: a review and analytic synthesis of the literature, *Genet Med* 1:315–322, 1999.

36. Zankl A, Brooks D, Boltshauser E, et al: Natural history of twin disruption sequence, *Am J Med Genet* 127:133–138, 2004.

37. Hunter AG: A pilot study of the possible role of familial defects in anticoagulation as a cause for terminal limb reduction malformations, *Clin Genet* 57:197–204, 2000.

# 50 Obstetric Procedure–Related Defects

## EARLY CVS, AMNIOCENTESIS NEEDLE INJURIES, INCOMPLETE D&C, FETAL REDUCTION PROCEDURES, PLACENTAL TRAUMA

### GENESIS

The underlying mechanism for most defects related to problems associated with obstetric procedures is vascular disruption. With chorionic villus sampling (CVS), removal of villi may result in embryonic hypotension, hypoxia, endothelial damage, hemorrhage, and necrosis with tissue loss.[1] Defects are more likely to involve distal structures in the upper body (hands and tongue) than proximal structures or the lower body, with middle digital rays more affected than medial or lateral rays (Fig. 50-1).[1-4] Following blunt trauma to the placenta, Quintaro et al[5] noted numerous ecchymoses that might be related to the increased frequency of hemangiomas in CVS-exposed infants. Limb defects caused by vascular disruption have a birth prevalence of 0.22 per 1000, accounting for 34% of all limb reduction defects (which occur with a prevalence rate of 0.69 per 1000).[6] The frequency of terminal transverse limb reduction defects is significantly higher after CVS than in nonexposed pregnancies, with earlier procedures resulting in more severe types of defects and a higher frequency of procedure-related defects.[7] The estimated risk for terminal transverse defects after CVS is estimated to be between 1:1000 and 1:3000.[8] Therefore, it is recommended that CVS only be performed after 10 weeks of gestation. Most experienced operators try to insert the CVS catheter into the chorion frondosum because if the catheter enters the decidua, it can cause hemorrhages. Loss rates after CVS increase with the number of insertions, and inexperienced operators usually require more insertions in order to obtain adequate samples.

Several case reports of infants born after failed attempts at dilatation and curettage (D&C) report vascular disruption defects such as limb reduction defects and amniotic band–related defects affecting limbs, facial clefts, and the cranium.[9,10] There is also a case report of a dichorionic-diamniotic twin born with hydrocephalus, clubfeet, and hypoplastic toes following myomectomy at 12 weeks of gestation for a 10-cm posterior retroplacental subserous uterine myoma.[11] Severe abdominal trauma at 52 days postconception has been hypothesized to cause blunt trauma to the abdomen, resulting in terminal transverse limb reduction defects and porencephaly.[12] Needle injuries from amniocentesis have been reported, primarily in the era prior to ultrasound-guided procedures (Figs. 50-2 and 50-3).[13-24] Contemporary midtrimester amniocen-

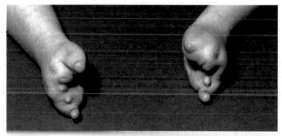
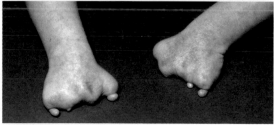

FIGURE 50-1. Disruptive loss of fingers in the hand (affecting central digits more severely). The mother of this fetus underwent CVS at 7 to 8 weeks, and, in addition to these digital reduction defects, there was a flank hemangioma.

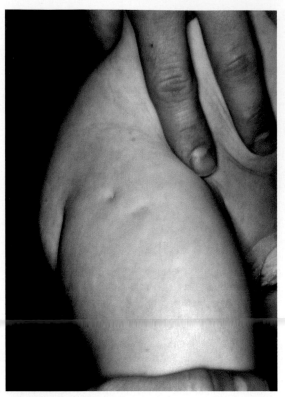

FIGURE 50-2. Amniocentesis puncture needle marks on an infant's thigh. The parent reported that the amniocentesis was done without ultrasound guidance and that the needle had to be repositioned several times before eventually drawing bloody amniotic fluid, which yielded a normal male karyotype.

tesis with concurrent ultrasound guidance in controlled studies appears to be associated with a procedure-related rate of excess pregnancy loss of 0.6% and reductions in the incidence of needle punctures and bloody amniotic fluid.[25] Early amniocentesis (i.e., at 11 to 12 weeks instead of 15 to 16 weeks) has been implicated as one cause of clubfoot. In the Canadian Early and Mid-Trimester Amniocentesis Trial (CEMAT), the risk of talipes equinovarus was increased from 0.1% with midtrimester amniocentesis to 1.4% with early amniocentesis.[26,27] Amniotic fluid leakage before 22 weeks was the only significant factor associated with clubfoot, there being a 15% risk with leakage but only a 1.1% risk without leakage (Fig. 50-4). None of the cases had persistent leakage at 18 to 20 weeks. In some circumstances, early amniocentesis might result in a developmental arrest of the foot as it transitions from a normal equinus position at 9 weeks to a neutral position at 12 weeks. The lateral side of the distal tibia grows faster than the

medial side, which perhaps results in pressure necrosis of the lateral distal tibia at 11 to 12 weeks.[27] An infant with vascular disruption defects has also been reported after a selective reduction of multiple gestations.[28]

## FEATURES

Defects in CVS-exposed pregnancies include terminal transverse limb reduction defects (with or without nubbins), amniotic band–like anomalies of the hands (digital fusion, syndactyly, constriction rings, loss of distal digits, and tapered fingers with stiff joints; digits 2 to 4 are especially affected) (see Fig. 50-1), hypoglossia, cranial nerve dysfunction, hemangiomas, intestinal atresia, clubfoot, and gastroschisis.[29-31] Amniocentesis is the presumed cause of many types of penetrating fetal injuries, including skin puncture marks (see Fig. 50-2), ocular perforation, limb, chest and abdominal trauma, cranial nerve injuries, porencephaly (see Fig. 50-3), and arteriovenous fistulae, with the vast majority of these injuries occurring in the era prior to ultrasound-guided amniocentesis. Early amniocentesis at 11 to 12 weeks has been associated with a 1% to 2% risk for talipes equinovarus (see Fig. 50-4).[26,27] Most of these injuries are due to direct trauma or a result of secondary vascular disruption or amniotic band disruption (Fig. 50-5).

## MANAGEMENT, PROGNOSIS, AND COUNSEL

Approximately 1% to 2% of twin pregnancies manifest a defect in one of the twins, causing prenatal care providers to consider selective feticide. In dichorionic pregnancy, the passage of substances and thromboembolic debris from one twin into the circulation of the co-twin is unlikely due to the lack of placental anastomoses; hence potassium chloride can be injected safely into the circulation of the affected twin to produce fetal asystole. In monochorionic twin pregnancies, selective termination can be performed only after complete and permanent occlusion of both the arterial and venous flows in the umbilical cord of the affected twin. Bipolar cord coagulation under ultrasound guidance is associated with a 70% to 80% survival rate in the unaffected co-twin.[32]

Surgery to improve limb function may be indicated for some terminal transverse limb reduction defects, and in some cases, the use of prostheses can be beneficial. In most cases, infants learn to use their deficient limbs more readily than those

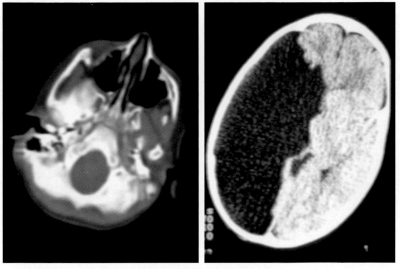

FIGURE 50-3. Amniocentesis-induced porencephaly following amniocentesis done on monozygotic twins during the 16th week without ultrasound guidance. This twin was the first to be tapped after ultrasound was used to identify a fluid pocket and then removed to prep the abdomen. Because the first two needle insertions went through apparent obstructions without yielding fluid, a third insertion was made, and chromosomally normal bloody fluid was obtained. The other twin had a separate amniotic sac and was tapped without incident. The first twin was born with porencephaly resulting from loss of flow in the right carotid artery, causing loss of tissue in the distribution of the right middle and posterior cerebral arteries. An external puncture site was evident just above the right ear, and she had severe mental retardation with seizures and a left hemiparesis. Magnetic resonance imaging confirmed the porencephaly and demonstrated normal carotid cranial foramina.

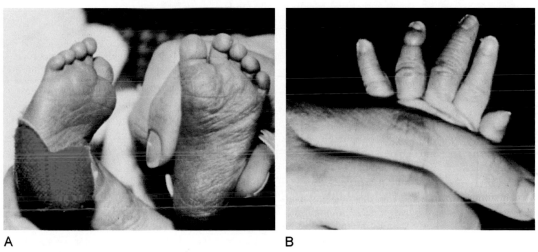

A                                                        B

FIGURE 50-4. This rigid equinovarus foot deformity **(A)** was associated with an amniotic band around a finger **(B)** and a history of amniotic fluid leakage at 11 to 12 weeks.

who experience traumatic amputations after birth. Such sporadic limb reduction defects due to obstetric procedures have no significant recurrence risk, and in many instances they can be prevented or minimized by performing procedures at the proper time and under real-time ultrasound guidance. A careful examination of the placenta is indicated to search for placental infarcts and clots, which might suggest that placental thrombosis contributed to the limb reduction defects (Fig. 50-6). In

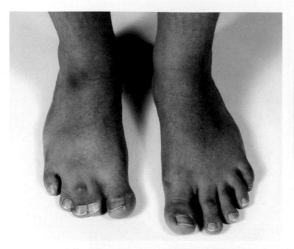

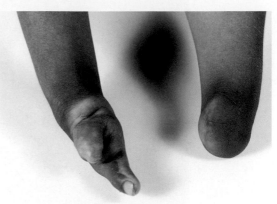

FIGURE 50-5. This boy was born with asymmetric terminal transverse limb reduction defects of the hand and wrist, short left lower leg and foot, syndactyly of the middle digits of the right foot, hypoglossia, and missing teeth. At 12 weeks' gestation, his mother went to an emergency department for vaginal bleeding, and a ring forceps was passed into the uterine cavity, resulting in passage of blood-tinged amniotic fluid and uterine cramping. The boy was diagnosed as having hypoglossia-hypodactyly due to vascular disruption.

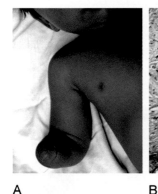

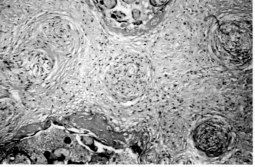

FIGURE 50-6. **A,** This boy was born at term with a right terminal transverse limb reduction defect. **B,** Examination of his placenta revealed multiple areas of occlusion and thrombosis of large fetal vessels with normal blood supply to the intervillous spaces.

(Courtesy of H. Eugene Hoyme, Stanford University Medical Center, Palo Alto, Calif.)

A                    B

addition, underlying inherited thrombophilias may predispose toward vascular disruption in some terminal transverse limb deficiency defects.[33] Because the risk of vascular disruption may be increased when certain common mutations within the coagulation pathway are present in the fetus and/or mother, and because such mutations can be inherited from an asymptomatic parent, a thrombophilia evaluation of the child and parents should be considered in any birth with an unexplained limb reduction defect.

## DIFFERENTIAL DIAGNOSIS

Occasionally, distal limb reduction defects occur with scalp vertex aplasia due to a genetic disorder, Adams-Oliver syndrome (see Fig. 39-7). Maternal hyperthermia during the late first trimester, resulting in fever over 39° C [102.2° F] for more than 2 days, can cause severe congenital limb disruption with hypoglossia, terminal transverse hemimelia, and Möbius sequence (Fig. 50-7).[34-37] The fetal death of a monozygotic co-twin can result in vasculodisruptive defects in the surviving co-twin. Finally, arthrogryposis has many different causes that are much more common than failed obstetric termination procedures. Such obstetric procedures are usually recorded in the medical records along with pathologic examination of the products of conception, so there should be little confusion as to the pathogenesis of such defects. There is some indication that the risk of fetal hemorrhage and resultant vascular disruption may be increased with

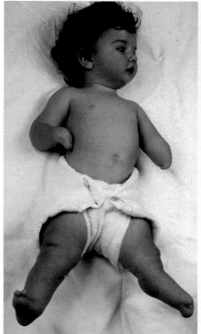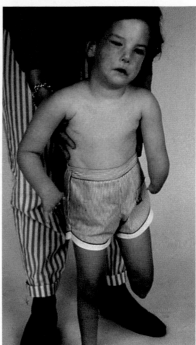

FIGURE 50-7. These children were born following prolonged high fever at 7 weeks' gestation with terminal transverse limb reduction defects, ankyloglossia, missing teeth, and bilateral 6th and 7th cranial nerve palsies. This same pattern of defects has been induced experimentally in animals following exposures to heat at an equivalent stage of gestation.

(Courtesy of Tony Lipson, Camperdown Children's Hospital, Sydney, Australia.)

certain common mutations within the coagulation pathway, which may be inherited from an asymptomatic parent, are present in the fetus.[33]

## References

1. Holmes LB: Teratogen-induced limb defects, *Am J Med Genet* 112:297–303, 2002.
2. Golden CM, Ryan LM, Holmes LB: Chorionic villus sampling: a distinctive teratogenic effect on fingers? *Birth Defects Res (Part A)* 67:557–562, 2003.
3. Los FJ, Brandenburg H, Niermeijer MF: Vascular disruptive syndromes after exposure to misoprostol or chorionic villus sampling, *Lancet* 353:843–844, 1999.
4. Light TR, Ogden JA. Congenital constriction band syndrome: pathophysiology and treatment, *Yale J Biol Med* 66:143–155, 1993.
5. Quintaro RA, Romero R, Mahoney MJ, et al: Fetal hemorrhagic lesions after chorionic villus sampling, *Lancet* 339:193, 1992.
6. McGuirk CK, Westgate M-N, Holmes LB: Limb deficiencies in newborn infants, *Pediatrics* 108:e64–c76, 2001.
7. Brumback BA, Holmes LB, Ryan LM: Adverse effects of chorionic villus sampling: a meta-analysis, *Stat Med* 18:2163–2175, 1999.
8. Olney RS, Khoury MG, Alo CJ, et al: Increased risk for terminal transverse digital deficiency after chorionic villus sampling: results of the United States Multistate Case-Control Study, 1988–1992, *Teratology* 51:20–29, 1995.
9. Holmes LB: Possible fetal effects of cervical dilatation and uterine curettage during the first trimester of pregnancy, *J Pediatr* 126:131–134, 1995.
10. Hall JG: Arthrogryposis (AMC) associated with unsuccessful attempts at termination of pregnancy, *Am J Med Genet* 63:293–300, 1996.
11. Danzer E, Hotzgreve W, Batukan P, et al: Myomectomy during the first trimester associated with fetal limb anomalies and hydrocephalus in a twin pregnancy, *Prenat Diagn* 21:848–851, 2001.
12. Viljoen DL: Porencephaly and terminal transverse limb defects following severe maternal trauma in early pregnancy, *Clin Dysmorphol* 4:75–78, 1995.
13. Broome DP, Wilson MG, Weiss B, et al: Needle puncture of fetus: a complication of second trimester amniocentesis, *Am J Obstet Gynecol* 126:247–252, 1976.
14. Naylor G, Roper JP, Willshaw HE: Ophthalmic complications of amniocentesis, *Eye* 4:845–849, 1990.
15. Rummelt V, Rummelt C, Naumann GOH: Congenital nonpigmented epithelial iris cyst after amniocentesis: clinicopathologic report on two children, *Ophthalmology* 100:776–781, 1993.
16. Creasman WT, Lawrence RA, Thiede HA: Fetal complications of amniocentesis, *JAMA* 204:949–952, 1968.
17. Epley SL, Hanson JW, Cruikshank DP: Fetal injury with midtrimester amniocentesis, *Obstet Gynecol* 53:77–80, 1979.
18. Egley CC: Laceration of fetal spleen during amniocentesis, *Am J Obstet Gynecol* 116:582–583, 1973.
19. Cromie WJ, Bates RB, Duckett JW: Penetrating renal trauma in the neonate, *J Urol* 119:259–260, 1978.
20. Patel CK, Taylor DSI, Russell-Eggitt IM, et al: Congenital third nerve palsy associated with mid-trimester amniocentesis, *Br J Ophthal* 77:530–533, 1993.
21. Chong SKF, Levitt GA, Lawson J, et al: Subarachnoid cyst with hydrocephalus—a complication of mid-trimester amniocentesis, *Prenat Diagn* 9:677–679, 1989.
22. Youroukos S, Papdelis F, Matsanoitis N: Porencephalic cyst after amniocentesis, *Arch Dis Child* 55:814–815, 1980.
23. Ledbetter DJ, Hall DG: Traumatic arteriovenous fistula; a complication of amniocentesis, *J Ped Surg* 27:720–721, 1992.

24. Williamson RA, Varner MW, Grant SS: Reduction in amniocentesis risks using a real-time needle guide procedure, *Obstet Gynecol* 65:751–755, 1985.

25. Seeds JW: Diagnostic midtrimester amniocentesis: how safe? *Am J Obstet Gynecol* 191:608–616, 2004.

26. Randomized trial to assess safety and fetal outcome of early and midtrimester amniocentesis: The Canadian Early and Mid-trimester Amniocentesis Trial (CEMAT) Group, *Lancet* 351:242–247, 1998.

27. Farrell SA, Summers AM, Dallaire L, et al: Club foot, an adverse outcome of early amniocentesis: disruption or deformation? CEMAT. Canadian Early and Mid-Trimester Amniocentesis Trial, *J Med Genet* 36:843–846, 1999.

28. Roze JM, Tschupp MJ, Arvis PL, et al: Interruption selective de grossesses et malformations embryonnaires des extremities, *J Gynecol Obstet Biol Reprod* 18:673–677, 1989.

29. Firth HV, Boyd PA, Chamberlain P, et al: Severe limb abnormalities after chorionic villus sampling at 56–66 days' gestation, *Lancet* 337:762–763, 1991.

30. Mahoney MJ: Limb abnormalities and chorionic villus sampling, *Lancet* 337:1422–1423, 1991.

31. Stoler JM, McGuirk CK, Lieberman E, et al: Malformations reported in chorionic villus sampling exposed children: a review and analytic synthesis of the literature, *Genet Med* 1:315–322, 1999.

32. Rustico MA, Baletti MG, Coviello D, et al: Managing twins discordant for fetal anomaly, *Prenat Diagn* 25:766–771, 2005.

33. Hunter AGW: A pilot study of the possible role of familial defects in anticoagulation as a cause for terminal limb reduction malformations, *Clin Genet* 57:197–204, 2000.

34. Lipson AH, Webster WS, Woodman-Brown PDC, et al: Moebius syndrome animal model—human correlations and evidence for brainstem vascular etiology, *Teratology* 40:339–350, 1989.

35. Superneau DW, Wertelecki W: Brief clinical report: similarity of effects—experimental hyperthermia as a teratogen and maternal febrile illness associated with oromandibular and limb defects, *Am J Med Genet* 21:575–580, 1985.

36. Martinez-Frias ML, Garcia Mazario MJ, Feito Caldas C, et al: High maternal fever during gestation and severe congenital limb disruptions, *Am J Med Genet* 98:201–203, 2001.

37. Graham JM Jr, Edwards MJ, Edwards MJ: Teratogen update: gestational effects of maternal hyperthermia due to febrile illnesses and resultant patterns of defects in humans, *Teratology* 58:209–221, 1998.

# Mechanics in Morphogenesis

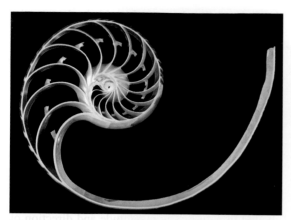

FIGURE 51-5. The growing nautilus mollusk outgrows one chamber after another, thus creating an equiangular, logarithmic spiral shell.

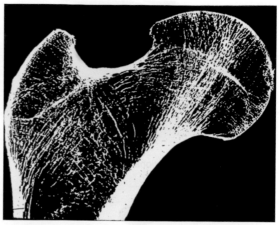

FIGURE 51-7. This section of the proximal human femur beautifully illustrates the relationship between function and form in the alignment of the bone spicules, which relate to the orientation of collagen fibrils.

(From Thompson D: *On growth and form. A new edition*, Cambridge, 1942, Cambridge University Press.)

Another beautiful example from nature of the impact of the size and direction of forces on form is the alignment of cellulose fibers in a tree. The reason the tree grows straight up relates to the alignment of cellulose fibers in the direction of the stress force of gravity. Extrinsic forces, such as compression by snow during the winter, may deform the young tree. However, once released from such temporary constraint, the sapling will again tend to grow in the direction of the force of gravity. The forces of prevailing winds may be sufficient to deform a tree (Fig. 51-6), and controlled external forces may be used to deform a young tree into a form that will be maintained after the tree is fully grown.

The collagen fibrils within developing bone may be compared with the cellulose fibers of a

Fish — shark

Reptile — ichthyosaur

Mammal — dolphin

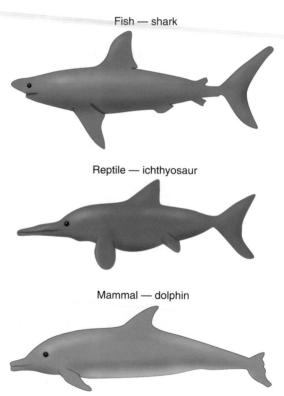

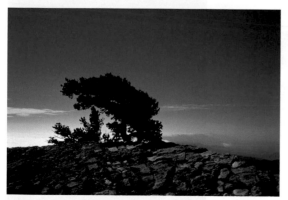

FIGURE 51-6. Ridgetop tree showing deformation by the prevailing winds that blow from right to left.

FIGURE 51-8. The adaptation of the form toward reducing turbulence and toward ease of free movement in water is beautifully exemplified by the similarities of form in a larger free-swimming fish, a reptile, and a mammal. In this environment, gravity is of less importance than is the buoyancy of the sea in shaping form.

(Adapted from Bunnell S, McIntyre J: *Mind in the water*, New York, 1974, Charles Scribner & Sons.)

tree. They are the basic structural elements, and they also align in the direction of stress in such a manner as to resist shear forces, as previously indicated. This is dramatically evidenced in the longitudinal section of the human femur shown in Fig. 51-7. The bone spicules are aligned in the direction of the stress of gravitational weight bearing and also in relation to muscle pull. The form of the upper femur relates to the combined forces of weight bearing plus the pull of major muscle groups. This results in a sloping "neck" of the femur and the two large promontories of bone in this region of the femur, the greater and lesser trochanters.

The force lines that are evident in the form of such a bone may be of value to the engineer in his or her design of somewhat similar structures. D'Arcy Thompson relates the story of a Zurich engineer, Professor Culmann, who became famous for his design of a mechanical crane. In the design of his crane, he used stress forces that he observed in a longitudinal section of the human femur in 1871. When shown the section of the femur by his friend, Professor Hermann von Meyer of the Anatomy Institute of the University of Zurich, Professor Culmann exclaimed, "There is my crane!" Possibly, there should be a closer interchange between biology and engineering, as the biomechanically determined "lines of stress" are naturally evident in many living creatures. The differences in these lines of stress will vary with the function of a bone. In the wings of a soaring bird, such as a vulture, the lines of stress relate to forces above and beneath the wing. The bone form in the pneumatized bone of a vulture is aligned accordingly and appears remarkably similar to the form that engineers learned to use in the wing girders of early airplanes, as well as in bridge trusses.

Mechanical forces play a major role in the form of an individual and relate to the function of that individual; for example, the pneumatized lightweight but strong bones of the larger soaring birds. The largest soaring mammal was the extinct

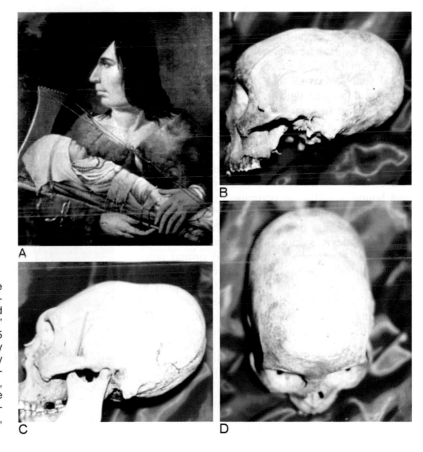

FIGURE 51-9. The Kwakiutl Native Americans of the Pacific Northwest used cedar boards and leather thongs to mold infants' heads. Boys were molded for 5 months, and girls were generally molded for 7 months. (**A,** Courtesy of Bill Holm, Burke Museum of Natural History and Culture, Seattle, Wash.; **B** to **D,** courtesy of Dr. Kate Donahue, Department of Anthropology, Plymouth State College, Plymouth, New Hampshire.)

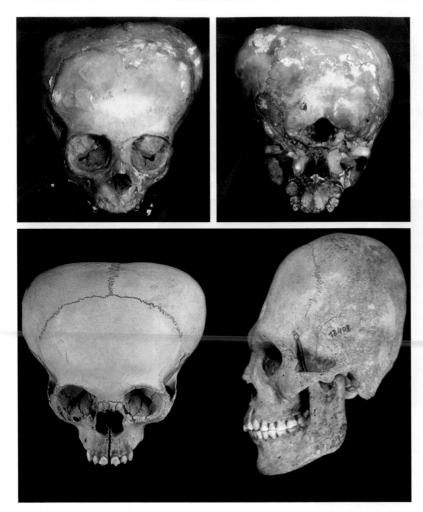

FIGURE 51-12. These bi-lobed, brachycephalic skulls from coastal Peru resulted from the application of boards to the occiput with pads to the frontal region and circumferential banding. Molding devices were applied until around age 8 months and then discarded because the desired deformation would persist.

(Courtesy of Dr. Kate Donahue, Department of Anthropology, Plymouth State College, New Hampshire.)

have achieved a combined weight of 4.0 kg, they become constrained, and their growth rate tends to slow, as also noted in animal studies. If only one animal is reared in a uterine horn, the newborn is appreciably larger at birth than when many are reared in the same uterine horn.[10] Situations other than multiple births may limit the available intrauterine space and cause it to yield a smaller baby, such as oligohydramnios, uterine malformation, and uterine fibroids (Fig. 51-15).

## Effects on Specific Tissues

### Bone

The early cartilage models of different long bones appear to be genetically specified, but the alignment of collagen fibrils and of bone trabeculae relate to mechanical forces, as do the bony promontories. Collagen fibrils align in the same direction as stress forces, thereby helping to resist shear forces, and sites of muscle attachment relate to muscle tension. For example, the size and shape of the greater trochanter relates to the relatively massive pull of five muscles at that site, including the very strong gluteus maximus muscle. The lesser trochanter only has one major muscle attaching at that site, the psoas minor. The combined forces of weight bearing plus muscle pull affect the form of the upper femur, including the normal configuration of the "neck" of the femur. Prolonged muscle weakness in the growing child may give rise to smaller trochanters and a straighter neck of the femur, termed the *coxa valga deformity* (Fig. 51-16). It is important that these bony findings be interpreted as secondary deformations due to a more primary neuromuscular

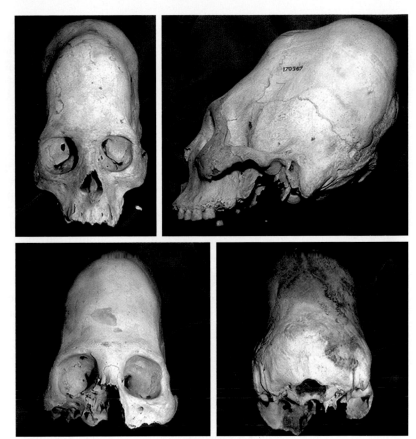

FIGURE 51-13. Highland Peruvians applied circumferential bandages to the calvarium to achieve a conic head shape. Coastal Peruvians applied boards to the occiput and pads to the frontal region along with circumferential banding.
(Courtesy of Dr. Kate Donahue, Department of Anthropology, Plymouth State College, New Hampshire.)

FIGURE 51-14. Among the Mangbetu people, circumferential binding was used to achieve a conic head shape that persisted throughout adulthood, as shown by this adult female as well as the skull.
(Courtesy of Dr. Tim Littlefield, Cranial Technologies, Tempe, Ariz.)

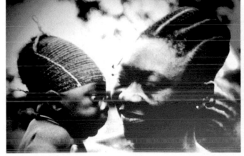
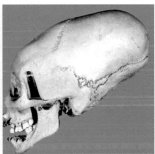

problem, rather than as additional malformations involving the skeletal system.

The impact of increasing weight is also evident in the breadth of bone, whereas linear growth is only mildly affected by muscle weakness. Thus paralysis or immobility of a limb results in only a 5% to 10% reduction in its rate of linear growth; however, subperiosteal growth in bone breadth is much more dramatically affected. Hence with muscle weakness or lack of use, the growing bone tends to become slender (Fig. 51-17).

The adaptive capacity of bone is beautifully exemplified by the realization that the amount of bone and its alignment are influenced by the very forces that the bone is required to withstand. Bone appears to have a critical strain or stress threshold, above which there tends to be bone deposition and below which there tends to be bone resorption.

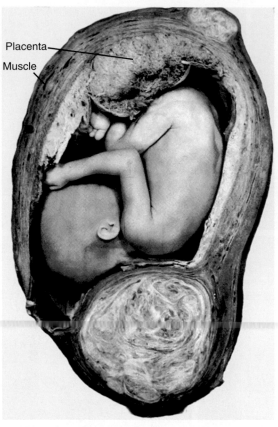

Placenta
Muscle

FIGURE 51-15. Diminished uterine cavity because of a large uterine fibroid.

Intermittent stress on a bone tends to foster local growth of bone, as exemplified in bony promontories at sites of muscle attachment. One example is the bony spurs that are liable to develop in the arch of the foot as a result of the strain of long-distance running. However, persistent stress on a bone, such as that caused by continuous external compression, can lead to a decrease in bone. This is dramatically exemplified by constraint-induced vertex craniotabes. This abnormality commonly results from prolonged pressure on the fetal vertex as a consequence of the head being forcibly "engaged" for a prolonged period of time prior to birth. A similar postnatal impact of persistent pressure on the calvarium was deduced by G. E. Smith from his evaluation of ancient Egyptian skulls.[11] He recognized that the upper-class Egyptians who lived during the 4th to 19th dynasties and wore heavy headdresses had a notable thinning of the calvarium. Smith deduced that this was the consequence of the *continuous pressure exerted by these heavy headdresses.*

### Joints

Joints develop secondarily within the condensed mesenchyme of the developing bones. Movement is an important factor in joint morphogenesis. Chronic lack of movement tends to give rise

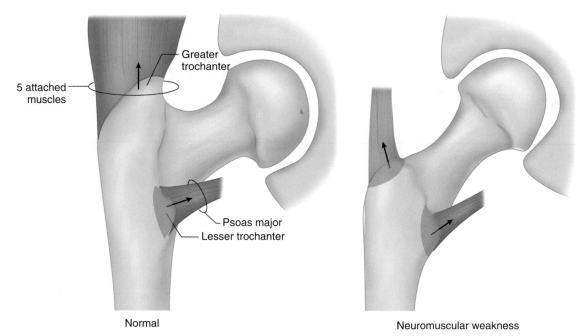

5 attached muscles

Greater trochanter

Psoas major
Lesser trochanter

Normal

Neuromuscular weakness

FIGURE 51-16. Impact of muscle weakness on the form of the proximal femur. The coxa valga and slimmer bone is secondary to the diminished forces exerted on the bone.

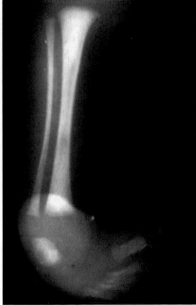

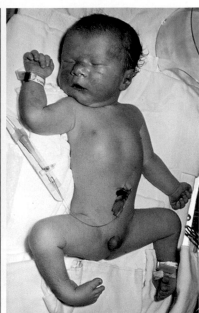

FIGURE 51-17. These slim lower leg bones are secondary to long-standing neuromuscular weakness in a newborn with myotonic dystrophy whose mother had this dominantly inheritable disorder.

to multiple joint contractures and a pattern of problems called the *fetal akinesia sequence* (Fig. 51-18).[12] One dramatic example was an infant with multiple joint contractures (termed *arthrogryposis*) whose mother had received tubocurarine for 19 days in early pregnancy for the treatment of tetanus.[13] Such medically induced early immobilization was considered to be the cause of the joint contractures in her fetus. Similar defects have been induced experimentally by the injection of curare into pregnant rats (Fig. 51-19).[14] Physical constraint due to prolonged oligohydramnios or fetal constraint may also cause joint contractures. Fig. 51-20 demonstrates the multiple consequences

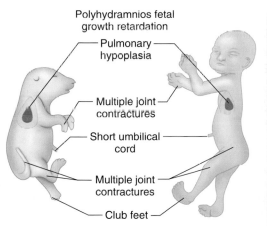

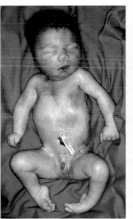

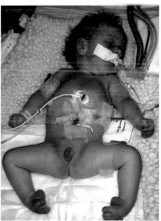

FIGURE 51-18. The fetal akinesia sequence results from decreased movement in utero. The consequent anomalies consisted of intrauterine growth retardation, micrognathia, multiple joint contractures, pulmonary hypoplasia, short umbilical cords, and polyhydramnios. These defects result from intrinsic deformation due to myoneural dysfunction, as shown in these brothers with the fetal akinesia deformation sequence due to type I Pena-Shokeir syndrome, a lethal autosomal recessive disorder resulting from pulmonary hypoplasia.

(Diagram from Moessinger AC: Fetal akinesia deformation sequence: an animal model. *Pediatrics* 72:857, 1983.)

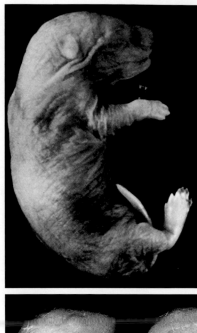
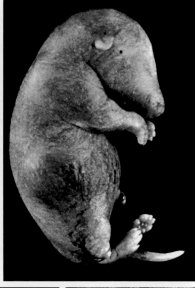
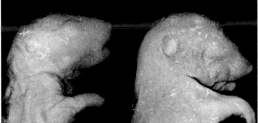
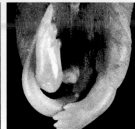

FIGURE 51-19. Moessinger modeled fetal akinesia sequence experimentally in rat fetuses, which were paralyzed by daily transuterine injections of curare from day 18 of gestation until term (day 21). Compared with the control fetuses *(left)*, the experimental fetuses demonstrated tight skin, micrognathia, and joint contractures.

(From Moessinger AC: Fetal akinesia deformation sequence: an animal model, *Pediatrics* 72:857, 1983.)

on bones and joint development in constrained twins carried to term by a small primigravida woman.

## Muscles

Muscle cells align in the direction of muscle pull, which has obvious importance to muscle function. The size of a muscle relates to the magnitude and frequency of the forces it exerts, and the larger the forces, the greater the muscle bulk. Conversely, with diminished function, a muscle becomes smaller in size, and lack of muscle function will result in a diminished, hypoplastic muscle. Based on a study of muscle tendon insertions in genetic limb reduction defects and sites of juncture in conjoined twins, in whom genetic instructions for such altered anatomy could not be predetermined, there appears to be a hierarchy for the determination of muscle-tendon attachment sites.[15] Tendons attach preferentially to bone, and in the absence of the bone to which a tendon would normally attach, the tendon attaches to the next closest bone. If no such bone is available, tendons may attach to other tendons or to the fascia of another muscle. If there is no connective tissue attachment site, then there is no muscle, which implies a need for muscle to function in the development and maintenance of muscle.[15] The biomechanical impact of muscle strength on bone form and growth has already been emphasized.

## Organ Capsules

Organ capsules may be viewed as exoskeletons that provide connective tissue support for particular tissues. Included within this category are the dura mater of the brain, the sclera and outer covering of the eye, the pericardium of the heart, the pleura of the lung, the peritoneum of the intestine, the capsule of the kidney, and the tunica albuginea of the testes. The skin may also be interpreted as an organ capsule, as it is the capsule for the entire organism. The only organ capsule that becomes ossified is that of the brain. The dura mater is responsible for the development and ossification

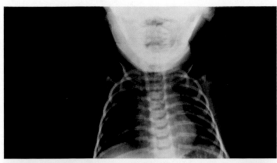

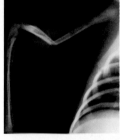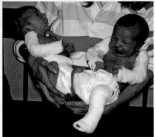

FIGURE 51-20. This 62-inch, 98-lb primiparous mother delivered these twins at term with a combined weight of 10 lb, 11 oz. There was marked fetal crowding during the last half of gestation to the extent that this small mother had such difficulty eating that she experienced a 2-lb weight loss during the course of her pregnancy. She noted very little fetal movement during the third trimester, and both twins were born with severe joint contractures, which resulted in 60- to 90-degree limitation of extension at the elbows and 30-degree limitation of extension at the knees. Twin A was born from a vertex presentation with thin bones, resulting in a fracture postnatally during routine handling. Twin B was delivered vaginally from a breech presentation with thin bones and fractured both humeri during delivery; he also had a right equinovarus foot deformity. Both twins had markedly redundant skin and large ears from prolonged compression. By the time photographs were taken at age 12 days, the joint contractures had shown marked improvement, and the twins were beginning to fill out their loose skin. The prognosis for continued improvement was excellent.

of the calvarium. (This will be considered in more depth in the craniofacial section of this chapter.) None of these organ capsules appear to have any basic impetus for growth. Rather, they grow in accordance with the mechanical forces imposed by the expansion of the particular organ or tissue that they envelop. All organ capsules are composed of connective tissues within which the collagen fibrils align, in accordance with the growth stretch imposed by the internal expansile growth of the respective organ. The direction of such forces is curvilinear, as is readily evident in the alignment of the collagen fibrils within these organ capsules.

## Skin and Its Derivatives

Skin does not appear to have any basic impetus for growth but instead grows in accordance with mechanical forces.[16] Normally, such forces are exerted by the growth of underlying tissues. If there is unusual growth of underlying tissues, the skin will respond accordingly. Thus, if hydrocephalus is present, the skin will grow in accordance with the enlarged head. The excessive skin of the pterygium colli that may occur in Turner's syndrome and certain other disorders is considered secondary to a more primary problem in the development of the lymphatic system, as shown in Figs. 51-21 and 51-22. A lag in the development of a channel between the juguloaxillary lymph sac and the internal jugular vein results in grossly distended jugular lymph sacs, which distend the overlying skin in the posterolateral regions of the neck.[17] This lymphaticovenous communication channel usually develops by the 40th day after conception, thus draining the distended lymphatic sacs. The excess skin remains as redundant folds of skin from the mastoid region toward the shoulder, a deformational clue to the nature of the problem that engendered the web neck. Another condition that may leave a residuum of redundant skin is the urethral obstruction malformation sequence. When the prostatic urethra fails to hollow out, back-up of urine can massively distend the bladder in early fetal life.[18] This will usually be lethal unless the bladder decompresses, which then yields a wrinkled "prune belly" abdomen with redundant folds of skin evident at birth.

The skin appears to respond to external pressure by growth in a fashion similar to its response to internal expansile stretch. For example, when there has been external pressure on the skin, such as occurs with oligohydramnios, there may be loose, redundant folds of skin at birth. Such accentuated folds in the face may account for the "Potter facies" noted with external constraint due to oligohydramnios. Redundant loose folds have also been noted on the back of the neck in infants who have been in prolonged breech presentation with the head hyperextended, yielding the breech head deformation sequence. This is presumed to be the consequence of excessive pressure of the basiocciput on the posterior neck resulting in localized overgrowth of the skin in this region. Similarly, skin overgrowth in the anterior neck and chin region may be noted with prolonged face presentation. Thus the finding of redundant excessive skin at birth may implicate either previous internal expansile growth stretch or previous external compression of considerable duration.

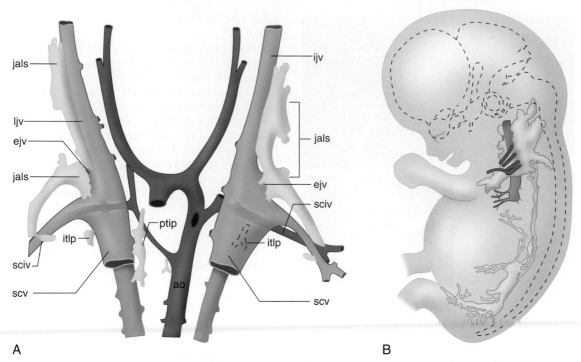

FIGURE 51-21. **A,** The early developing lymph channels drain into the venous system. In the cervical region the jugular lymph sac *(jals)* drains into the jugular vein *(ejv* and *ijv)*. **B,** This occurs at 40 days of development, by which time the jugular and axillary lymph sacs (in yellow) empty into the jugular vein (in blue). (**A,** From van de Putte SC: The development of the lymphatic system in man, *Adv Anat Embryol* 51:1, 1975. **B,** From Töndury G, Kubik S: *Zur ontogenese des lymphatischen systems. Handbuch der Allgemeinen Pathologie*, Berlin, 1975, Springer-Verlag.)

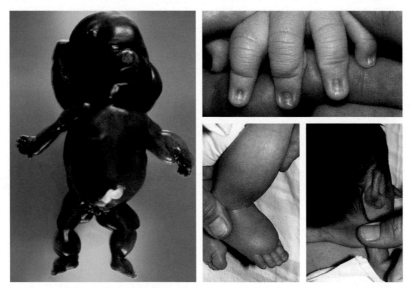

FIGURE 51-22. If there is a delay or failure in the development of the communication between the lymphatic system and the venous system, the lymphatic system distends to cause lymphedema, as is evident in this fetus with 45,X Turner's syndrome. Such lymphedema is the major reason why most fetuses with Turner's syndrome fail to survive. In newborn infants with Turner's syndrome, the distended jugular lymph sacs result in excess skin in the lateral neck (pterygia coli). Distended lymphatic sacs can also interfere with the developing aorta, thus, infants with Turner's syndrome and a web neck should be closely examined for aortic coarctation. Lymph accumulation may also cause peripheral lymphedema that results in puffy hands and feet, and prior lymph accumulation may yield such residual features as loose skin in the face and a lax abdomen.

An occasional finding in a normal baby is a small, raw, punched-out lesion in the skin of the scalp (Fig. 51-23). Such lesions also are a frequent feature in babies with trisomy 13 syndrome, as shown in Fig. 51-23, *B*, but they can also occur in otherwise normal individuals as an autosomal dominant trait (Fig. 51-23, *A*). These areas of aplasia cutis congenita tend to occur in close proximity to the parietal hair whorl. The parietal hair whorl may represent the apical point from which growth stretch is exerted by the domelike outgrowth of the brain. This point in the developing skin of the scalp would therefore be the most liable to break down during the period of rapid brain growth, which stretches the skin away from this point. Using this hypothesis, the ulceration would be the result of the interaction of mechanical forces plus a greater-than-average liability to breakdown of the skin at this point of maximal stretch.[19] The development of dermal appendages and dermal ridges also follows mechanical principles, as follows:

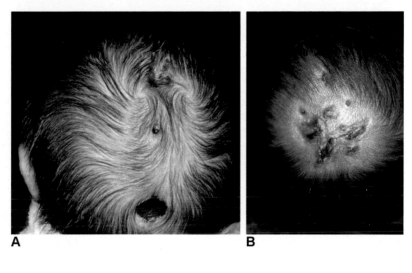

FIGURE 51-23. Small areas of vertex cutis aplasia resembling ulcerations can occur in otherwise normal newborns as an autosomal dominant trait (**A**) and in newborns with trisomy 13 syndrome (**B**). Note that these lesions tend to occur at or near the site of the parietal hair whorl, the location of maximal stretch exerted on the developing skin of the scalp by the domelike outgrowth of the brain.

**A**                    **B**

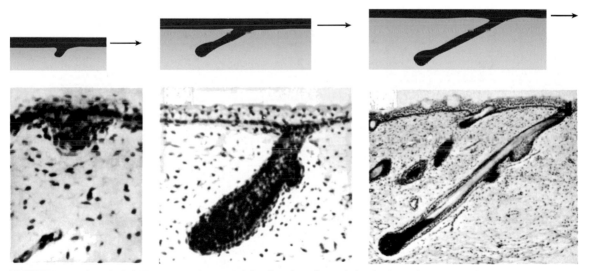

FIGURE 51-24. As a hair follicle grows downward, its direction of angulation is determined by the forces exerted via the underlying growth of the brain. These stretch forces, which are greater at the surface than in deeper tissues, affect the hair directional patterning, which is usually set by about 16 weeks.

(From Smith DW, Gong BT: Scalp-hair patterning: its origin and significance relative to early brain and upper facial development, *Teratology* 9:17, 1974.)

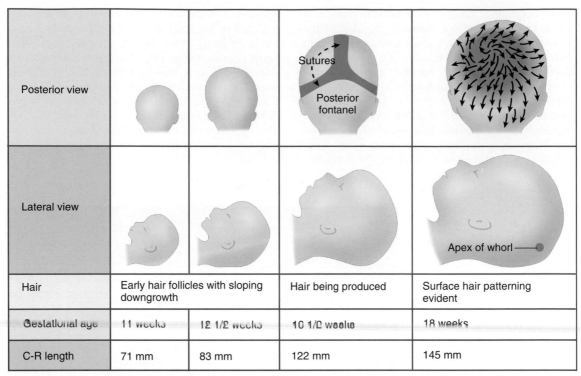

| | | | | |
|---|---|---|---|---|
| Posterior view | | | Sutures<br>Posterior<br>fontanel | |
| Lateral view | | | | Apex of whorl—— |
| Hair | Early hair follicles with sloping downgrowth | | Hair being produced | Surface hair patterning evident |
| Gestational age | 11 weeks | 12 1/2 weeks | 10 1/2 weeks | 18 weeks |
| C-R length | 71 mm | 83 mm | 122 mm | 145 mm |

FIGURE 51-25. The rapid domelike projection of the brain during the period of hair follicle downgrowth is evident in these proportionate drawings of the early fetal head at this time.

(From Smith DW, Gong BT: Scalp-hair patterning: its origin and significance relative to early brain and upper facial development, *Teratology* 9:17, 1974.)

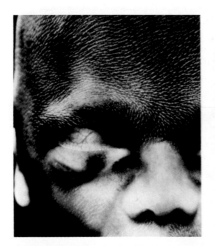

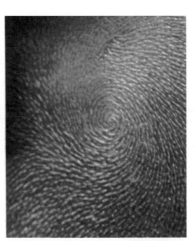

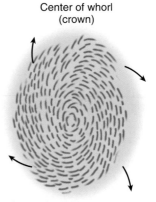

Center of whorl
(crown)

Center from which asymmetric
growth stretch is away from

FIGURE 51-26. As the fetal hairs emerge at about 18 weeks, the hair directional patterns are beautifully evident. Over the forehead the "frontal hair stream" emanating from the fixed skin points of the ocular puncta meets with the down-sweeping parietal hair stream, which emanates from the parietal hair whorl (crown). On any expanding sphere or hemisphere there must be at least one fixed point from which all other points are moving. Presumably, it is the mild asymmetry of forces that conveys the whorl pattern.

(From Smith DW, Gong BT: Scalp-hair patterning: its origin and significance relative to early brain and upper facial development, *Teratology* 9:17, 1974.)

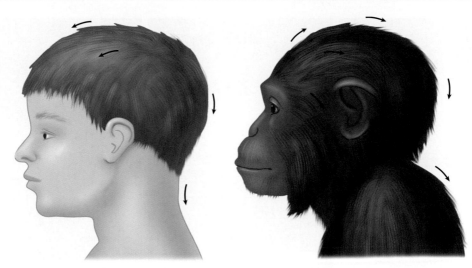

FIGURE 51-27. Head hair patterning in a boy compared with that in a young chimpanzee. In the human, the large domelike brain has generated a parietal whorl and the hair "streams" from that spot, with the parietal hair stream sweeping forward to meet with the frontal hair stream on the forehead. Because the chimpanzee has a much smaller brain, the frontal hair stream simply sweeps directly back over the head with no parietal whorl or parietal hair stream.
(From Kidd W: *The direction of hair in animals and man*, London, 1903, Adam and Charles Black.)

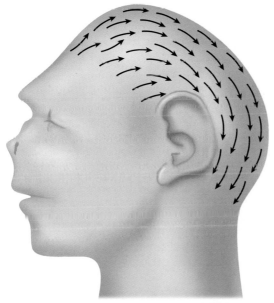

FIGURE 51-28. Child with severe microcephaly and midfacial defect. There is no parietal hair whorl, and the frontal hair stream sweeps back over the scalp in a fashion similar to that found in the chimpanzee.
(From Smith DW, Gong BT: Scalp-hair patterning: its origin and significance relative to early brain and upper facial development, *Teratology* 9:17, 1974.)

1. *Hair directional patterning:* As the hair follicles grow downward from the germinative layer of the skin at 10 to 18 weeks of development, they take on a sloping angulation (Fig. 51-24).[20] This angulation is considered to be the consequence of the direction and magnitude of growth stretch exerted on the surface skin during the period of downgrowth of the hair follicles, which have a sloping angulation as a result of differential lag. When the keratinized rods of hair are extruded at 16 to 18 weeks of development, the direction of the hair appears to be set for life and reflects the magnitude and direction of growth stretch exerted on the skin during the 11- to 16-week period (Figs. 51-25 and 51-26). On any expanding sphere or hemisphere there is one immobile point, away from which all other points are moving. Over the scalp, this point is usually in the parietal region; this is considered to result in the parietal hair whorl, or crown. This is a beautiful example of the impact of mechanical forces on form. Thus, differences in brain growth and form are considered the reason for most differences in

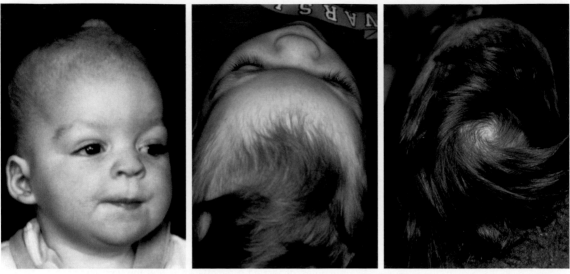

FIGURE 51-29. This profoundly retarded child was exposed to 40- to 60-mg Accutane per day from the 2nd through the 20th week of gestation and had microcephaly, a brain hamartoma protruding from the scalp, and a markedly altered scalp hair pattern.

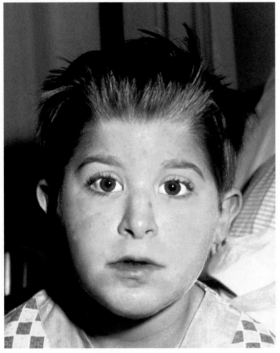

FIGURE 51-30. Frontal brain deficiency may result in the frontal hair stream sweeping upward into the scalp region and giving rise to a frontal upsweep, more commonly referred to as a "cowlick." This occurs in mild degrees in about 3% of normal individuals. This figure represents an unusual degree in a child with Rubinstein-Taybi syndrome.

(From Smith DW, Gong BT: Scalp-hair patterning: its origin and significance relative to early brain and upper facial development, *Teratology* 9:17, 1974.)

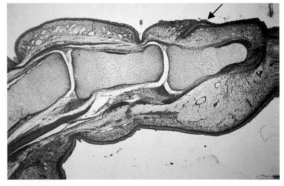

FIGURE 51-31. Longitudinal section of the finger in an 11-week fetus showing the orientation of the early nail plate *(arrow)* to the distal phalanx. The growing cells of the nail plate become a keratinized nail that generally reflects the form of the underlying distal bony phalanx.

(Courtesy of Gian Töndury, University of Zurich, Zurich, Switzerland.)

scalp hair directional patterning, including those that exist between humans and other primates (Fig. 51-27). Of special clinical relevance are the aberrant hair directional patterns that may be secondary to early problems of brain morphogenesis, examples of which are shown in Figs. 51-28 to 51-30. Such findings not only tend to implicate a problem in brain morphogenesis but also suggest that the disorder had its advent prior to 16 weeks of fetal life.

2. *Nails:* Each nail is a keratinized plate derived from the germinative layer of skin, similar to what is seen with hair follicles. The nail tends to conform to the shape of the distal phalanx (Fig. 51-31). Thus, if the distal phalanx is short and broad, then the nail is short and broad, as seen in brachydactyly D (Fig. 51-32). If the distal phalanx is hypoplastic, the nail is hypoplastic, as seen in fetal alcohol syndrome and fetal dilantin syndrome (Fig. 51-33). If the distal phalanx is bifid, the nail is bifid. The impact of forces on the early form of the nails due to peripheral lymphedema in Turner syndrome is illustrated in Fig. 51-34.

3. *Dermal ridge patterning:* As with other primates, humans have dermal ridges on the thickened skin of the volar surfaces of the hands and feet. This parallel ridging provides an important frictional surface for the palms and soles. These ridges develop at 13 to 19 weeks of fetal life and appear to form at right angles to the plane of growth stretch in the skin.[21] Dermal ridges resemble the ridges of sand that develop on the beach at right angles to the direction of the flow of water or wind. The surface characteristics over underlying pads give rise to curvilinear dermal ridge patterns that reflect the shape of the pads at the time of dermal ridge development (Figs. 51-35 and 51-36). If the fingertip pad is low, the pattern forms an arch; however, if the pads are very prominent, a whorl develops, with the center of the whorl representing the apex of the pad. A high proportion of loops, the most common fingertip pattern, has little clinical relevance. The finding of 6 or more arches on the 10 fingertips is unusual (found in only 3% of normal individuals), and the finding of 8 or more whorls on the fingertips is also unusual. Altered dermal ridge patterning is generally a nonspecific deformation, providing evidence of the nature of the topographic growth dynamics in the volar surfaces of the hands and feet at 13 to 19 fetal weeks.

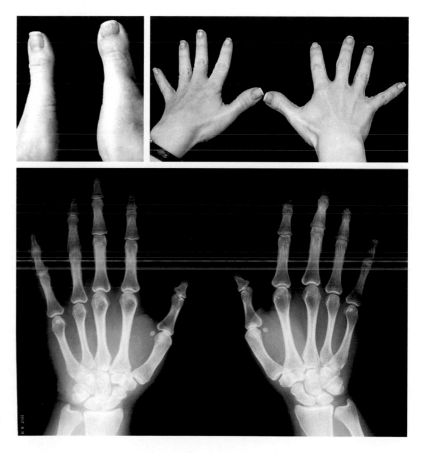

FIGURE 51-32. This figure compares the short, wide distal nail and phalanx in the thumb of an woman with brachydactyly D (an autosomal dominant trait) with that of a normal woman *(left).*

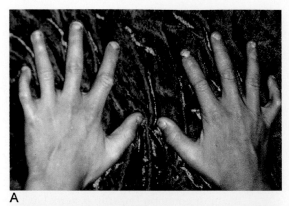

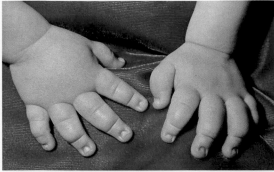

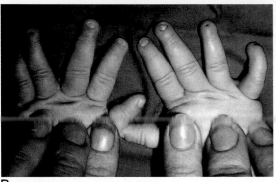

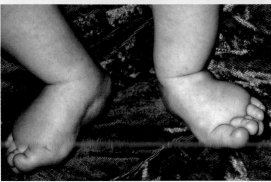

FIGURE 51-34. Fetal lymphedema may distort the form of the nails, as exemplified in a newborn with peripheral lymphedema due to Turner syndrome. The narrow, hyperconvex nails with the appearance of a deep-set nail base are the residual consequences of prior lymphedema.

FIGURE 51-33. Distal phalangeal and nail hypoplasia in the hands of a person with fetal alcohol syndrome **(A)** and fetal hydantoin syndrome **(B)**.

**4.** *Dermal creases:* The dermal creases (Fig. 51-37) are simply deep wrinkles that reflect the flexional planes of functional folding in the thickened skin of the palms and soles.[22] They occur in relation to joints and provide evidence of the functional movement at such joints. Over the palm, the thenar flexion crease relates to the flexional plane of oppositional flexion of the thumb and first metacarpal. The upper palmar crease reflects the sloping plane of flexional folding of the third, fourth, and fifth metacarpophalangeal joints, and the mid-palmar crease simply reflects the folding plane in the skin between the other two palmar creases. Small differences in the shape or form of the hand can result in a single upper palmar crease, sometimes termed a *simian crease* (Fig. 51-38, *A*). This highly nonspecific finding is found unilaterally in 4% and bilaterally in 1% of normal individuals, and it is also observed in more than 50% of individuals with Down syndrome.

Absent creases often reflect absent or deficient function of a flexional plane across the surface of a joint (see Fig. 51-38).

### Craniofacial Region

The normal formation of the brain is genetically determined. The growth of the brain in size (magnitude) and shape (direction) exerts a major mechanical impact on the form of the tissues that surround and relate to the brain in the craniofacial region. The early neural structures have a major impact. Thus the brain affects the development of the calvarium and its sutures,[23] the outgrowth of the optic cup has a major impact on the development of the orbit,[24] the invaginating olfactory placodes are primarily responsible for the subsequent formation of the nose, and the invaginating auditory placodes form the inner ear structures and determine the orientation of the temporal wing of the sphenoid bone. The role of pressure on the regulation of craniofacial bone growth

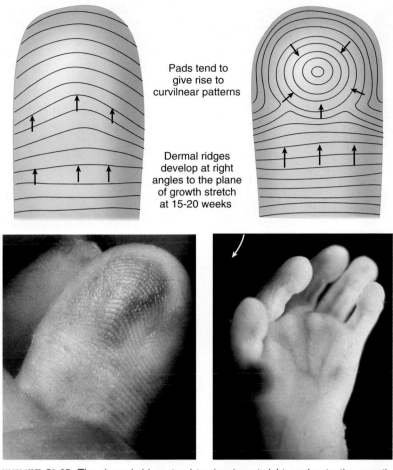

Pads tend to give rise to curvilnear patterns

Dermal ridges develop at right angles to the plane of growth stretch at 15-20 weeks

FIGURE 51-35. The dermal ridges tend to develop at right angles to the growth stretch exerted on the skin by the development of the underlying tissues. Where there are pads, such as those shown in the fingertips and interdigital areas of the palm of an 8.5 week fetus *(right)*, the result is the development of curvilinear ridge patterns.

was beautifully demonstrated by comparing the orbital growth in 8-week-old kittens, which were evenly divided into three surgical groups for unilateral operations. (1) orbital evisceration alone; (2) orbital evisceration followed by a silastic implant; and (3) orbital evisceration followed by a tissue expander. Only group 3 experienced normal orbital growth, whereas group 1 showed a 23.4% reduction in size and group 2 showed a 9% reduction in size.[25] Therefore the statement that the "face reflects the brain" has much evidence to support it. Particular features in the craniofacial region are summarized in this section. Fig. 51-39 emphasizes the integral relationship that exists between the face and the brain. Beyond the mechanical impacts of brain development on

facial form, there are indirect effects of neuromuscular function on facial form. Such effects are depicted in Figs. 51-40 and 51-41.

## Calvarium

The growth and shape of the brain normally determines the shape of the calvarium. Thus in the absence of problems of calvarial development, such as constraint molding and/or craniosynostosis, it is the brain that determines the shape of the calvarium. For example, a narrow forehead means a narrow forebrain, and a brachycephalic skull (that is not excessively widened due to deformation) means a brain of short length. The

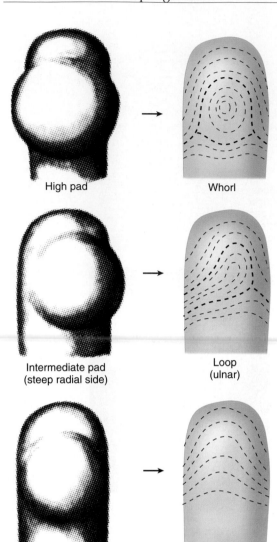

High pad

Whorl

Intermediate pad
(steep radial side)

Loop
(ulnar)

Low pad

Arch

FIGURE 51-36. The fingertip dermal ridge patterning appears to relate to the form of the fingertip pads at the time of development of the dermal ridges.

(From Mulvihill JJ, Smith DW: Genesis of dermatoglyphics, *J Pediatr* 75:579, 1969.)

organ capsule of the brain, the dura mater, is literally the mother tissue in the development of the bony calvarium and its sutures (Figs. 51-42 to 51-44). The calvarium consists of bony plates joined by strips of unmineralized dura, the sutures. These sutures relate directly to the form of the early brain and reflect dural folds into the surface of the brain. As the brain grows, it stretches the overlying dura mater. The brain is not a smooth hemisphere, and dural reflections occur into the

recesses of the brain. These dural reflections are shown in Figs. 51-42 and 51-43. Normally, no ossification overlies these dural reflections as long as growth stretch continues (Fig. 51-44), and these are the usual sites of the sutures.[23] The metopic and sagittal sutures relate to the sites of the dural reflections into the interhemispheral fissure and the falx cerebri. The lambdoid sutures relate to the sites of the dural reflection between the cerebrum and cerebellum, the falx cerebelli. The coronal sutures relate to the insular sulci of the brain, with its dural reflections off the sphenoid wings, which faithfully fills in this sulcus in the brain.[23] Between the sites of dural reflection, ossification begins within the membranous dura as niduses of ossification spread outward toward the sites of the sutures. The radial orientation of the spreading ossification appears to relate to tensile forces within the dura. At the sites of initial ossification in the calvarium, there may be small external promontories, which are most evident in infancy and childhood. These promontories may be noted toward the center of each frontal bone, each parietal bone, and each lateral portion of the occipital bone. They appear to be normal features. The major era for the early development of the calvarium is from 12 to 16 weeks. In areas of the developing calvarium where the stretch forces may be diminished, such as in the region of the parietal bone near the posterior fontanelle and along the lambdoid sutures, multiple small centers of ossification may develop and then coalesce. These are referred to as *wormian bones*. When posterior occipital pressure occurs due to molding or when the skull is demineralized, the dura may become relaxed, and wormian bones will form in increased numbers, especially within the posterior sutures.

The implication of these principles is that early brain form determines the sites of dural reflections and thereby the location of sutures. This thesis is supported by aberrations of early brain morphogenesis that give rise to altered dural reflections and thereby affect the location of sutures, as shown in Figs. 51-45 and 51-46. The sutures of the calvarium may be altered by several means, including primary defects of brain morphogenesis, problems in suture development, metabolic problems, and external constraint.[26] A serious deficit of brain growth with a lack of growth stretch at suture sites, whether in primary microcephaly or overshunted hydrocephalus, may allow for mineralization of one or more sutures. This secondary craniosynostosis may then lead to further problems. A primary defect of brain formation may affect the presence or site of dural reflections and thus the

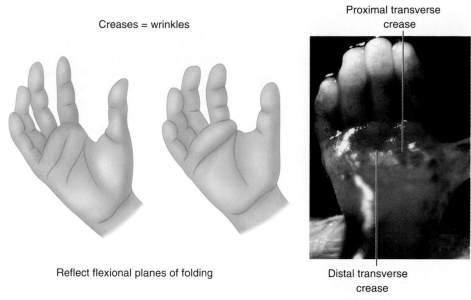

Creases = wrinkles

Proximal transverse crease

Reflect flexional planes of folding

Distal transverse crease

FIGURE 51-37. Creases relate to flexional planes of folding, always being secondary to mechanical forces. The upper palmar crease relates to the sloping plane of folding of the third, fourth, and fifth metacarpophalangeal joints, the thenar crease relates to the flexion of the thenar region, and the midpalmar crease represents the folding plane between these two.

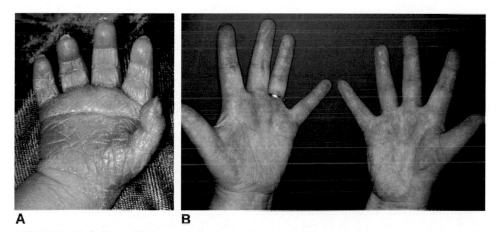

**A**                    **B**

FIGURE 51-38. **A,** Minor differences in the form of the hand in Down syndrome can result in a single crease across the upper palm (simian crease). This hand also has a short fifth finger and a single crease as a consequence. **B,** These hands have absent or hypoplastic thenar creases with absent interphalangeal thumb creases, indicating a functional deficit in oppositional flexional folding of the thenar region (which was inherited as a variably expressed autosomal dominant trait).

presence and site of the sutures. One example is holoprosencephaly, in which a primary failure of diverticulation of the two cerebral vesicles may result in a single cerebral ventricle and no interhemispheral fissure. This is usually, but not always, accompanied by the lack of a metopic suture (see Fig. 51-46).

External constraint of the developing fetal head may result in a lack of growth stretch at a given suture, thereby causing craniosynostosis. This appears to be the most common cause for this problem.[26,27] The impact of craniosynostosis on craniofacial form depends on the age of onset of sutural closure and the suture(s) involved. Sagittal craniosynostosis limits lateral growth of the calvarium, resulting in a narrow, elongated, scaphocephalic head shape. Coronal synostosis limits anteroposterior growth, resulting in a short and

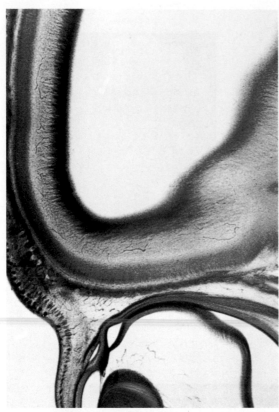

FIGURE 51-39. At 10 weeks, the cerebrum, which has only one cortical layer at this stage, is molding the forehead. The upper face is influenced by the early brain derivatives, the eyes. The mesenchymal tissues will soon condense and organize the supportive skeletal framework in accordance with these neural tissues. The growth of the cranial base anterior to the pituitary will occur in relationship to the frontal growth of the brain.

wide (brachycephalic) head shape. Early coronal synostosis also prevents the forward growth of the brain and hence the anterior growth of the cranial base. Because the cranial base is the roof of the face, the midface tends to be retrusive, the orbits become shallow, the eyes become more widely spaced, and the forehead becomes high and wide.

Craniosynostosis of both the sagittal and coronal sutures will limit the capacity for brain growth and will usually result in increased intracranial pressure. Radiographs of the skull may show a "beaten-copper" appearance, partially due to a more vertical orientation of the bone fibrils within the calvarium, which tend to align in relation to the altered stress forces. The head tends to become tower shaped, which leads to oxycephaly, acrocephaly, or turricephaly. The head is quite malleable, especially during fetal life. This is a normal and

obviously necessary phenomenon during vaginal delivery. During delivery, the bony plates of the calvarium overlap at the sutures, sometimes to a surprising degree. Such normal vertex molding is usually transient and limited in duration to a few days. Prolonged uterine constraint with compression of the fetal head during late fetal life may give rise to deformations of the head that usually slowly resolve over time; cases of extensive molding may require management to achieve a more normal resolution.[26,27]

### Cranial Base

The anterior cranial base develops from cartilage that becomes ossified, with persisting growth centers posterior and anterior to the sella turcica. The region anterior to the sella turcica, which is designated as the anterior cranial base, tends to grow forward in accordance with frontal brain growth. Hence cranial base growth parallels normal brain growth. The modern human brain is only 25% of its adult size at birth and continues to grow at a rapid rate throughout the first year of life, when it reaches 50% of its adult size.[28] Human brains are 95% of adult size by age 10 years. In comparison, a chimpanzee brain is already 40% of its adult size by birth and reaches 80% of the adult volume by the end of the first year. A 1-year-old *Homo erectus* brain was closer to apes in its growth pattern and measured 72% to 84% of adult size at that age, which implies differences in the development of *Homo erectus'* cognitive abilities when compared with modern humans.[28] It is important to appreciate that the anterior cranial base is the roof of the face, from which the maxilloethmoid complex projects downward to form the anterior portion of the nasal bridge. A deficit of frontal brain growth may yield a shorter cranial base and a less-prominent nasal bridge. A shorter cranial base will generally yield a flatter facial profile with a tendency toward a small, retrusive midface.

### Eyes

Early outpouchings from the diencephalon, the optic cups, induce the formation of the lenses in the overlying ectoderm; thus begins the formation of the eye. Zones of periocular hair growth suppression determine the frontal hair pattern and are strongly influenced by the size and location of the eyes (Fig. 51-47). Surrounding mesenchymal cells condense to form the globular eye

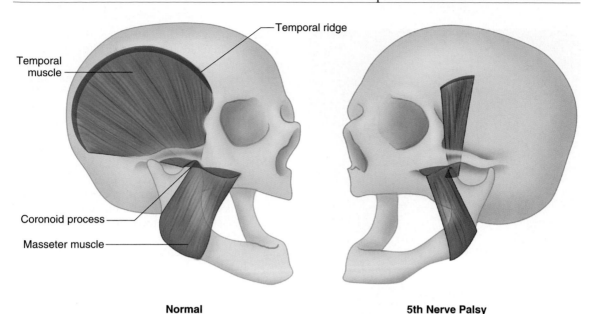

**Normal**                                                         **5th Nerve Palsy**

FIGURE 51-40. Mechanical force relationships between function and form as illustrated in a 60-year-old man who had a unilateral 5th nerve palsy from early in life. On the affected side the facial muscles are quite small, and all the sites of muscle attachment were less prominent on the affected side.

capsule within which the collagen fibrils align in relation to fluid pressure from within the eye. Around the eye, the mesenchymal tissues condense to form the bony orbit, which conforms to and is shaped in relation to the eye.[24] Excessive fluid pressure within the eye may result in increased glaucoma. This tends to distort the shape of the tense eye toward increased anterior globular prominence. It may also result in cloudiness of the cornea and destructive changes within the eye, which can lead to eventual blindness. A small eye (microphthalmia) yields a small orbit. A lack of any optic cup results in no orbit, and loss of an eye in early childhood arrests orbital growth unless a tissue expander is maintained in the eye socket.[24,25] The accessory tissues around the eye, which consist of muscles, lacrimal ducts, eyebrows, eyelids, and eyelashes, all relate to the development of the early optic cup.[24] For example, an altered position of the early orbit is accompanied by predictable secondary development of all these accessory structures in the aberrant position of the optic vesicle (see Fig. 51-47).

### Ears

The different parts of the ear are derived from different areas of the developing embryo, as follows:

1. *Inner ear:* The otic placode, which is neural tissue, invaginates from the surface ectoderm to become the otocyst. The differential growth of the otocyst leads to the beautiful spiral form of the cochlea and the form of the vestibular apparatus. The mesenchyme around the otic placode is induced to form cartilage that faithfully conforms to its shape and exerts a major role in the development of the sphenoid wing.

2. *Middle ear:* The derivatives of the second and third branchial arches form the malleus, incus, and stapes as a connecting functional link between the tympanic membrane and the round window of the cochlea, thus transmitting auditory vibrations to the cochlea. Any ankylosis within the joints between these bones may result in a problem of conductive deafness.

3. *External ear:* The external auricle forms from the cartilaginous cores of the six auricular-hillocks, which blend into a sheet of cartilage that grows throughout life. Mild to moderate deformations of the external auricle are common in the newborn due to constraint of the pliable auricle in late fetal life. Oligohydramnios accentuates such deformation and may result in an "accordion" ear and/or an ear that is

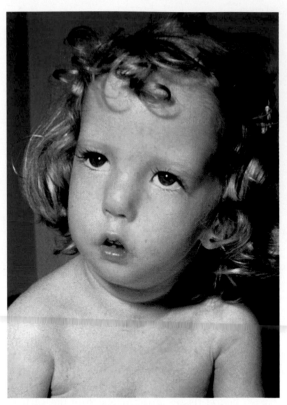

FIGURE 51-41. This girl is lacking sixth and seventh nerve function (Möbius malformation sequence). The facial impact is secondary to the longstanding deficit of forces in the developing face. The almond-shaped eye is interpreted as being secondary to a deficiency of orbicularis oculi function, the small alae nasae to a deficit in the muscles that attach to this cartilage, and the small mouth to a lack of orbicularis oris muscle function. The shallow temporal region is ascribed to weakness of the temporal muscle, the shallow malar region to deficit of masseter function, and the small mandible to a diminished function of the mandible.

enlarged and flattened against the skull. The shoulder may be pressed up under the auricle in such situations as breech presentation, resulting in uplifting of the lower auricle. These distortions tend to resolve toward normal form after birth and are benign deformations. Localized compression that affects one ear more than the other may result in overgrowth of the compressed ear.[29] Distended jugular lymph sacs, such as frequently occurs in the fetus with Turner's syndrome, may distort the auricles, making them more prominent and slanted than usual (see Fig. 51-22).[17]

The position and form of the cartilaginous folds of the auricle relate largely to the sites of insertion and origin of the auricular muscles.[30] Therefore some defects in the form of the external auricle may be the consequence of aberrant development and/or function of particular ear muscles (Fig. 51-48). Absence of the posterior auricular ear muscle, which normally holds the ear against the calvarium, results in a protruding auricle. On the other hand, absence of the superior auricular ear muscle results in a folded-over "lop" ear that may appear low in placement. The inner conchal plical folds appear to relate to the intrinsic auricular ear muscles, and defects in their development may result in varying degrees of a simplified conchal form. Experimental studies in the rodent have shown that early denervation of the seventh nerve, which supplies the auricular ear muscles, will result in a simple auricle that lacks the usual conchal folds. Similar effects are seen with the ears in CHARGE syndrome (coloboma, heart disease, atresia choanae, retarded growth and development, genital hypoplasia, and ear anomalies and/or deafness) due to seventh nerve weakness. With profound muscular hypotonia or lax connective tissues, the ears may protrude (Fig. 51-49).

## Nose and Nasopharynx

The neural olfactory pits invaginate from the surface ectoderm and then send axons to synapse with those of the olfactory lobes. Later, when the base of the skull becomes cartilage and bone, these axons create the sites of "perforation" in the cribriform plate. Around the edges of the olfactory pit, the medial and lateral nasal swellings rapidly grow out and coalesce with the maxillary swelling to form much of the external nose and fuse inferiorly to form the upper lip. The invaginating olfactory pits meet posteriorly with the foregut, and the epithelium between them breaks down, thus providing ready communication between the nasal and oral cavities. The cartilaginous nasal septum is in direct continuity with the anterior base of the skull, and hence alterations in growth of the base of the skull may secondarily affect nasal morphogenesis. The fusion of the maxillary palatal shelves and the nasal septum separates the nasal cavity from the mouth proper. Cartilaginous plates develop in the ala nasi, which have muscle attachments that allow for constriction of the nares. Within the nose, the cartilaginous turbinates grow, and evaginations from the nasal cavity occur into the surrounding bone. These

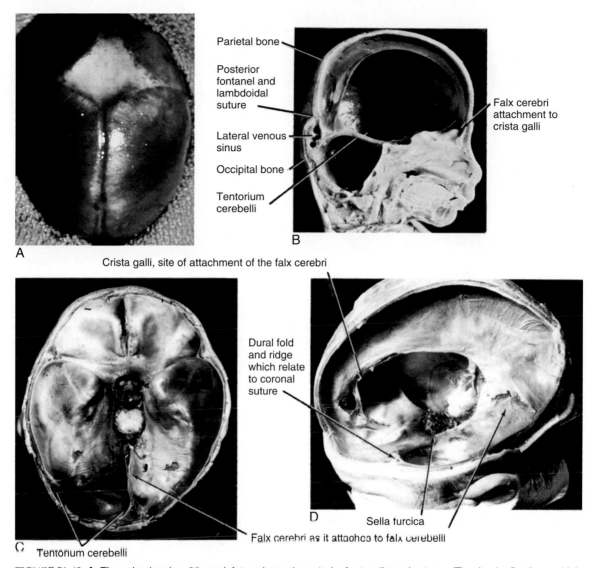

Parietal bone

Posterior fontanel and lambdoidal suture

Lateral venous sinus

Occipital bone

Tentorium cerebelli

Falx cerebri attachment to crista galli

B

A

Crista galli, site of attachment of the falx cerebri

Dural fold and ridge which relate to coronal suture

D          Sella turcica

Falx cerebri as it attaches to falx cerebelli

C   Tentorium cerebelli

FIGURE 51-42. **A,** The calvarium in a 20-week fetus shows the anterior fontanelle and sutures. The dural reflections, which relate mechanically to the recesses in the developing brain, are shown in a 16-week fetus **(B)** and in a term baby **(C, D).** Note how the lines of growth stretch are evident in the alignment of collagen fibrils within the dura. (Courtesy of Prof. Gian Töndury, University of Zurich, Zurich, Switzerland.)

evaginations become sinuses, which aerate the surrounding bones. This substantially reduces their weight while still providing excellent structural support. Sinus development is largely incomplete at birth. The first pharyngeal pouch persists as the eustachian tube and middle ear. Evaginations from the middle ear aerate the mastoid portion of the temporal bone, in a fashion similar to that of the sinuses.

Late uterine constraint may distort the nose. Most commonly it becomes compressed to one side during the neonate's transition through the birth canal. After birth, this usually resolves spontaneously, although some manual pulling and remolding may be merited. Persisting compression may limit the growth of the nose, as in a face presentation. However, postnatal catch-up growth will usually result in a restoration toward normal form. As previously mentioned, aberrations of the growth of the cranial base, such as occur with problems of frontal brain growth, may alter both the relative position of the nasal bridge and the size and form

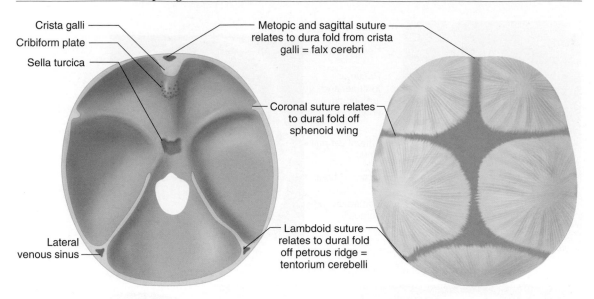

FIGURE 51-43. Conceptual drawing from a 17-week fetus, by which time the early calvarium is formed. **A,** The basilar view shows the sites of dural reflection from the crista galli, sphenoid wings, and petrous ridges. These dural reflections are the sites of passive sutural development, as shown on the right. **B,** The top view of the early calvarium shows how ossification begins in the central spots between the dural reflections and spreads centrifugally toward the sutures. (From Smith DW, Töndury G: Origins of the calvarium and its sutures, *Am J Dis Child* 132:662, 1978.)

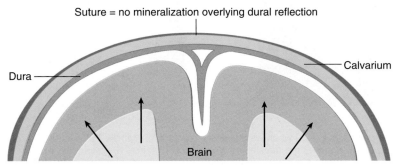

FIGURE 51-44. As long as there is continued growth stretch from the expanding brain, the sites over the dural reflections remain unossified, thereby forming the sutures.

of the nose. Problems with the development and/or function of the musculature of the ala nasi may result in a narrow nose with small alar wings. The sinuses tend to extend well into the solid bone that surrounds them. If there is a loss of permanent teeth from the upper jaw, the maxillary sinus will extend farther than usual, coming into close proximity with the alveolar ridge at the sites of the missing teeth.

## Palate and Tongue

The palatal shelves, which initially project downward alongside the tongue, undergo a shift into their horizontal position and then fuse from front to back with each other and with the nasal septum. If the mandible is unusually small, there may be posterior displacement of the tongue, which will tend to occlude closure of the palatal

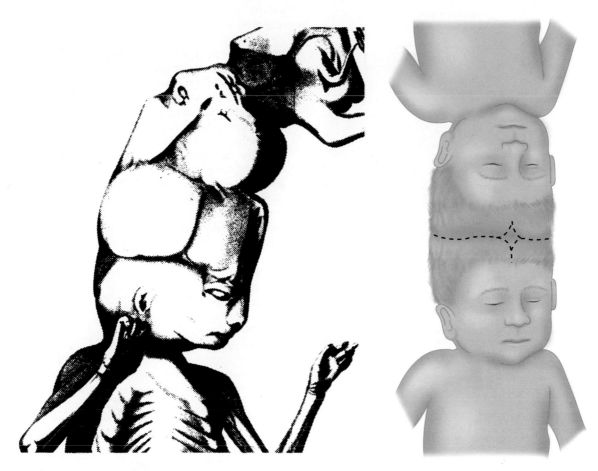

FIGURE 51-45. Conjoined twins provide an experiment of nature to demonstrate that the suture sites relate to the dural reflections. At the sites of juncture of the two brains, there are dural reflections, and at these locations, sutures and fontanelles are observed in positions where they would not normally be present.
(From Smith DW, Töndury G: Origins of the calvarium and its sutures, *Am J Dis Child* 132:662, 1978.)

shelves, giving rise to a U-shaped palatal defect[31] (Fig. 51-50). The posteriorly displaced tongue may obstruct the posterior pharynx, giving rise to partial upper airway obstruction at birth. The initiating problem in mandibular size may be a malformation, and thus the consequences are termed the *early micrognathia malformation sequence*, or the *Robin malformation sequence.*[32] The small mandible could also be the result of early fetal constraint with limitation of mandibular growth (in such an instance the anomaly could be termed the *early micrognathia deformation sequence*), which possibly explains why isolated Robin sequence is associated with twinning and discordantly expressed.[32]

Not only does the tongue play a significant mechanical role in palatal closure, but it also exerts a major impact on palatal form. Normally, lateral palatine ridges extend from the palate on the lingual side of the alveolar ridges (Fig. 51-51).[33] These ridges are prominent in fetal life and are composed of mucopolysaccharide-rich connective tissue and numerous small salivary glands. The force of tongue thrust tends to smooth out these ridges during fetal life. Any disorder that limits tongue thrust into the palate (e.g., hypotonia, other neurologic deficits, or microglossia) will result in prominent lateral palatine ridges (see Fig. 51-51), often giving the appearance of a narrow, high-arched palate. At the other extreme, an enlarged tongue may result in relative flattening and broadening of the hard palate. Thus, the tongue, a very strong muscle, exerts a major impact on the palate. A narrow palate that appears highly arched is common in

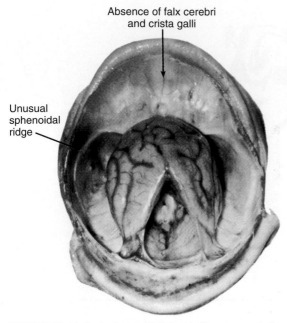

Absence of falx cerebri and crista galli

Unusual sphenoidal ridge

FIGURE 51-16. An instance of alobar holoprosencephaly. Because there was no interhemispheral fissure, there is no dural reflection at this site (falx cerebri), and as a consequence there is no metopic suture. There is also an aberrant alignment of the sphenoid wings relating to the altered brain impact in this location. This was associated with a comparable aberrant alignment of the coronal sutures.

(From DeMeyer W, White PT: EEG in holoprosencephaly (arhinencephaly), *Arch Neurol* 11:507–520, 1964).

children with mental deficiency. The reason for this is not clear, but it may relate to a deficit in functional usage of the facial musculature.

### Alveolar Ridge, Teeth, and Mandible

The tooth anlagen develop as ectodermal downgrowths that interact with the underlying mesenchyme to form the teeth, which then erupt, usually through the channel of their original downgrowth. If there is a failure of tooth development, then the alveolar ridge lacks prominence at that region. Thus the major mass of the alveolar ridges relates to the presence of teeth. The form of the enamel and the crown of a tooth, which is produced by the ectodermal component, are genetically determined and allow for amazing interdigitation between the upper and lower teeth. The forces of biting and chewing tend to foster alignment of the teeth. The growth of the mandible tends to follow the lead of the upper jaw. This applies to lateral

growth as well. Thus if the maxilla is narrow, the mandible also tends to be narrow. If there is a deficit of mandibular function, the mandible will slow its growth rate and remain hypoplastic. The muscles of the mandible are powerful, and their sites of attachment give rise to bony promontories. Fig. 51-40 shows the impact of a unilateral fifth nerve palsy on these muscles and therefore on the bony form of the face. The impact of the facial muscles on bony promontories is dramatically exemplified by experimental studies in rodents. For example, early resection of the masseter muscle results in a complete lack of the coronoid process, its site of insertion on the mandible (Fig. 51-52). If the teeth are crowded, one or more may erupt in an aberrant alignment. Usually the easiest management is removal of the "crowded-out" tooth. Malalignment of the teeth is common, and orthodontic methods of constraint have become a common practice for the realignment of teeth and jaws during childhood.

### Thorax and Lung

The growth of the ribs and thoracic cage is integral to the normal development of the lungs. The lungs develop as progressive arborizations from outbuddings of the foregut. The septation of the thoracic and abdominal cavities by the diaphragm allows the fetus to make respiratory movements. Adequate growth of the thoracic cage is important during the latter phases of lung development, when the lung progresses from a solid organ tissue to one with alveolar sacs capable of aeration. Restrictive crowding of the lungs during late fetal lung growth may result in the lung being incompletely developed by birth, causing respiratory insufficiency at birth. Deficient lung growth may be due to a number of different causes, as summarized in Table 51-3. External constraint of an unusual degree, such as may occur within a bicornuate uterus, may cause thoracic restriction. With oligohydramnios, the lack of fluid within the developing lung combined with early constraint to thoracic growth impairs normal lung development.[34] As a consequence, respiratory insufficiency is the predominant cause of death in newborn babies affected by the oligohydramnios deformation sequence. Crowding of the lung during growth may be intrinsic, as in diaphragmatic hernia, which allows variable amounts of abdominal contents to gain access to the thoracic cavity and thereby limits the capacity for normal lung growth. Hence, the newborn with a diaphragmatic hernia may die of respiratory insufficiency, even

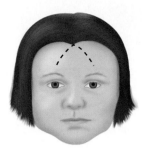
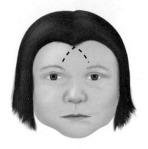
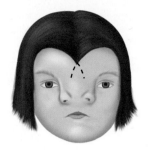

| Periocular fields | Normal | Decreased | Normal |
|---|---|---|---|
| Interocular distance | Normal | Normal | Increased |

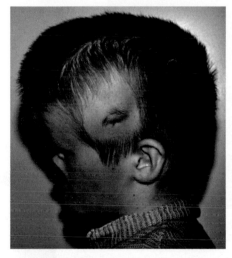
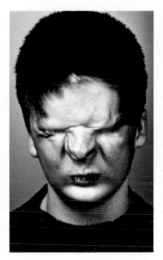
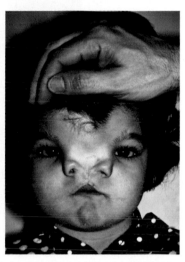

FIGURE 51-47. Zones of periocular hair growth suppression determine the frontal hair pattern, and with microphthalmia, hair extends onto the face, whereas ocular hypertelorism results in a widow's peak. A rudimentary eye projected to an unusual temporal location in the individual on the bottom left. At this site the early optic vesicle gave rise to the development of a small optic cup. Furthermore, there was the development of periocular muscles, lacrimal apparatus, and eyelids, plus the growth of the hair at the eyebrow location and a zone of periocular hair growth suppression.

(From Smith DW, Gong BT: Scalp-hair patterning: its origin and significance relative to early brain and upper facial development, *Teratology* 9:17, 1974.)

if diaphragmatic repair is performed promptly in order to displace abdominal contents from the thoracic cage soon after birth. Because of this problem, fetal surgery for diaphragmatic hernia has helped to improve survival by allowing for more normal lung development. The thoracic cage is malleable and may show alterations of form in relation to constraint. If the fetus has its chin forced into the chest, for example, there may be both a small mandible and a mild "impression" on the chest wall.

## Cardiovascular

The early heart tubes fuse to become one tube, which then undergoes contortions to become the four-chambered heart. The growth of specific ridges within the developing heart gives rise to the separations between the blood channels and the development of the valves. Thus, the growth of the atrioventricular cushions assists in the separation of the atria and ventricles and the formation of the tricuspid and mitral valves. The growth of

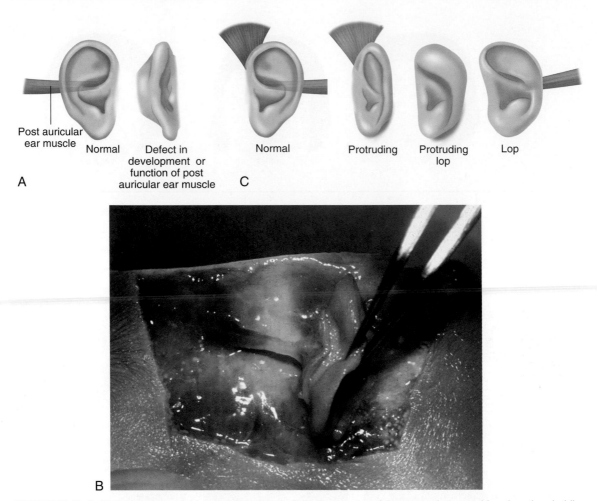

Post auricular
ear muscle

Normal        Defect in
            development or
            function of post
            auricular ear muscle

A

Normal        Protruding    Protruding    Lop
                            lop

C

B

FIGURE 51-48. **A,** The posterior auricular muscle attaches from the concha of the ear to the mastoid region, thus holding the auricle toward the head. A protruding ear can result from absence or deficient function of the posterior auricular muscle. A lop ear is a secondary deformation due to a defect in development of function of the superior auricular ear muscle, which attaches the superior auricle to the head. **B,** Photo from a 16-week fetus. **C,** Drawings summarize the relationship between the extrinsic ear muscles and ear form.
  (**B,** From Smith DW, Takashima H: Protruding auricle: a neuromuscular sign, *Lancet* 1:747, 1978. **C,** Courtesy of Thomas Stebbins, University of Washington School of Medicine, Seattle, Wash.)

the conotruncal pads separates the single outlet truncus into the aorta and pulmonary arteries with the development of aortic and pulmonary valves. Throughout cardiac morphogenesis the direction and force of the streams of blood play a major role in the development of cardiac form. For example, the blood coming from the placenta through the ductus venosus flows across the right atrium and maintains the patency of the foramen ovale, directly shunting the blood into the left atrium. As soon as placental blood flow ceases at birth, other changes take place, such as closure of the ductus arteriosus and the increase in blood flow to the pulmonary vascular bed. The direction and magni-

tude of blood flow changes results in the closure of the foramen ovale.

Any anatomic change in early heart development usually has a major effect on subsequent cardiac morphogenesis by changing the biomechanics within the developing heart. For example, a ventricular septal defect results in excessive shunting of blood into the right ventricle and the pulmonary system, thus causing enlargement of the right ventricle. The excessive pressure on the pulmonary circulation eventually causes increased vascular resistance, further increasing the load on the right ventricle, which may then begin to fail in its function. Early intervention, with closure of the

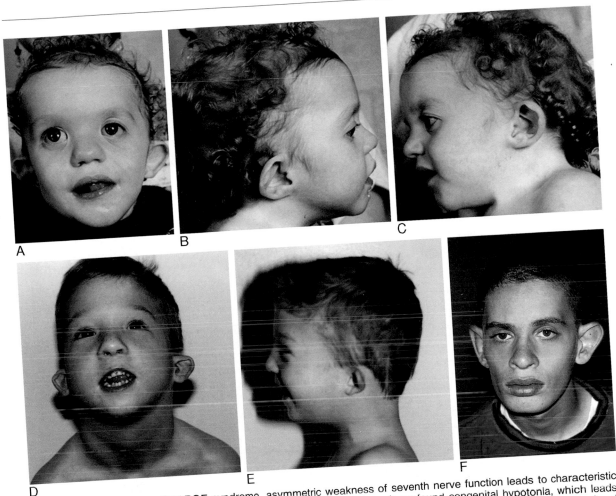

FIGURE 51-49. **A** to **C**, In CHARGE syndrome, asymmetric weakness of seventh nerve function leads to characteristic abnormal folding and prominence of the concha. In FG syndrome there is profound congenital hypotonia, which leads to small prominent cupped ears (**D** and **E**), while in fragile X syndrome (**F**), the ears tend to be large and prominent due to the combination of hypotonia and lax connective tissues.

ventricular septal defect, may prevent such biomechanical consequences, all of which may be interpreted as *deformations* in the cardiovascular system. Interference with the early flow patterns may be a primary cause for problems in cardiac morphogenesis. Ishikawa produced defects of the heart and great vessels in 42% of chick embryos by placing them in a centrifuge for 9 hours during the period of cardiac morphogenesis.[35] These cardiac defects were presumed to be the consequence of alterations in cardiac flow patterns during this critical time in heart development. Similar alterations in chick heart morphogenesis have been induced by Clark,[36] using mechanical alterations in early vascular flow patterns. The peripheral blood vessels develop as a coalescence of multiple small lacunae into vessels. Initially there tends to be a general network of small vessels. The magnitude and direction of flow will result in enlargement of some of these minute vessels in a particular direction, whereas a diminished flow will result in regression of vessels. Hence the vascular patterns develop to a major extent in relation to the needs of a particular region and to its form. If there is hypoplasia of a region, the vascular channels in that region are generally smaller than usual.

## Intestines

The endoderm outpouches in a forward direction as the foregut and in a posterior direction as the hindgut. As the intestines enlarge, they extend beyond the abdominal wall into the allantoic sac and then later return to the abdominal cavity. This enlargement gives rise to multiple foldings of the

Once upon a time, there was a family of pigs. A huge family.
A family that was outgrowing its house.

"I'm sorry, you three, but you're old enough to be on your
own now," Mama Pig said. "I need the room."

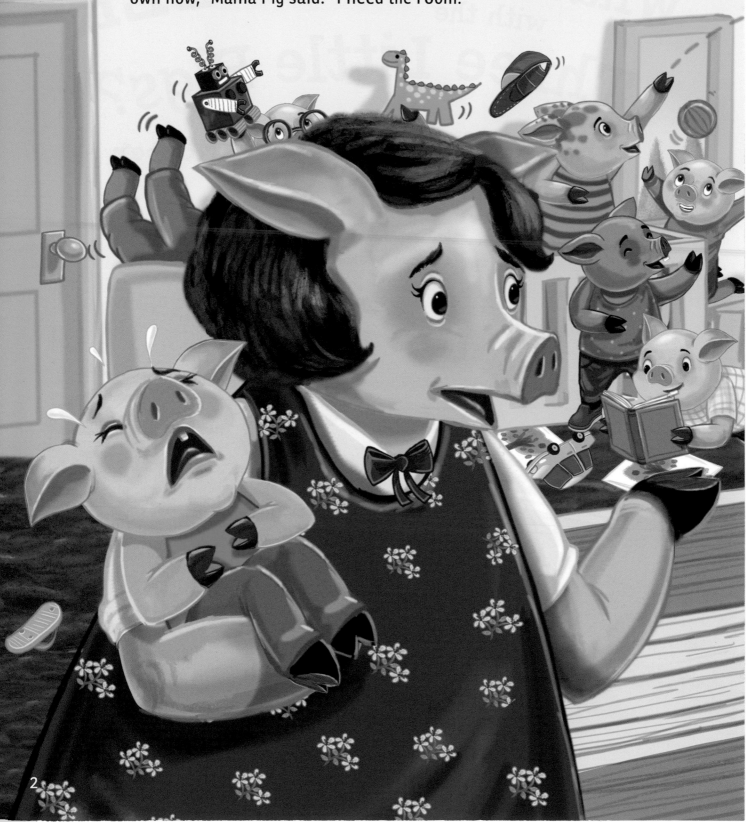

2

Steve, Hector, and Alice were sad. But they knew Mama was right. It was time for them to go.

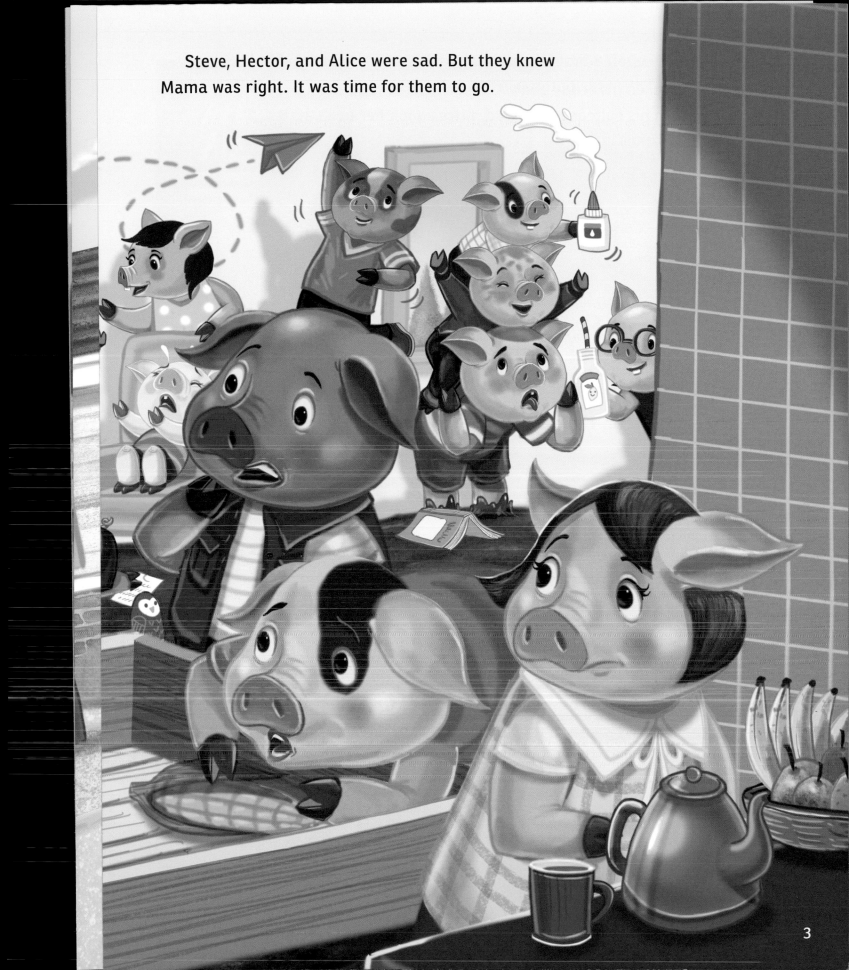

Hector looked through the peephole.

"Oh, mud. It's that Wulf guy," he said.

"You can't escape me one way or another," B.B. Wulf called. "Now I'll eat you *and* your piggy brother!"

"You'll never get in. We're surrounded by icy, ice, ice!" Steve shouted.

The wolf smiled, took out his cell phone, and tapped a few times.

"Oh, that's fine. You can stop your yipping," B.B. Wulf said. "I've just placed an order with next-day shipping."

Steve and Hector couldn't imagine what that awful wolf was up to.

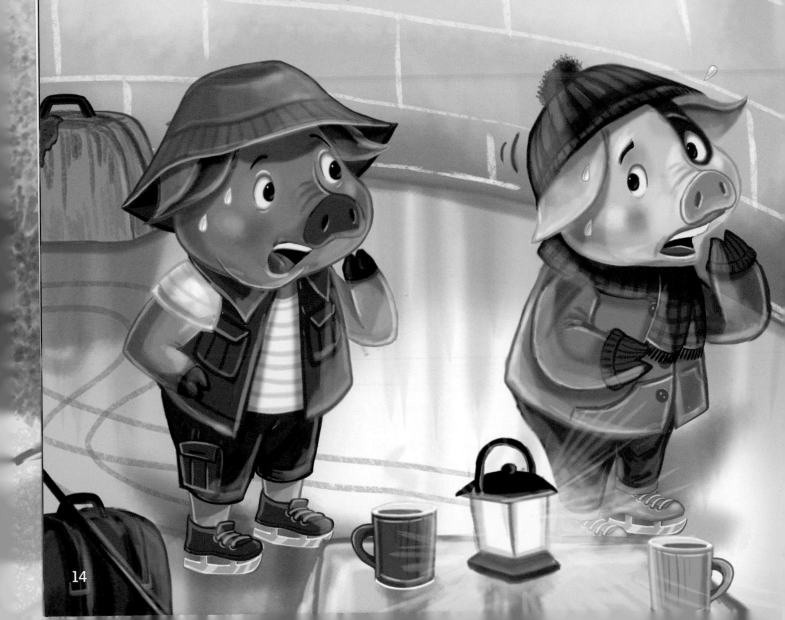

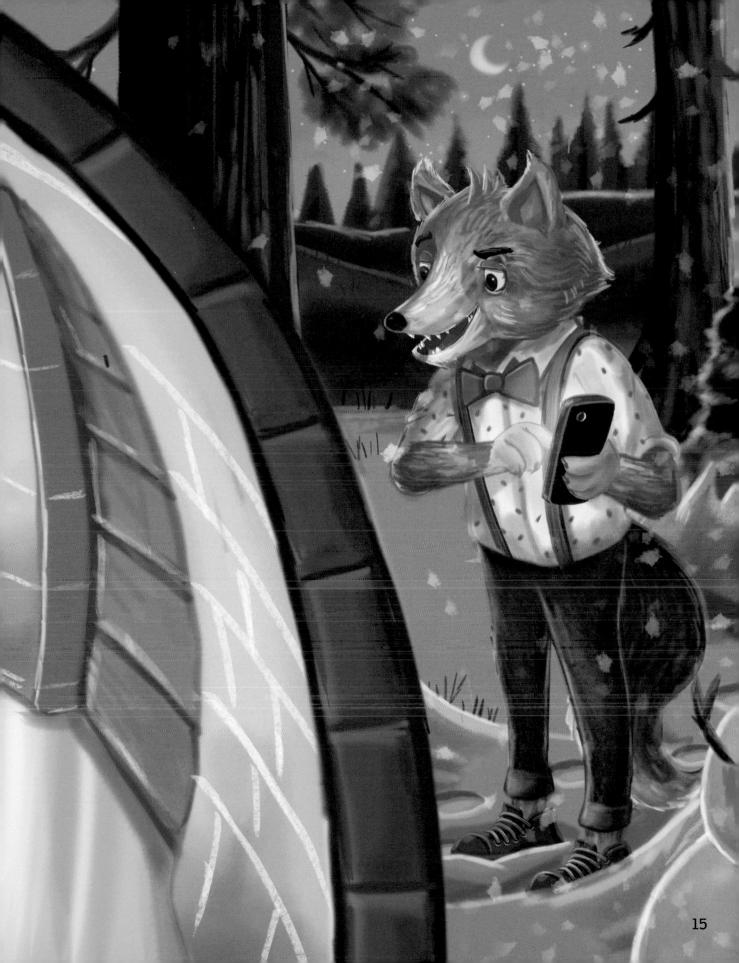

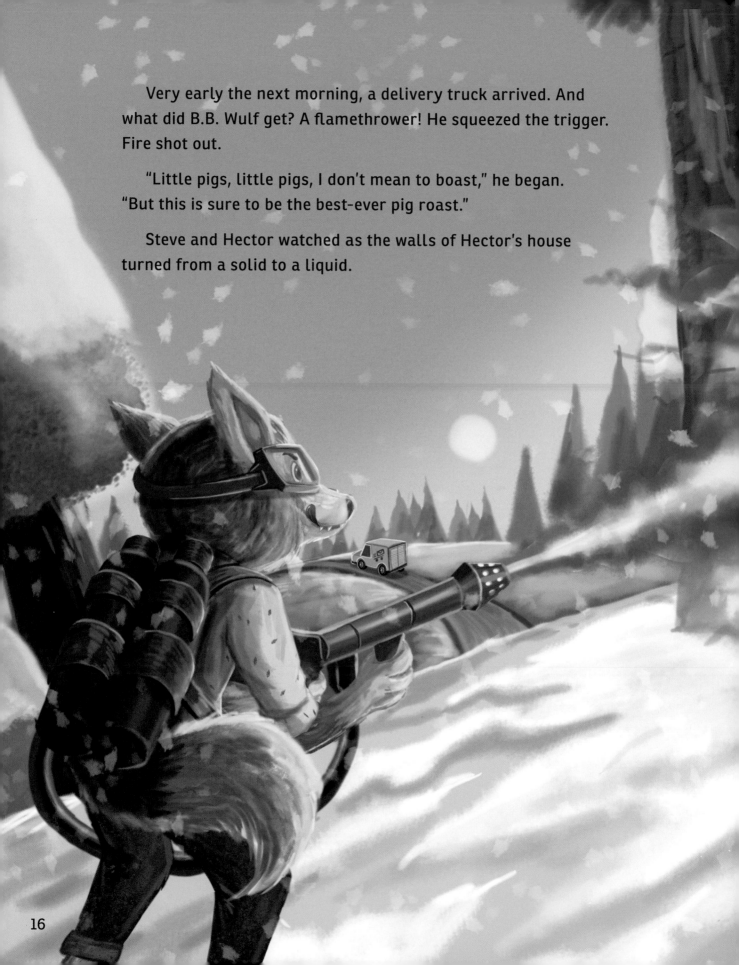

Very early the next morning, a delivery truck arrived. And what did B.B. Wulf get? A flamethrower! He squeezed the trigger. Fire shot out.

"Little pigs, little pigs, I don't mean to boast," he began. "But this is sure to be the best-ever pig roast."

Steve and Hector watched as the walls of Hector's house turned from a solid to a liquid.

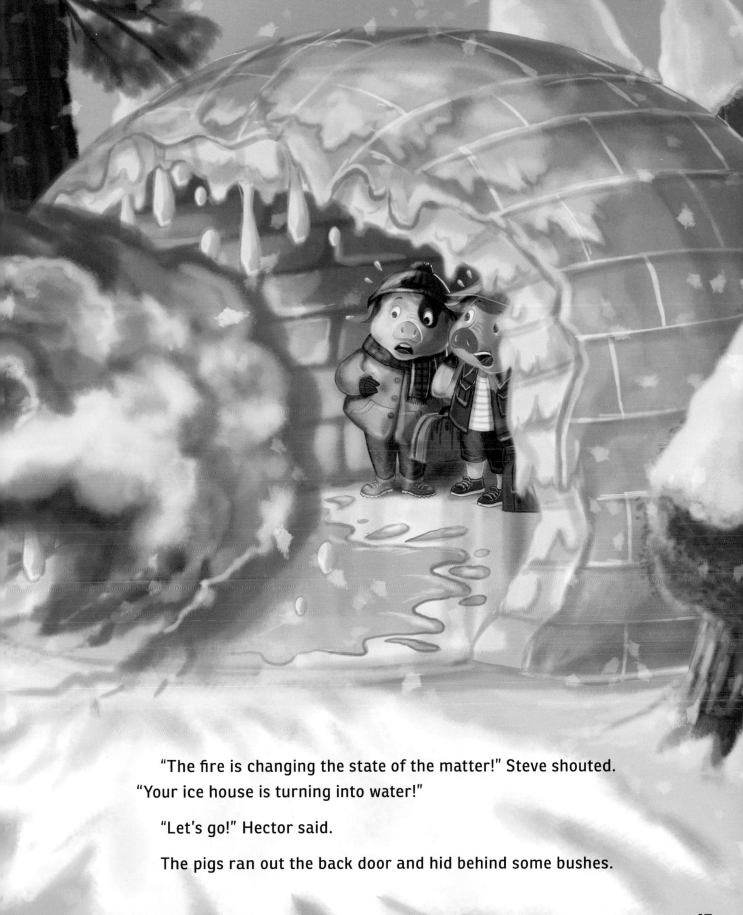

"The fire is changing the state of the matter!" Steve shouted.
"Your ice house is turning into water!"

"Let's go!" Hector said.

The pigs ran out the back door and hid behind some bushes.

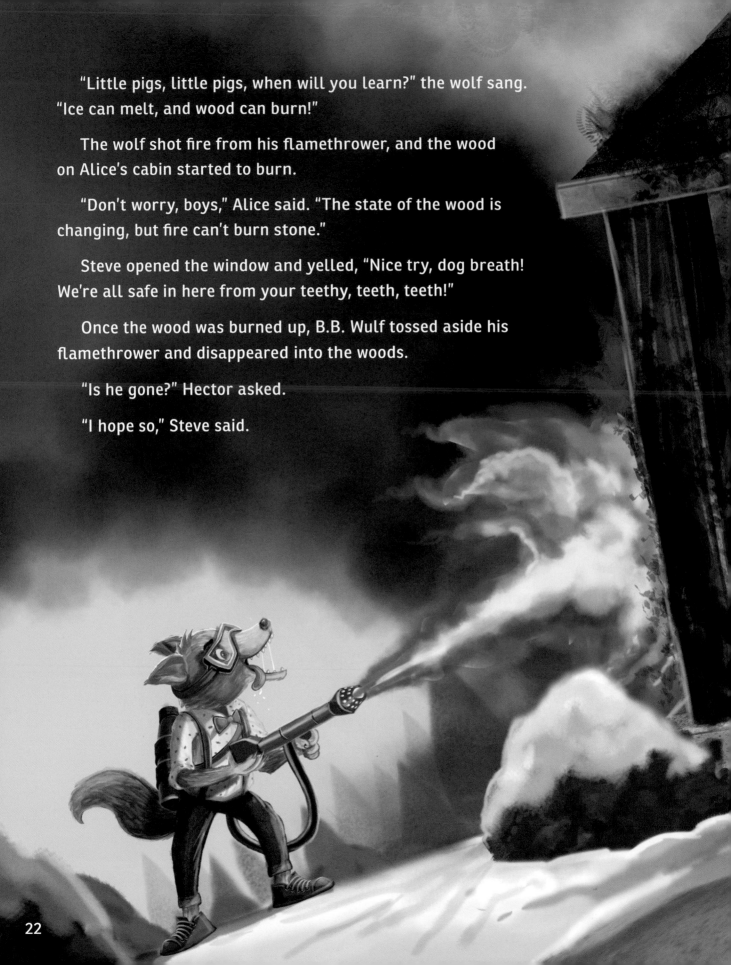

"Little pigs, little pigs, when will you learn?" the wolf sang. "Ice can melt, and wood can burn!"

The wolf shot fire from his flamethrower, and the wood on Alice's cabin started to burn.

"Don't worry, boys," Alice said. "The state of the wood is changing, but fire can't burn stone."

Steve opened the window and yelled, "Nice try, dog breath! We're all safe in here from your teethy, teeth, teeth!"

Once the wood was burned up, B.B. Wulf tossed aside his flamethrower and disappeared into the woods.

"Is he gone?" Hector asked.

"I hope so," Steve said.

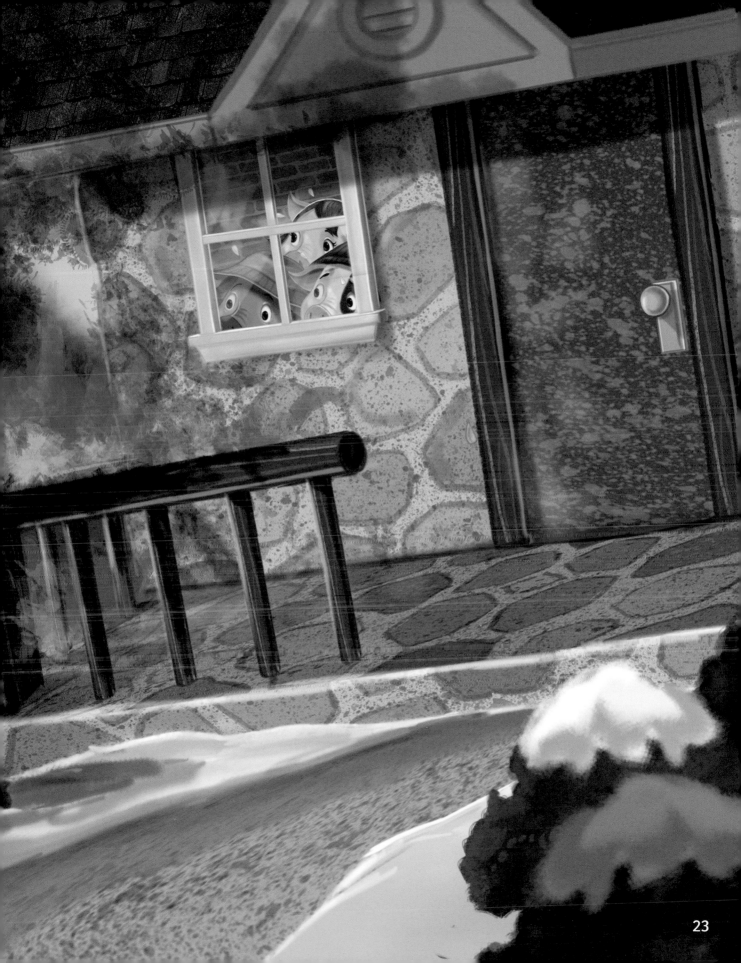

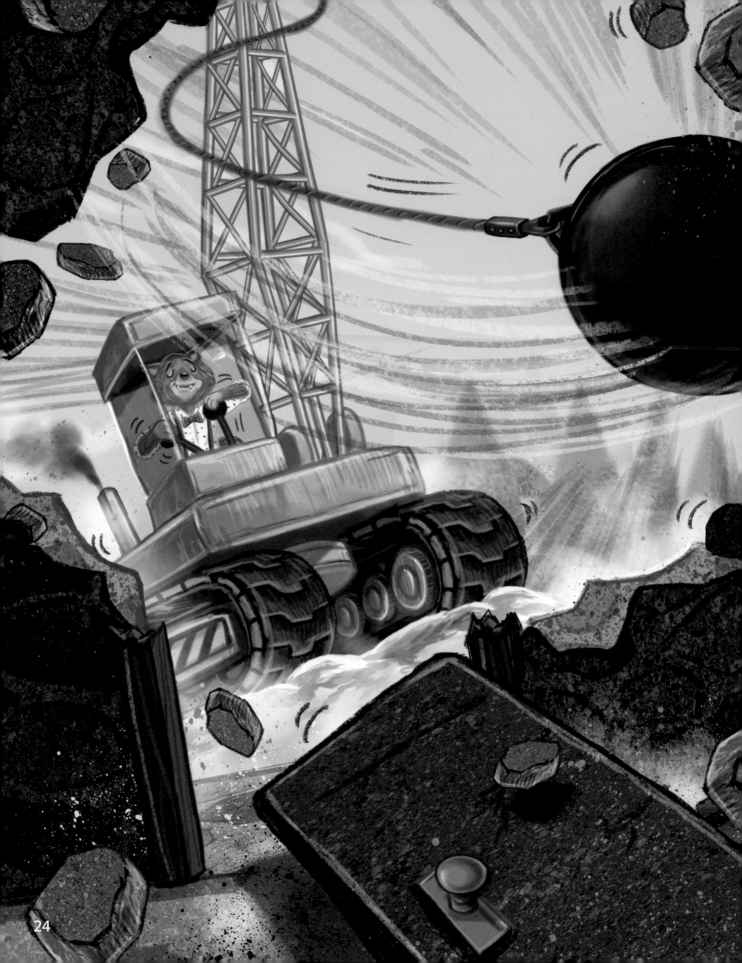

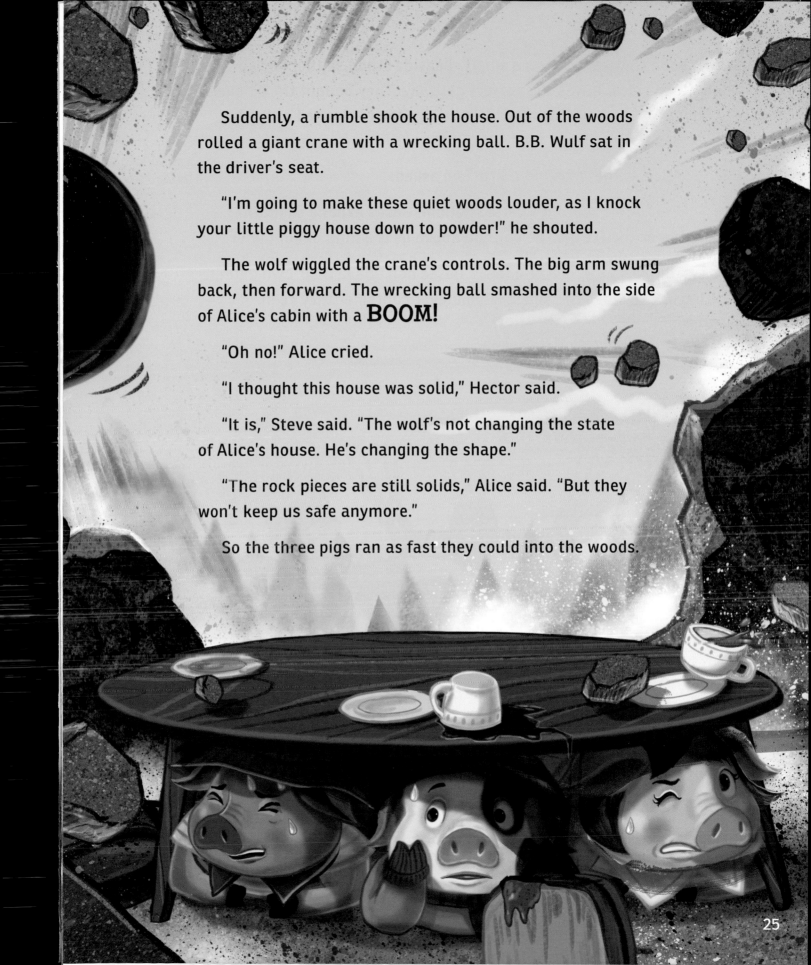

Suddenly, a rumble shook the house. Out of the woods rolled a giant crane with a wrecking ball. B.B. Wulf sat in the driver's seat.

"I'm going to make these quiet woods louder, as I knock your little piggy house down to powder!" he shouted.

The wolf wiggled the crane's controls. The big arm swung back, then forward. The wrecking ball smashed into the side of Alice's cabin with a **BOOM!**

"Oh no!" Alice cried.

"I thought this house was solid," Hector said.

"It is," Steve said. "The wolf's not changing the state of Alice's house. He's changing the shape."

"The rock pieces are still solids," Alice said. "But they won't keep us safe anymore."

So the three pigs ran as fast they could into the woods.

# Index

Special thanks to our adviser, Darsa Donelan, Professor of Physics,
Gustavus Adolphus College, Saint Peter, Minnesota, for her expertise.

Editor: Jill Kalz
Designer: Lori Bye
Premedia Specialist: Tori Abraham
The illustrations in this book were created digitally.

Picture Window Books
1710 Roe Crest Drive
North Mankato, MN 56003
www.mycapstone.com

Library of Congress Cataloging-in-Publication data is available on the Library of Congress website.
ISBN 978-1-5158-2896-9 (library binding)
ISBN 978-1-5158-2900-3 (paperback)
ISBN 978-1-5158-2904-1 (eBook PDF)
Summary: What's the matter with the three little pigs? They're being tormented by a hungry wolf, that's what!
And no matter what kind of matter they use to build their homes, it doesn't matter. The STEM-savvy, rhyme-
loving wolf in this fractured fairy tale always seems to spoil the day.

Printed and bound in the United States of America.
102018   000052